The New Complete
MEDICAL
and HEALTH
ENCYCLOPEDIA

The New Complete
MEDICAL
and HEALTH
ENCYCLOPEDIA

EDITED BY
Richard J. Wagman, M.D., F.A.C.P.
Assistant Clinical Professor of Medicine
Downstate Medical Center
New York, New York

AND BY
the J. G. Ferguson Editorial Staff

Volume 3

J. G. FERGUSON PUBLISHING COMPANY / CHICAGO

Acknowledgments

Grateful acknowledgment is made of the courtesy of the following organization:

Holt, Rinehart and Winston, Inc., New York, New York, for permission to reprint art and caption material from *Field & Stream Guide to Physical Fitness* with illustrations by Alex Orr.

Portions of *The New Complete Medical and Health Encyclopedia* have been previously published under the title of *The Complete Illustrated Book of Better Health* and *The Illustrated Encyclopedia of Better Health*, edited by Richard J. Wagman, M.D.

Contributors to The New Complete Medical and Health Encyclopedia

Editor
RICHARD J. WAGMAN, M.D., F.A.C.P.
Assistant Clinical Professor of Medicine
Downstate Medical Center
New York, New York

Consultant in Surgery
N. HENRY MOSS, M.D., F.A.C.S.
Associate Clinical Professor of Surgery
Temple University Health Sciences Center
and Albert Einstein Medical Center;
Past President, American Medical Writers Association;
Past President, New York Academy of Sciences

Consultant in Gynecology
DOUGLASS S. THOMPSON, M.D.
Clinical Professor of Obstetrics and Gynecology
and Clinical Associate Professor of Community Medicine
University of Pittsburgh School of Medicine
Pittsburgh, Pennsylvania

Consultant in Pediatrics
CHARLES H. BAUER, M.D.
Clinical Associate Professor of Pediatrics
and Chief of Pediatric Gastroenterology
The New York Hospital-Cornell Medical Center
New York, New York

Consultants in Psychiatry
JULIAN J. CLARK, M.D.
Assistant Professor of Psychiatry
and
RITA W. CLARK, M.D.
Clinical Assistant Professor of Psychiatry
Downstate Medical Center
New York, New York

Consulting Editor
KENNETH N. ANDERSON
Formerly Editor
Today's Health

BRUCE O. BERG, M.D.
  Associate Professor
  Departments of Neurology
    and Pediatrics
  Director, Child Neurology
  University of California
  San Francisco, California

D. JEANNE COLLINS
  Assistant Professor
  College of Allied Health
    Professions
  University of Kentucky
  Lexington, Kentucky

ANTHONY A. DAVIS
  Vice President and
    Education Consultant
  Metropolitan X-Ray and
    Medical Sales, Inc.
  Olney, Maryland

PETER A. DICKINSON
  Editor Emeritus
  Harvest Years/Retirement
    Living

GORDON K. FARLEY, M.D.
  Associate Professor of Child Psychiatry
  Director, Day Care Center
  University of Colorado Medical Center
  Denver, Colorado

ARTHUR FISHER
  Group Editor
  Science and Engineering
  Popular Science

EDMUND H. HARVEY, JR.
  Editor
  Science World

HELENE MacLEAN
  Medical writer

BEN PATRUSKY
  Science writer

STANLEY E. WEISS, M.D.
  Assistant Attending Physician,
    Renal Service
  Beth Israel Hospital and Medical
    Center
  New York, New York

JEFFREY S. WILLNER, M.D.
  Attending Radiologist
  Southampton Hospital
  Southampton, New York

Contents

CHAPTER 13

Nutrition and Weight Control

Food and meals are man's best friends. His health and his social life are tied intimately and everlastingly to what he eats and how he eats it. Of all the physiological functions which maintain his life, eating and all that it entails is the one in which he most expresses his personal preferences and the cultural traditions of his ancestors.

Most people develop eating habits early in life that accord with family patterns and modify them only slightly over the years. Sometimes these habits conform to ideal food recommendations from the viewpoint of maintaining and fostering good health. More often, however, they do not.

Knowledge about food, eating, and their relationship to health is the best way to change inappropriate eating patterns of adults and to introduce youngsters to good eating habits that should last a lifetime.

Basic Nutritional Requirements

In a somewhat oversimplified way, a person can be compared with a working mechanism such as a car. The material of which each is made —tissue cells for the person, metal for the car—has to come from somewhere: the human's, from conception to birth, comes from the food eaten by his mother; after birth, from what he himself eats.

During growth and thereafter, the person's cells must be repaired and replaced just as a car must have new tires, parts, and paint from time to time. And like the car, the human has an engine—his muscular activity—which requires fuel. This fuel is provided by food in the form of calories.

In humans, the process by which food is used by the body is called *metabolism*. It begins with chemi-

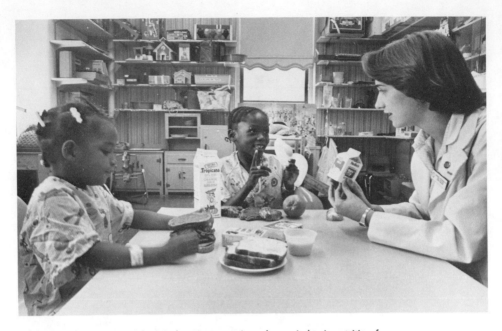

Young hospital patients receive a lesson in basic nutrition from a
dietitian who uses props to explain which foods are essential.

cal processes in the gastrointestinal tract which change plant and animal food into less complex components so that they can be absorbed to fulfill their various functions in the body.

Protein

Of the several essential components of food, *protein* is in many ways the most important. This is so because much of the body's structure is made up of proteins. For example, the typical 160-pound man is composed of about 100 pounds of water, 29 pounds of protein, 25 pounds of fat, 5 pounds of minerals, 1 pound of carbohydrate, and less than an ounce of vitamins. Since the muscles, heart, brain, lungs, and gastrointestinal organs are made up largely of protein, and since the protein in these organs is in constant need of replacement, its importance is obvious.

Chemically, proteins are mixtures of amino acids which contain various elements, including nitrogen. There are 20 different amino acids that are essential for the body's protein needs. Eight of these must be provided in the diet; the rest can be synthesized by the body itself.

Meat, fish, eggs, and milk or milk products are the primary protein foods and contain all of the necessary amino acids. Grains and vegetables are partly made up of protein, but more often than not, they do not provide the whole range of amino acids required for proper nourishment.

Carbohydrates

Carbohydrates are another essential food component. They are also called *starches* or *sugars* and are present in large quantities in grains, fruits, and vegetables. They serve as the primary source of calories for muscle contraction and must be available in the body constantly for this purpose.

It takes one pound of carbohydrates to provide a 160-pound man with fuel for about half a day. Therefore, if he isn't getting new carbohydrate supplies during the day from his food, he will begin to convert his body fat or protein into sugar. This isn't desirable unless he has an excess of body fat, and in any event, could not go on indefinitely.

Fats

Fats are a chemically complex food component composed of *glycerol* (a sweet, oily alcohol) and fatty acids. Fats exist in several forms and come from a variety of sources. One way to think of them is to group them as visible fats, such as butter, salad oil, or the fat seen in meat, and as invisible fats, which are mingled, blended, or absorbed into food, either naturally, as in nuts, meat, or fish, or during cooking. Another way is to think of them as solid at room temperature (fats), or as liquid at room temperature (oils).

SATURATED AND UNSATURATED: Fats are also classified as *saturated* or *unsaturated.* This is a chemical distinction based on the differences in molecular structure of different kinds of fat. If the carbon atoms in a fat molecule are surrounded or boxed in by hydrogen atoms, they are said to be saturated. This type of fat seems to increase the cholesterol content of the blood. *Polyunsaturated* fats, such as those found in fish and vegetable oils, contain the least number of hydrogen atoms and do not add to the blood cholesterol content. In general, fats in foods of plant origin are more unsaturated

than in those of animal origin.

Fats play several essential roles in the metabolic process. First of all, they provide more than twice the number of calories on a comparative weight basis than do proteins and carbohydrates. They also can be stored in the body in large quantities and used as a later energy source. They serve as carriers of the fat-soluble vitamins A, D, E, and K, and—of no little importance—they add to the tastiness of food.

Vitamins

Vitamins, which are present in minute quantities in foods in their natural state, are essential for normal metabolism and for the development and maintenance of tissue structure and function. In addition to the fat-soluble vitamins noted above, there are a number of B vitamins, as well as vitamin C, also called *ascorbic acid.* If any particular vitamin is missing from the diet over a sufficiently long time, a specific disease will result.

The understanding of the subtle and complicated role of vitamins in maintaining life and health has come about during this century with the development of highly refined research methods. It is likely that continuing research will shed more light on their importance.

Minerals

Minerals are another component of basic nutritional needs. All living things extract them from the soil, which is their ultimate source. Like vitamins, they are needed for normal metabolism and must be present in the diet in sufficient amounts for the maintenance of good health. The essential minerals are copper, iodine, iron, manganese, zinc, molybdenum, fluorine, and cobalt.

When the normal diet is deficient in certain minerals, these minerals need to be specially added to the diet: iodine for thyroid function, and fluorine for protection against dental cavities. Additional iron for hemoglobin formation may be indicated when the diet is deficient in it, or when there has been an excessive loss of red blood cells, as some women experience with their menstrual periods.

Water

Water is not really a food in the fuel or calorie-producing sense, but it is in many ways a crucial component of nutrition. It makes up from 55 to 65 percent of the body's weight, and is constantly being eliminated in the form of urine, perspiration, and expired breath. It must therefore be replaced regularly, for while a person can live for

METRIC EQUIVALENTS OF TRADITIONAL FOOD MEASURES		
1 teaspoon	=	5 milliliters
1 tablespoon	=	15 milliliters
1/4 cup	=	60 milliliters
1/3 cup	=	80 milliliters
1/2 cup	=	120 milliliters
2/3 cup	=	160 milliliters
3/4 cup	=	180 milliliters
1 cup	=	240 milliliters or 0.24 liter

NUTRIENTS IN COMMON FOODS

	Food energy	Protein	Fat	Carbohydrate
	Calories	Grams	Grams	Grams
Milk and Milk Products				
Milk; 1 cup:				
Fluid, whole	165	9	10	12
Fluid, nonfat (skim)	90	9	trace	13
Buttermilk, cultured (from skim milk)	90	9	trace	13
Evaporated (undiluted)	345	18	20	24
Dry, nonfat (regular)	435	43	1	63
Yoghurt (from partially skimmed milk); 1 cup	120	8	4	13
Cheese; 1 ounce:				
Cheddar, or American	115	7	9	1
Cottage:				
From skim milk	25	5	trace	1
Creamed	30	4	1	1
Cream cheese	105	2	11	1
Swiss	105	7	8	1
Desserts (largely milk):				
Custard, baked; 1 cup, 8 fluid ounces	305	14	15	29

Adapted from *Nutritive Value of American Foods* by Catherine F. Adams, Agriculture Handbook No. 456, U.S. Department of Agriculture, issued November 1975. The cup measure used in the following table refers to the standard 8-ounce measuring cup of 8 fluid ounces or one-half liquid pint. When a measure is indicated by ounce, it is understood to be by weight—1/16 of a pound avoirdupois—unless a fluid ounce is indicated. All weights and measures in the table are in U.S. System units. To find the metric equivalents, see the table on this page.

NUTRIENTS IN COMMON FOODS

	Food energy	Protein	Fat	Carbohydrate
	Calories	Grams	Grams	Grams
Ice cream, plain, factory packed:				
1 slice or individual brick, ⅛ quart .	130	3	7	14
1 container, 8 fluid ounces . . .	255	6	14	28
Ice milk; 1 cup, 8 fluid ounces . .	200	6	7	29
Eggs				
Egg, raw, large:				
1 whole	80	6	6	trace
1 white	15	4	trace	trace
1 yolk	60	3	5	trace
Egg, cooked; 1 large:				
Boiled	80	6	6	trace
Scrambled (with milk and fat) . . .	110	7	8	1
Meat, Poultry, Fish, Shellfish				
Bacon, broiled or fried, drained,				
2 medium thick slices	85	4	8	trace
Beef, cooked without bone:				
Braised, simmered, or pot-roasted;				
3-ounce portion:				
Entire portion, lean and fat . .	365	19	31	0
Lean only, approx. 2 ounces . .	140	17	4	0
Hamburger patties, made with				
Regular ground beef; 3-ounce patty .	235	21	17	0
Lean ground round; 3-ounce patty .	185	23	10	0
Roast; 3-ounce slice from cut having				
relatively small amount of fat:				
Entire portion, lean and fat . . .	255	22	18	0
Lean only, approx. 2.3 ounces . .	115	19	4	0
Steak, broiled; 3-ounce portion:				
Entire portion, lean and fat . . .	375	19	32	0
Lean only, approx. 1.8 ounces . .	105	17	4	0
Beef, canned: corned beef hash: 3 ounces .	155	8	10	9
Beef and vegetable stew: 1 cup . . .	220	16	11	15
Chicken, without bone: broiled; 3 ounces .	115	20	3	0
Lamb, cooked:				
Chops; 1 thick chop, with bone,				
4.8 ounces:				
Lean and fat, approx. 3.4 ounces . .	340	21	28	0
Lean only, 2.3 ounces	120	18	5	0
Roast, without bone:				
Leg; 3-ounce slice:				
Entire slice, lean and fat . . .	265	20	20	0
Lean only, approx. 2.3 ounces . .	120	19	5	0
Shoulder; 3-ounce portion, without				
bone:				
Entire portion, lean and fat . .	300	18	25	0
Lean only, approx. 2.2 ounces . .	125	16	6	0

weeks without food, he can live for only a few days without water.

Normally, the best guide to how much water a person needs is his sense of thirst. The regulating mechanism of excretion sees to it that an excessive intake of water will be eliminated as urine. The usual water requirement is on the order of two quarts a day in addition to whatever amount is contained in the solids which make up the daily diet. Information on the protein, fat, and carbohydrate content in specific foods, as well as the number of calories, may be obtained by consulting the table *Nutrients in Common Foods,* pp. 698-716. The Metric Equivalents table converts spoon and cup measures into metric measures.

Basic Daily Diets

Everyone should have at least the minimal amount of basic nutrients for resting or basal metabolism. The specific needs of each individual are determined by whether he is still growing, and by how much energy is required for his normal activities. All those who are still growing— and growth continues up to about 20 years of age—have relatively high food needs.

For Infants

That food needs of an infant are especially acute should surprise no one. The newborn baby normally triples his birth weight during his first year and is very active in terms of calorie expenditure.

For his first six months, breast milk or formula, or a combination of both, fills his nutritional needs. The amount of milk he should get each day is about two and a half ounces per pound of his body weight. This

A sixteenth century artist used figures of fruit, vegetables, grains, and flowers to make up his portrait of a woman at harvest time.

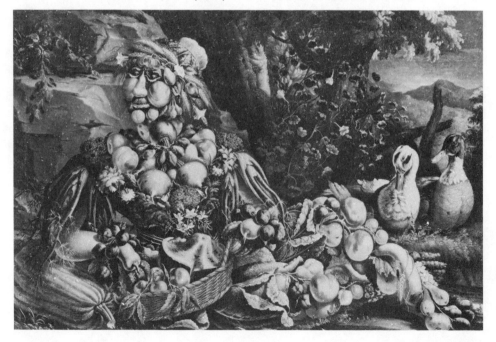

NUTRIENTS IN COMMON FOODS

	Food energy	Protein	Fat	Carbohydrate
	Calories	Grams	Grams	Grams
Liver, beef, fried; 2 ounces	120	13	4	6
Pork, cured, cooked:				
Ham, smoked; 3-ounce portion,				
without bone	245	18	19	0
Luncheon meat:				
Boiled ham; 2 ounces	130	11	10	0
Canned, spiced; 2 ounces . . .	165	8	14	1
Pork, fresh, cooked:				
Chops; 1 chop, with bone, 3.5 ounces:				
Lean and fat, approx. 2.4 ounces . .	295	15	25	0
Lean only, approx. 1.6 ounces .	120	14	7	0
Roast; 3-ounce slice, without bone:				
Entire slice, lean and fat . . .	340	19	29	0
Lean only, approx. 2.2 ounces . .	160	19	9	0
Sausage:				
Bologna; 8 slices (4.1 by 0.1 inches				
each), 8 ounces	690	27	62	2
Frankfurter; 1 cooked, 1.8 ounces . .	155	6	14	1
Tongue, beef, boiled; 3 ounces . .	205	18	14	trace
Veal, cutlet, broiled; 3-ounce portion,				
without bone	185	23	9	0
Fish and shellfish:				
Bluefish, baked or broiled; 3 ounces .	135	22	4	0
Clams: raw, meat only; 3 ounces . .	70	11	1	3
Crabmeat, canned or cooked; 3 ounces .	90	14	2	1
Fishsticks, breaded, cooked, frozen;				
10 sticks (3.8 by 1.0 by 0.5 inches				
each), 8 ounces	400	38	20	15
Haddock, fried; 3 ounces . . .	135	16	5	6
Mackerel: broiled; 3 ounces . . .	200	19	13	0
Oysters, raw, meat only; 1 cup (13–19				
medium-size oysters, selects) . .	160	20	4	8
Oyster stew: 1 cup (6–8 oysters) . .	200	11	12	11
Salmon, canned (pink); 3 ounces . .	120	17	5	0
Sardines, canned in oil, drained				
solids; 3 ounces	180	22	9	1
Shrimp, canned, meat only; 3 ounces .	110	23	1	—
Tuna, canned in oil, drained solids;				
3 ounces	170	25	7	0
Mature Beans and Peas, Nuts				
Beans, dry seed:				
Common varieties, as Great Northern,				
navy, and others, canned; ` cup:				
Red	230	15	1	42
White, with tomato or molasses:				
With pork	330	16	7	54
Without pork	315	16	1	60

NUTRIENTS IN COMMON FOODS

	Food energy	Protein	Fat	Carbohydrate
	Calories	Grams	Grams	Grams
Beans, dry seed:				
Lima, cooked; 1 cup	260	16	1	48
Cowpeas or black-eyed peas,				
dry, cooked; 1 cup	190	13	1	34
Peanuts, roasted, shelled; 1 cup	840	39	71	28
Peanut butter; 1 tablespoon	90	4	8	3
Peas, split, dry, cooked; 1 cup	290	20	1	52
Vegetables				
Asparagus:				
Cooked; 1 cup	35	4	trace	6
Canned; 6 medium-size spears	20	2	trace	3
Beans:				
Lima, immature, cooked; 1 cup	150	8	1	29
Snap, green:				
Cooked; 1 cup	25	2	trace	6
Canned: solids and liquid; 1 cup	45	2	trace	10
Beets, cooked, diced; 1 cup	70	2	trace	16
Broccoli, cooked, flower stalks; 1 cup	45	5	trace	8
Brussels sprouts, cooked; 1 cup	60	6	1	12
Cabbage; 1 cup:				
Raw, coleslaw	100	2	7	9
Cooked	40	2	trace	9
Carrots:				
Raw: 1 carrot (5½ by 1 inch)				
or 25 thin strips	20	1	trace	5
Cooked, diced; 1 cup	45	1	1	9
Canned, strained or chopped; 1 ounce	5	trace	0	2
Cauliflower, cooked, flower buds; 1 cup	30	3	trace	6
Celery, raw: large stalk, 8 inches long	5	1	trace	1
Collards, cooked; 1 cup	75	7	1	14
Corn, sweet:				
Cooked; 1 ear 5 inches long	65	2	1	16
Canned, solids and liquid; 1 cup	170	5	1	41
Cucumbers, raw, pared; 6 slices				
(⅛-inch thick, center section)	5	trace	trace	1
Lettuce, head, raw:				
2 large or 4 small leaves	5	1	trace	1
1 compact head (4¾-inch diameter)	70	5	1	13
Mushrooms, canned, solids and				
liquid; 1 cup	30	3	trace	9
Okra, cooked; 8 pods (3 inches long,				
⅝-inch diameter)	30	2	trace	6
Onions: mature raw; 1 onion (2½-inch				
diameter)	50	2	trace	11
Peas, green; 1 cup:				
Cooked	110	8	1	19
Canned, solids and liquid	170	8	1	32

provides 50 calories per pound, and in the early months is usually given in six feedings a day at four-hour intervals.

If his weight gain is adequate and he appears healthy, and if his stomach is not distended by swallowed air, his appetite is normally a satisfactory guide to how much he needs. The formula-fed baby should get a supplement of 35 milligrams of ascorbic acid each day and 400 international units of vitamin D if the latter has not been added to the milk during its processing.

SOLID FOODS: Between two and six months of age, the baby should begin to eat solid foods such as cooked cereals, strained fruits and vegetables, egg yolk, and homogenized meat. With the introduction of these foods, it is not really necessary to calculate the baby's caloric intake. Satisfaction of appetite, proper weight gain, and a healthy appearance serve as the guides to a proper diet.

By one year of age, a baby should be getting three regular meals a day, and as his teeth appear, his food no longer needs to be strained. By 18 to 24 months, he should no longer need baby foods. For further information on the care and feeding of infants, see under *Birth, Infancy, and Maturation,* p. 426.

NUTRIENTS IN COMMON FOODS

	Food energy	Protein	Fat	Carbohydrate
	Calories	Grams	Grams	Grams
Peppers, sweet:				
Green, raw; 1 medium	15	1	trace	3
Red, raw; 1 medium	20	1	trace	4
Potatoes:				
Baked or boiled; 1 medium, 2½-inch diameter (weight raw, about 5 ounces):				
Baked in jacket	90	3	trace	21
Boiled; peeled before boiling	90	3	trace	21
Chips; 10 medium (2-inch diameter)	110	1	7	10
French fried:				
Frozen, ready to be heated for serving; 10 pieces (2 by ½ by ½ inch)	95	2	4	15
Ready-to-eat, deep fat for entire process; 10 pieces (2 by ½ by ½ inch)	155	2	7	20
Mashed; 1 cup:				
Milk added	145	4	1	30
Milk and butter added	230	4	12	28
Radishes, raw; 4 small	10	trace	trace	2
Spinach:				
Cooked; 1 cup	45	6	1	6

Basic Food Groups

The recommended daily amounts of food for people over the age of two have been established with reasonable accuracy. They are called minimal daily amounts, but they always contain a fairly generous safety factor.

THE FOUR GROUP DIVISION: In general, foods are divided into four major groups:

- Meat, fish, eggs
- Dairy products
- Fruits and vegetables
- Breads and cereals.

THE SEVEN GROUP DIVISION: For purposes of planning daily requirements, a more detailed way of considering food groupings is the following:

- Leafy green and yellow vegetables
- Citrus fruits, tomatoes, and raw cabbage
- Potatoes and other vegetables and fruits
- Milk, cheese, and ice cream
- Meat, poultry, fish, eggs, dried peas, and beans
- Bread, flour, and cereals
- Butter and fortified margarine

The *Daily Food Guide* (see p. 705) is a general guide to planning nutritionally balanced meals for preteens, teens, and adults of any age.

The Years of Growth

Even though a child will never again triple his weight in a single year as he did during his first, a proper diet is crucial during the

NUTRIENTS IN COMMON FOODS

	Food energy	Protein	Fat	Carbohydrate
	Calories	Grams	Grams	Grams
Spinach:				
Canned, creamed, strained; 1 ounce .	10	1	trace	2
Squash:				
Cooked, 1 cup:				
Summer, diced	35	1	trace	8
Winter, baked, mashed . . .	95	4	1	23
Canned, strained or chopped; 1 ounce .	10	trace	trace	2
Sweet potatoes:				
Baked or boiled; 1 medium, 5 by				
2 inches (weight raw, about				
6 ounces):				
Baked in jacket	155	2	1	36
Boiled in jacket	170	2	1	39
Candied; 1 small, 3½ by 2 inches . .	295	2	6	60
Canned, vacuum or solid pack; 1 cup .	235	4	trace	54
Tomatoes:				
Raw; 1 medium (2 by 2½ inches),				
about ⅓ pound	30	2	trace	6
Canned or cooked; 1 cup . . .	45	2	trace	9
Tomato juice, canned; 1 cup . . .	50	2	trace	10
Tomato catsup; 1 tablespoon . . .	15	trace	trace	4
Turnips, cooked, diced; 1 cup . . .	40	1	trace	9
Turnip greens, cooked; 1 cup . . .	45	4	1	8

DAILY FOOD GUIDE

	Child	Pre-teen and Teen	Adult	Aging Adult
Milk or milk products (*cups*)	2–3	3–4 or more	2 or more	2 or more
Meat, fish, poultry, and eggs (*servings*)	1–2	3 or more	2 or more	2 or more
Green and yellow vegetables (*servings*)	1–2	2	2	at least 1
Citrus fruits and tomatoes (*servings*)	1	1–2	1	1–2
Potatoes, other fruits, vegetables (*servings*)	1	1	1	0–1
Bread, flour, and cereal (*servings*)	3–4	4 or more	3–4	2–3
Butter or margarine (*tablespoons*)	2	2–4	2–3	1–2

1. The need for the nutrients in 1 or 2 cups of milk daily can be satisfied by cheeses or ice cream. (1 cup of milk is approximately equivalent to 1½ cups of cottage cheese or 2–3 large scoops of ice cream.)

2. It is important to drink enough fluid. The equivalent of 3–5 cups daily is recommended.

3. The recommended daily serving of meat, fish, and poultry (3 oz.) may be alternated with eggs or cheese, dried peas, beans, or lentils.

4. Iron-rich foods should be selected as frequently as possible by teen-age and adult females to help meet their high requirement for this mineral (liver, heart, lean meats, shellfish, egg yolks, legumes, green leafy vegetables, and whole grain and enriched cereal products).

From *Your Age and Your Diet* (1971), reprinted with permission from the American Medical Association

NUTRIENTS IN COMMON FOODS

	Food energy	Protein	Fat	Carbohydrate
	Calories	Grams	Grams	Grams
Fruits				
Apples, raw; 1 medium (2½ inch diameter), about ⅓ pound	70	trace	trace	18
Apple juice, fresh or canned; 1 cup	125	trace	0	34
Apple sauce, canned:				
Sweetened; 1 cup	185	trace	trace	50
Unsweetened; 1 cup	100	trace	trace	26
Apricots, raw; 3 apricots (about ¼ pound)	55	1	trace	14
Apricots, canned in heavy syrup; 1 cup	200	1	trace	54
Apricots, dried; uncooked; 1 cup (40 halves, small)	390	8	1	100
Avocados, raw, California varieties: ½ of a 10-ounce avocado (3½ by 3¼ inches)	185	2	18	6
Avocados, raw, Florida varieties: ½ of a 13-ounce avocado (4 by 3 inches)	160	2	14	11
Bananas, raw; 1 medium (6 by 1½ inches), about ⅓ pound	85	1	trace	23
Blueberries, raw; 1 cup	85	1	1	21
Cantaloupes, raw, ½ melon (5-inch diameter)	40	1	trace	9

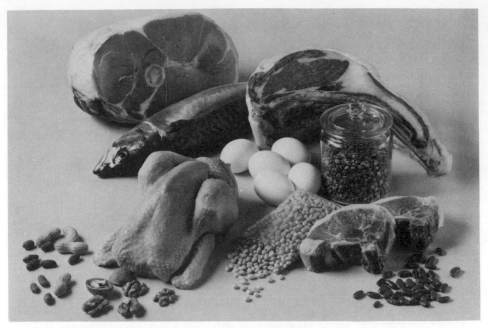

The meat group includes fish, poultry, dry beans and peas, nuts, and eggs.

NUTRIENTS IN COMMON FOODS

	Food energy	Protein	Fat	Carbohydrate
	Calories	Grams	Grams	Grams
Cherries, sour, sweet, and hybrid, raw; 1 cup	65	1	1	15
Cranberry sauce, sweetened; 1 cup . .	550	trace	1	142
Dates, "fresh" and dried, pitted and cut; 1 cup	505	4	1	134
Figs:				
Raw; 3 small (1½-inch diameter), about ¼ pound	90	2	trace	22
Dried; 1 large (2 by 1 inch) . . .	60	1	trace	15
Fruit cocktail, canned in heavy syrup, solids and liquid; 1 cup	175	1	trace	47
Grapefruit:				
Raw; ½ medium (4¼-inch diameter, No. 64's)	50	1	trace	14
Canned in syrup; 1 cup	165	1	trace	44
Grapefruit juice:				
Raw; 1 cup	85	1	trace	23
Canned:				
Unsweetened; 1 cup	95	1	trace	24
Sweetened; 1 cup	120	1	trace	32
Frozen concentrate, unsweetened:				
Undiluted; 1 can (6 fluid ounces) .	280	4	1	72
Diluted, ready-to-serve; 1 cup . .	95	1	trace	24

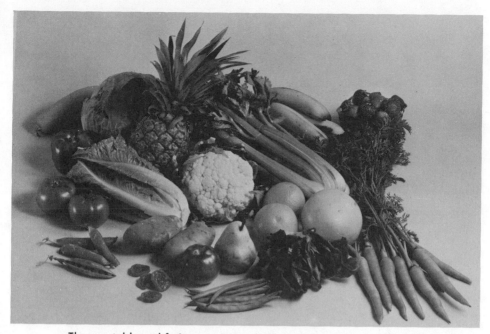

The vegetable and fruit group is a rich source of vitamins and minerals.

NUTRIENTS IN COMMON FOODS

	Food energy	Protein	Fat	Carbohydrate
	Calories	Grams	Grams	Grams
Grapefruit juice:				
Frozen concentrate, sweetened:				
Undiluted; 1 can (6 fluid ounces) .	320	3	1	85
Diluted, ready-to-serve; 1 cup . .	105	1	trace	28
Grapes, raw; 1 cup:				
American type (slip skin) . . .	70	1	1	16
European type (adherent skin) . .	100	1	trace	26
Grape juice, bottled; 1 cup	165	1	1	42
Lemonade concentrate, frozen, sweetened:				
Undiluted; 1 can (6 fluid ounces) . .	305	1	trace	113
Diluted, ready-to-serve; 1 cup . .	75	trace	trace	28
Oranges, raw; 1 large orange				
(3-inch diameter)	70	1	trace	18
Orange juice:				
Raw; 1 cup:				
California (Valencias)	105	2	trace	26
Florida varieties:				
Early and midseason . . .	90	1	trace	23
Late season (Valencias) . . .	105	1	trace	26
Canned, unsweetened; 1 cup . . .	110	2	trace	28
Frozen concentrate:				
Undiluted; 1 can (6 fluid ounces) .	305	5	trace	80
Diluted, ready-to-serve; 1 cup . .	105	2	trace	27

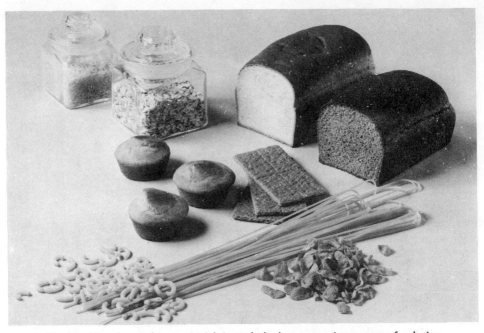

The bread and cereal group is rich in carbohydrates, a prime source of calories.

NUTRIENTS IN COMMON FOODS

	Food energy	Protein	Fat	Carbohydrate
	Calories	Grams	Grams	Grams
Peaches:				
Raw:				
1 medium (2½-inch diameter), about ¼ pound	35	1	trace	10
1 cup, sliced	65	1	trace	16
Canned (yellow-fleshed) in heavy syrup; 1 cup	185	1	trace	49
Dried: uncooked; 1 cup	420	5	1	109
Pears:				
Raw; 1 pear (3 by 2½-inch diameter) .	100	1	1	25
Canned in heavy syrup; 1 cup . .	175	1	trace	47
Pineapple juice; canned; 1 cup . . .	120	1	trace	32
Plums:				
Raw; 1 plum (2-inch diameter), about 2 ounces	30	trace	trace	7
Canned (Italian prunes), in syrup; 1 cup	185	1	trace	50
Prunes, dried:				
Uncooked; 4 medium prunes . . .	70	1	trace	19
Cooked, unsweetened; 1 cup (17–18 prunes and ⅓ cup liquid) . . .	295	3	1	78
Prune juice, canned; 1 cup	170	1	trace	45
Raisins, dried; 1 cup	460	4	trace	124

years from 2 to 18, since this is a period of tremendous growth.

Other food goals that should be realized during the childhood and adolescent years are an awareness of what a balanced diet is, a reasonable tolerance for a variety of foods, decent manners at the table, and a sense of timing about when to eat and when not to eat.

These are also the years that a young person should begin to learn something about how to buy and prepare food, how to serve it attractively, and how to clean up after a meal.

CREATING A PLEASANT ATMOSPHERE AT MEALTIME: Although a child's attitudes about food and eating can often be exasperating, it is up to the parent to make mealtime as pleasant as possible, and above all, to avoid any battles of will.

If a young child is too tired, too excited, or too hungry to cope with a meal without ending up in tears or a tantrum, he should not be forced to eat. There are several ways to help children develop a wholesome attitude towards food and eating; here are a few suggestions:

• Children should never be bribed with candy, money, or the promise of special surprises as a way of getting them to eat properly.

• They should not be given the idea that dessert is a reward for finishing the earlier part of the meal.

Coaxing a tired toddler to eat can be a challenging task for his mother. Nutritionists advise against forcing an upset child to eat.

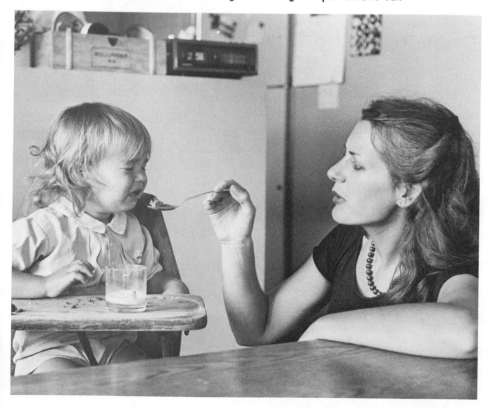

BEEF CHART

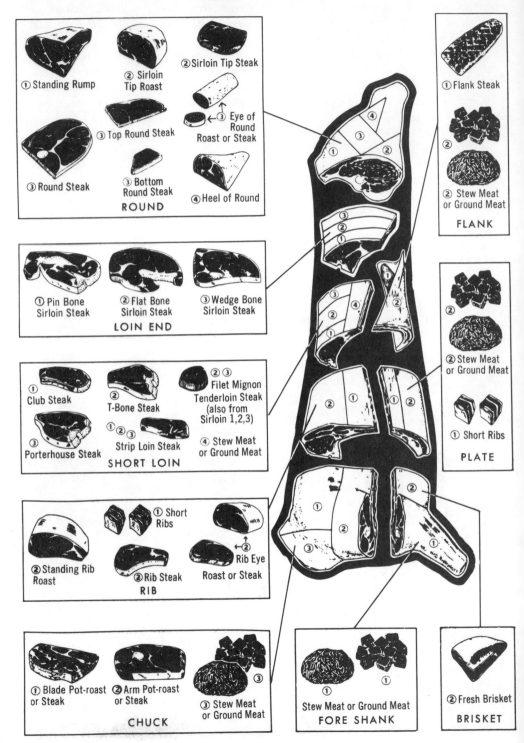

ROUND
① Standing Rump
② Sirloin Tip Roast
② Sirloin Tip Steak
③ Top Round Steak
③ Eye of Round Roast or Steak
③ Round Steak
③ Bottom Round Steak
④ Heel of Round

LOIN END
① Pin Bone Sirloin Steak
② Flat Bone Sirloin Steak
③ Wedge Bone Sirloin Steak

SHORT LOIN
① Club Steak
② T-Bone Steak
②③ Filet Mignon Tenderloin Steak (also from Sirloin 1,2,3)
③ Porterhouse Steak
①②③ Strip Loin Steak
④ Stew Meat or Ground Meat

RIB
② Standing Rib Roast
① Short Ribs
② Rib Steak
② Rib Eye Roast or Steak

CHUCK
① Blade Pot-roast or Steak
② Arm Pot-roast or Steak
③ Stew Meat or Ground Meat

FORE SHANK
① Stew Meat or Ground Meat

BRISKET
② Fresh Brisket

FLANK
① Flank Steak
② Stew Meat or Ground Meat

PLATE
② Stew Meat or Ground Meat
① Short Ribs

NUTRIENTS IN COMMON FOODS

	Food energy	Protein	Fat	Carbohydrate
	Calories	Grams	Grams	Grams
Raspberries, red:				
Raw; 1 cup	70	1	trace	17
Frozen; 10-ounce carton	280	2	1	70
Strawberries:				
Raw; 1 cup	55	1	1	12
Frozen; 10-ounce carton	300	2	1	75
Tangerines; 1 medium (2½-inch				
diameter), about ¼ pound . . .	40	1	trace	10
Watermelon: 1 wedge (4 by 8 inches),				
about 2 pounds (weighed with rind) .	120	2	1	29

Grain Products

Biscuits, baking powder, enriched flour;				
1 biscuit (2½-inch diameter) . . .	130	3	4	20
Bran flakes (40 percent bran) with				
added thiamine; 1 ounce	85	3	1	22
Breads:				
Cracked wheat:				
1 pound (20 slices)	1,190	39	10	236
1 slice (½ inch thick)	60	2	1	12
Italian; 1 pound	1,250	41	4	256
Rye:				
American (light):				
1 pound (20 slices)	1,100	41	5	236
1 slice (½ inch thick) . . .	55	2	trace	12
Pumpernickel; 1 pound . . .	1,115	41	5	241
White:				
1–2 percent nonfat dry milk:				
1 pound (20 slices)	1,225	39	15	229
1 slice (½ inch thick) . . .	60	2	1	12
3–4 percent nonfat dry milk:				
1 pound (20 slices)	1,225	39	15	229
1 slice (½ inch thick) . . .	60	2	1	12
5–6 percent nonfat dry milk:				
1 pound (20 slices)	1,245	41	17	228
1 slice (½ inch thick) . . .	65	2	1	12
Whole wheat, graham, or entire wheat:				
1 pound (20 slices)	1,105	48	14	216
1 slice (½ inch thick) . . .	55	2	1	11
Cakes:				
Angelfood: 2-inch sector (1/12 of cake,				
8-inch diameter)	160	4	trace	36
Butter cakes:				
Plain cake and cupcakes without				
icing:				
1 square (3 by 3 by 2 inches) . .	315	4	12	48
1 cupcake (2¾-inch diameter) . .	120	2	5	18

LAMB CHART

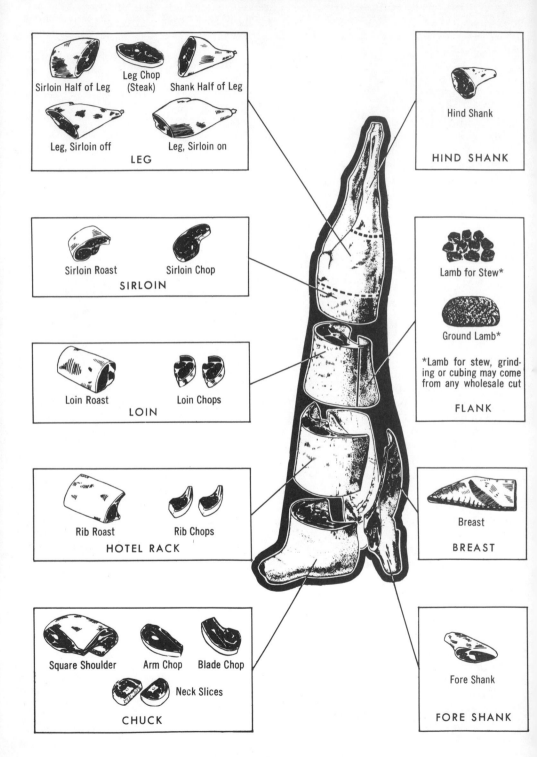

LEG
Sirloin Half of Leg
Leg Chop (Steak)
Shank Half of Leg
Leg, Sirloin off
Leg, Sirloin on

SIRLOIN
Sirloin Roast
Sirloin Chop

LOIN
Loin Roast
Loin Chops

HOTEL RACK
Rib Roast
Rib Chops

CHUCK
Square Shoulder
Arm Chop
Blade Chop
Neck Slices

HIND SHANK
Hind Shank

FLANK
Lamb for Stew*
Ground Lamb*
*Lamb for stew, grinding or cubing may come from any wholesale cut

BREAST
Breast

FORE SHANK
Fore Shank

• Relatively small portions should be served and completely finished before anything else is offered.

• Between-meal snacks should be discouraged if they cut down on the appetite at mealtime.

• From time to time, the child should be allowed to choose the foods that he will eat at a meal.

Parents should keep in mind that the atmosphere in which a child eats and the attitudes instilled in him toward food can be altogether as basic as the nourishment for his body.

TEEN-AGE DIET: From the start of a child's growth spurt, which begins at age 10 or 11 for girls and between 13 and 15 for boys, and for several years thereafter, adolescent appetites are likely to be unbelievably large and somewhat outlandish. Parents should try to exercise some control over the youngster who is putting on too much weight as well as over the one who is attracted by a bizarre starvation diet.

Adult Nutrition

Adult nutrition is concerned with more than 50 years of an individual's life span. In typical cases, there is a slow but steady weight gain that may go unnoticed at first; for some, there is an obesity problem that begins at about age 40.

Since it is never easy to lose weight, it is especially important for adults to eat sensibly and avoid excess calories. See under *Weight*, p. 718, for a discussion of weight control and obesity.

NUTRIENTS IN COMMON FOODS

	Food energy	Protein	Fat	Carbohydrate
	Calories	Grams	Grams	Grams
Butter cakes:				
Plain cake with icing:				
2-inch sector of iced layer cake ($^1/_{16}$ of cake, 10-inch diameter)	320	5	6	62
Rich cake:				
2-inch sector layer cake, iced ($^1/_{16}$ of cake, 10-inch diameter)	490	6	19	76
Fruit cake, dark; 1 piece (2 by $1^1/_2$ by $^1/_4$ inches)	60	1	2	9
Sponge; 2-inch sector ($^1/_{12}$ of cake, 8-inch diameter)	115	3	2	22
Cookies, plain and assorted; 1 cookie (3-inch diameter)	110	2	3	19
Cornbread or muffins made with enriched, degermed cornmeal; 1 muffin ($2^3/_4$-inch diameter)	105	3	2	18
Cornflakes: 1 ounce	110	2	trace	24
Corn grits, degermed, cooked: 1 cup	120	3	trace	27
Crackers:				
Graham; 4 small or 2 medium	55	1	1	10
Saltines; 2 crackers (2-inch square)	35	1	1	6
Soda, plain: 2 crackers ($2^1/_2$-inch square)	45	1	1	8

PORK CHART

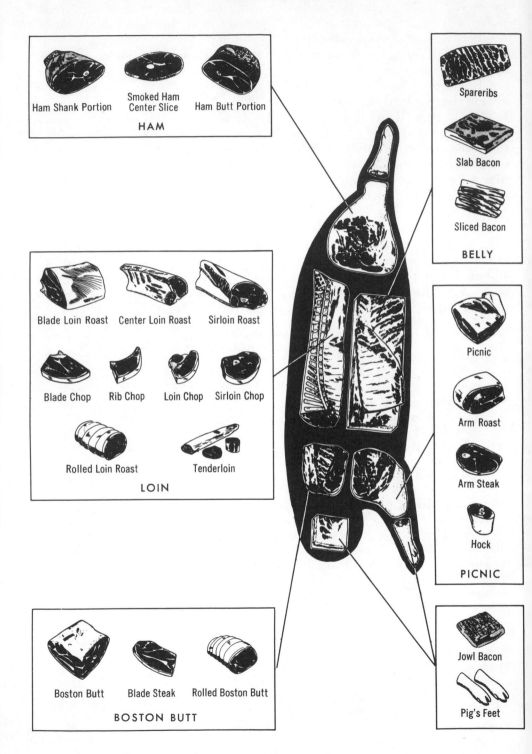

HAM
Ham Shank Portion · Smoked Ham Center Slice · Ham Butt Portion

BELLY
Spareribs · Slab Bacon · Sliced Bacon

LOIN
Blade Loin Roast · Center Loin Roast · Sirloin Roast · Blade Chop · Rib Chop · Loin Chop · Sirloin Chop · Rolled Loin Roast · Tenderloin

PICNIC
Picnic · Arm Roast · Arm Steak · Hock

BOSTON BUTT
Boston Butt · Blade Steak · Rolled Boston Butt

Jowl Bacon · Pig's Feet

NUTRIENTS IN COMMON FOODS

	Food energy Calories	Protein Grams	Fat Grams	Carbohydrate Grams
Doughnuts, cake type; 1 doughnut . .	135	2	7	17
Farina, cooked; 1 cup	105	3	trace	22
Macaroni, cooked; 1 cup:				
Cooked 8–10 minutes (undergoes additional cooking as ingredient of a food mixture)	190	6	1	39
Cooked until tender	155	5	1	32
Noodles (egg noodles), cooked: 1 cup .	200	7	2	37
Oat cereal (mixture, mainly oat flour), ready-to-eat; 1 ounce	115	4	2	21
Oatmeal or rolled oats, regular or quick cooking, cooked; 1 cup	150	5	3	26
Pancakes, baked; 1 cake (4-inch diameter):				
Wheat (home recipe)	60	2	2	7
Buckwheat (with buckwheat pancake mix)	45	2	2	6
Pies; 3½-inch sector (⅛ of 9-inch diameter pie):				
Apple	300	3	13	45
Cherry	310	3	13	45
Custard	250	7	13	27
Lemon meringue	270	4	11	40
Mince	320	3	14	49
Pumpkin	240	5	13	28
Pretzels; 5 small sticks	20	trace	trace	4
Rice, cooked; 1 cup:				
Converted	205	4	trace	45
White	200	4	trace	44
Rice, puffed or flakes; 1 ounce . . .	110	2	trace	25
Rolls:				
Plain, pan (16 ounces per dozen); 1 roll .	115	3	2	20
Hard, round (22 ounces per dozen); 1 roll	160	5	2	31
Sweet, pan (18 ounces per dozen); 1 roll	135	4	4	21
Spaghetti, cooked until tender; 1 cup .	155	5	1	32
Waffles, baked, with enriched flour: 1 waffle (4½ by 5½ by ½ inches) . .	215	7	8	28
Wheat, puffed: 1 ounce	100	4	trace	22
Wheat, rolled, cooked; 1 cup . . .	175	5	1	40
Wheat flakes; 1 ounce	100	3	trace	23
Wheat flours:				
Whole wheat; 1 cup, sifted . . .	400	16	2	85
All purpose or family flour: 1 cup, sifted	400	12	1	84
Wheat germ; 1 cup, stirred . . .	245	17	7	34

NUTRIENTS IN COMMON FOODS

	Food energy	Protein	Fat	Carbohydrate
	Calories	Grams	Grams	Grams
Fats, Oils, Related Products				
Butter; 1 tablespoon	100	trace	11	trace
Fats, cooking:				
Vegetable fats:				
1 cup	1,770	0	200	0
1 tablespoon	110	0	12	0
Lard:				
1 cup	1,985	0	220	0
1 tablespoon	125	0	14	0
Margarine; 1 tablespoon	100	trace	11	trace
Oils, salad or cooking; 1 tablespoon . .	125	0	14	0
Salad dressings; 1 tablespoon:				
Blue cheese	90	1	10	1
Commercial, plain (mayonnaise type) .	60	trace	6	2
French	60	trace	6	2
Mayonnaise	110	trace	12	trace
Thousand Island	75	trace	8	1
Sugars, Sweets				
Candy; 1 ounce:				
Caramels	120	1	3	22
Chocolate, sweetened, milk . . .	145	2	9	16
Fudge, plain	115	trace	3	23
Hard	110	0	0	28
Marshmallow	90	1	0	23
Jams, marmalades, preserves; 1				
tablespoon	55	trace	trace	14
Jellies; 1 tablespoon	50	0	0	13
Sugar; 1 tablespoon	50	0	0	12
Syrup, table blends; 1 tablespoon . .	55	0	0	15
Miscellaneous				
Beverages, carbonated, cola types; 1 cup .	105	—	—	28
Bouillon cubes; 1 cube	2	trace	trace	0
Chocolate, unsweetened; 1 ounce . .	145	2	15	8
Gelatin dessert, plain, ready-to-serve;				
1 cup	155	4	0	36
Sherbet, factory packed; 1 cup (8-fluid-ounce container)	235	3	trace	58
Soups, canned, prepared with equal amount of water; 1 cup:				
Bean with pork	168	8	6	22
Beef noodle	140	8	5	14
Bouillon, broth, and consomme . .	30	5	0	3
Chicken consomme	44	7	trace	4
Clam chowder, Manhattan style . .	80	2	3	12
Tomato	90	2	3	16
Vegetable beef	80	5	2	10
Vinegar; 1 tablespoon	2	0	—	1

FOR OLDER PEOPLE: People over 60 tend to have changes in their digestive system that are related to less efficient and slower absorption. Incomplete chewing of food because of carelessness or impaired teeth can intensify this problem. Avoiding haste at mealtimes ought to be the rule.

In cases where a dental disorder makes proper chewing impossible, food should be chopped or pureed. Older people occasionally have difficulty swallowing and may choke on a large piece of unchewed meat.

Food for older people should be cooked simply, preferably baked, boiled, or broiled rather than fried, and menus excessively rich in fats should be avoided. A daily multivitamin capsule is strongly recommended for those over 60. A poor appetite can be stimulated by an ounce or two of sherry before a meal unless there are medical reasons for avoiding alcoholic beverages of any kind. See under *Aging and What to Do About It*, p. 654, for a discussion of diet and eating habits in the later years.

DURING PREGNANCY: A pregnant woman needs special foods to maintain her own health as well as to safeguard the health of her baby. She should have additional vitamin D and iron, usually recommended as dietary supplements. More important for most women is the provision of adequate protein in the diet to prevent toxemia of pregnancy or underweight babies. Between 70 and 85 grams of protein a day should be eaten during pregnancy, even if this results in a weight gain of as much as 25 pounds. Adequate nutrition is more important than restricting weight gain to 20 pounds or less.

NURSING MOTHERS: A nursing mother has special dietary needs in addition to those satisfied by the normal adult diet. She should drink an extra quart of milk and eat two more servings of citrus fruit or tomatoes, one more serving of lean meat, fish, poultry, eggs, beans, or cheese, and one more serving of leafy green or yellow vegetables.

Malnutrition

The classic diseases of nutritional deficiency, or malnutrition, such as scurvy and pellagra, are now rare, at least in the United States. The chief reason for their disappearance is the application of scientific knowledge gained in this century of the importance of vitamins and minerals in the diet. Thus most bread is fortified with vitamins and minerals, and in addition, commercial food processing has made it possible for balanced diets of an appealing variety to be eaten all year round.

Many people do not get an adequate diet, either through ignorance or because they simply cannot afford it. A number of food programs have been created to assist them, but unfortunately, the programs don't reach everyone who needs help.

Causes of Malnutrition

Some people, either because of ignorance or food faddism, do not eat a balanced diet even though they can afford to. There are also large numbers of people with nutritional deficiency diseases who can be described as abnormal, at least in regard to eating. Some are alcoholics; others live alone and are so depressed that they lack sufficient drive to feed themselves properly.

Combination of any of these factors increase the likelihood of poor nutrition and often lead to health-damaging consequences.

DISEASE: People can also develop nutritional deficiencies because they have some disease that interferes with food absorption, storage, and utilization, or that causes an increased excretion, usually in the urine, of substances needed for nutrition. These are generally chronic diseases of the gastrointestinal tract including the liver, or of the kidneys or the endocrine glands.

MEDICATIONS: Nutritional deficiencies can also result from loss of appetite caused by medications, especially when a number of different medications are taken simultaneously. This adverse affect on the appetite is a strong reason for not taking medicines unless told to do so by a doctor for a specific purpose.

Most people are not aware of inadequacies in their diet until there are some dramatic consequences. Nor is it easy to recognize the presence of a disorder that might be causing malnutrition. A doctor should be consulted promptly when there is a persistent weight loss, especially when the diet is normal. He should also be informed of any changes in the skin, mucous membranes of the mouth or tongue, or nervous system function, since such symptoms can be a warning of dietary deficiency.

The family or friends of a person with a nutritional deficiency can often detect his condition because they become aware of changes in his eating patterns. They can also note early signs of a deficiency of some of the B vitamins, such as cracks in the mucous membranes at the corners of the mouth, or some slowing of intellectual function.

Correction of Nutritional Deficiencies

Nutritional deficiencies are among the most easily preventable causes of disease. It is important to realize that even mild deficiencies can cause irreparable damage, particularly protein deprivation in young children, which can result in some degree of mental retardation. Periodic medical checkups for everyone in the family are the best way to make sure that such deficiencies are corrected before they snowball into a chronic disease. In most cases, all that is required is a change in eating habits.

Weight

Probably the most important dietary problem in the United States today is obesity. It is certainly the problem most talked about and written about, not only in terms of good looks, but more important, in terms of good health.

All studies indicate that people who are obese have a higher rate of disease and a shorter life expectancy than those of average weight. From a medical point of view, people who are too fat may actually suffer from a form of malnutrition, even though they look overnourished.

Being too fat and being overweight are not necessarily the same. Heavy bones and muscles can make a person overweight in terms of the charts, but only an excess amount of

TABLE 1

| Desirable Weights for Men and Women Aged 25 and Over[1] (in pounds by height and frame, in indoor clothing) | | | | | | | |
| MEN (in shoes, 1-inch heels) | | | | WOMEN (in shoes, 2-inch heels) | | | |
Height	Small Frame	Medium Frame	Large Frame	Height	Small Frame	Medium Frame	Large Frame
5' 2"	112–120	118–129	126–141	4' 10"	92– 98	96–107	104–119
5' 3"	115–123	121–133	129–144	4' 11"	94–101	98–110	106–122
5' 4"	118–126	124–136	132–148	5' 0"	96–104	101–113	109–125
5' 5"	121–129	127–139	135–152	5' 1"	99–107	104–116	112–128
5' 6"	124–133	130–143	138–156	5' 2"	102–110	107–119	115–131
5' 7"	128–137	134–147	142–161	5' 3"	105–113	110–122	118–134
5' 8"	132–141	138–152	147–166	5' 4"	108–116	113–126	121–138
5' 9"	136–145	142–156	151–170	5' 5"	111–119	116–130	125–142
5' 10"	140–150	146–160	155–174	5' 6"	114–123	120–135	129–146
5' 11"	144–154	150–165	159–179	5' 7"	118–127	124–139	133–150
6' 0"	148–158	154–170	164–184	5' 8"	122–131	128–143	137–154
6' 1"	152–162	158–175	168–189	5' 9"	126–135	132–147	141–158
6' 2"	156–167	162–180	173–194	5' 10"	130–140	136–151	145–163
6' 3"	160–171	167–185	178–199	5' 11"	134–144	140–155	149–168
6' 4"	164–175	172–190	182–204	6' 0"	138–148	144–159	153–173

[1]Adapted from Metropolitan Life Insurance Co., New York. New weight standards for men and women. *Statistical Bulletin* 40:3.

fat tissue can make someone obese. However, height and weight tables are generally used to determine obesity.

Table 1 lists standard desirable weights for people of various heights, calculated with indoor clothing and shoes on. Frame sizes are estimated in a general way. This table applies to anyone over the age of 25, indicating that weight gain for the rest of the life span is unnecessary for biological normalcy.

Table 2 gives average weights of American men and women, according to height and age. These measurements are made without clothing or shoes. Note that the weights are considerably higher than the corresponding ones of Table 1. There is a modest weight gain until the middle years and then a gradual loss.

To determine whether a person is obese according to the tables, the percent that he is overweight has to be calculated. An individual is usually considered obese in the clinical sense if he weighs 20 percent more than the standard tables indicate for his size and age.

THE PINCH TEST: Another method of determining obesity is to use the "pinch" test. In most adults under 50 years of age, about half of the body fat is located directly under the skin. There are various parts of the body, such as the side of the lower torso, the back of the upper arm, or directly under the shoulder blade, where the thumb and forefinger can pinch a fold of skin and fat away from the underlying bone structure.

If the fold between the fingers—which is, of course, double thickness when it is pinched—is thicker than one inch in any of these areas, the likelihood is that the person is obese.

TABLE 2

	MEN						
	\textbf{Average Weights for Men and Women[1]} \textit{(in pounds by age and height, in paper gown and slippers)}						
Height	18–24 Years	25–34 Years	35–44 Years	45–54 Years	55–64 Years	65–74 Years	75–79 Years
5' 2"	137	141	149	148	148	144	133
5' 3"	140	145	152	152	151	148	138
5' 4"	144	150	156	156	155	151	143
5' 5"	147	154	160	160	158	154	148
5' 6"	151	159	164	164	162	158	154
5' 7"	154	163	168	168	166	161	159
5' 8"	158	168	171	173	169	165	164
5' 9"	161	172	175	177	173	168	169
5' 10"	165	177	179	181	176	171	174
5' 11"	168	181	182	185	180	175	179
6' 0"	172	186	186	189	184	178	184
6' 1"	175	190	190	193	187	182	189
6' 2"	179	194	194	197	191	185	194

	WOMEN						
4' 9"	116	112	131	129	138	132	125
4' 10"	118	116	134	132	141	135	129
4' 11"	120	120	136	136	144	138	132
5' 0"	122	124	138	140	149	142	136
5' 1"	125	128	140	143	150	145	139
5' 2"	127	132	143	147	152	149	143
5' 3"	129	136	145	150	155	152	146
5' 4"	131	140	147	154	158	156	150
5' 5"	134	144	149	158	161	159	153
5' 6"	136	148	152	161	164	163	157
5' 7"	138	152	154	165	167	166	160
5' 8"	140	156	156	168	170	170	164

[1]Adapted from National Center for Health Statistics: Weight by Height and Age of Adults, United States. *Vital Health Statistics.* PHS Publication No. 1000–Series 11, No. 14.

The Problem of Overweight

The percentage of overweight people in this country has been increasing steadily, chiefly because people eat more and use less physical energy than they used to. Americans do very little walking because of the availability of cars; they do very little manual labor because of the increasing use of machines. They may eat good wholesome meals, but they have the time for nibbling at all hours, especially when sitting in front of the television screen.

These patterns usually begin in childhood. Youngsters rarely walk to school any more; they get there by bus or car. They often have extra money for snacks and soft drinks, and frequently parents encourage them to overeat without realizing that such habits do them more harm than good.

Most overweight children remain overweight as adults. They also have greater difficulty losing fat, and if they do lose it, tend to regain it more

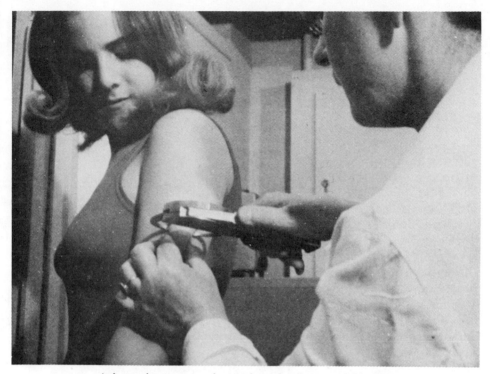

A doctor demonstrates the pinch test for obesity. A fold of skin and fat of the upper arm should be no thicker than one inch.

easily than overweight adults who were thin as children. Many adults become overweight between the ages of 20 and 30. Thus, by age 30, about 12 percent of American men and women are 20 percent or more overweight, and by age 60, about 30 percent of the male population and 50 percent of the female are at least 20 percent overweight. As indicated above, the phenomenon of weight gain while aging does not represent biological normalcy.

Why People Put On Weight

Why does weight gain happen? Excess weight is the result of the imbalance between caloric intake as food and caloric expenditure as energy, either in maintaining the basic metabolic processes necessary to sustain life or in performing physical activity. Calories not spent in either of these ways become converted to fat and accumulate in the body as fat, or *adipose* tissue.

A *calorie* is the unit of measurement that describes the amount of

		Calories
	Sedentary	2,500
	Moderately active	3,000
	Active	3,500
	Very active	4,250
	Sedentary	2,100
	Moderately active	2,500
	Active	3,000
	Very active	3,750

Guidelines for average daily calorie consumption by men and women. With increasing use of labor-saving devices, most Americans fall into the sedentary category.

energy potentially available in a given food. It is also used to describe the amount of energy the body must use up to perform a given function.

An ounce of protein contains 130 calories, as does an ounce of carbohydrate. An ounce of fat, by contrast, contains 270 calories. This biochemical information isn't too helpful in calculating the calories in a particular piece of meat, slice of bread, or pat of butter. For such practical figures, there are useful pocket guides, such as *Calories and Weight,* a U.S. Government publication that can be obtained by sending $1.00 to the Superintendent of Documents, U.S. Government Printing Office, Washington, D. C. 20401, and asking for the Agriculture Information Bulletin No. 364.

Counting Calories

If an adult gets the average 3,000 calories a day in his food from the age of 20 to 70, he will have consumed about 55 million calories. About 60 percent of these calories will have been used for his basic metabolic processes. The rest—22 million calories—might have resulted in a gain of about 6,000 pounds of fat, since each group of 3,500 extra calories could have produced one pound of fat.

In some ways, it's a miracle that people don't become more obese than they do. The reason, of course, is that most or all of these extra calories are normally used to provide energy for physical activity. On this page are some examples of calorie expenditure during various activities.

A reasonably good way for an adult to figure his daily caloric

TYPE OF ACTIVITY	CALORIES PER HOUR
Sedentary: reading, sewing, typing, etc.	30–100
Light: cooking, slow walking, dressing, etc.	100–170
Moderate: sweeping, light gardening, making beds, etc.	170–250
Vigorous: fast walking, hanging out clothes, golfing, etc.	250–350
Strenuous: swimming, bicycling, dancing, etc.	350 and more

needs for moderate activities is to multiply his desirable weight (as noted in Table 1) by 18 for men and by 16 for women. If the typical day includes vigorous or strenuous activities, extra calories will, of course, be required.

Parental Influences and Hereditary Factors

Although there are exceptions, almost all obese people consume more calories than they expend. The reasons for this imbalance are complex. One has to do with parental weight. If the weight of both parents is normal, there is only a 10 percent likelihood that the children will be obese. If one parent is obese, there is a 50 percent probability that the children will be too, and if both are, the probability of obese offspring is 80 percent.

No one knows for certain why this is so. It is probably a combination of diet habits acquired in youth, conditioning during early years to react to emotional stress by eating, the absence of appropriate exercise patterns, and genetic inheritance.

Some obese people seem to have

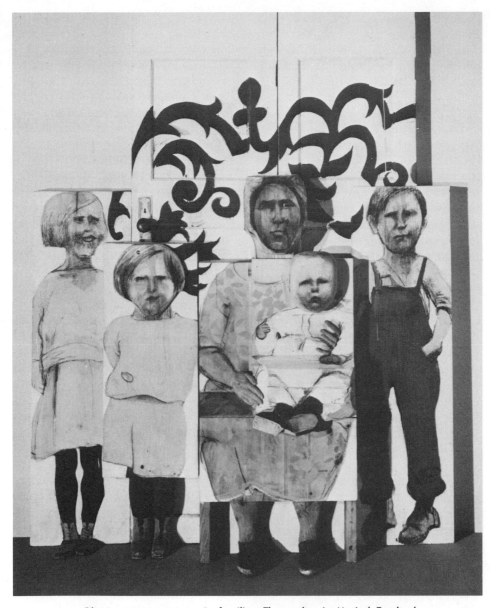

Obesity appears to run in families. The mother in Marisol Escobar's sculpture "The Family" has two children who resemble her in body type.

an impairment in the regulatory mechanism of the area of the central nervous system that governs food intake. Simply put, they do not know when to stop eating. Others, particularly girls, may eat less than their nonobese counterparts, but they are considerably less active. Some researchers think that obese people have an inherent muscle rhythm deficiency. A few people appear to have an abnormality in the metabolic process which results in the accumulation of fat even when the balance between calories taken in and expended is negative and should lead to weight loss.

Obesity and Health

There are many reasons why obesity is a health hazard. The annual death rate for obese people between the ages of 20 and 64 is half again as high as that for people whose weight is close to normal. This statistical difference is due primarily to the increased likelihood that the obese person will suffer from diabetes mellitus and from diseases of the digestive and circulatory systems, especially of the heart.

One possible reason for the increased possibility of heart disease is that there are about two-thirds of a mile of blood vessels in each pound of adipose tissue. Thus 20 or more pounds of excess weight are likely to impose a great additional work load on the heart.

Obese people are also poorer surgical risks than the nonobese, and it is often more difficult to diagnose and therefore to treat their illnesses correctly.

Permanent loss of excess weight makes the formerly obese person come closer to matching the life expectancy of the nonobese. However, losing and regaining weight as a repeated pattern is even more hazardous in terms of health than consistent obesity.

Psychological Consequences of Obesity

In ways that are both obvious and subtle, obesity often has damaging psychological consequences. This is particularly true for obese children,

who tend to feel isolated and rejected by their peers. They may consider themselves victims of prejudice and blame their obesity for everything that goes wrong in their lives. In many cases, the destructive relationship between obesity and self-pity keeps perpetuating itself.

Obese adults are likely to experience the same feelings, but to a somewhat lesser degree. For some, obesity is an escape which consciously or unconsciously helps them to avoid situations in which they feel uncomfortable—those that involve active competition or relationships with the opposite sex.

Avoiding Excess Weight

Clearly, obesity is a condition that most people would like to avoid. Not putting on extra pounds does seem to be easier, in theory at least, then taking them off. One possible explanation for this is that additional adipose tissue consists of a proliferation of fat cells. Shrinking these cells is one thing, eliminating them is another. Our present lack of fundamental knowledge about the regulatory and metabolic mechanisms relating to obesity limits the technique of preventing overweight to recommending a balance between caloric intake and expenditure.

The real responsibility for preventing the onset of obesity in childhood rests with parents. All of the fundamentals of good nutrition and healthy eating habits are of the utmost importance in this connection. Caloric expenditure in the form of regular exercise is equally important.

EXERCISING BY HABIT: This does not necessarily mean that exercise should be encouraged for its own

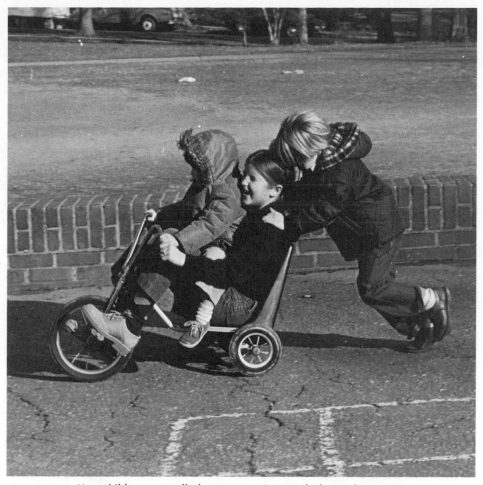

Most children naturally love to exercise regularly in play. Maintaining the habit of exerting oneself is the secret of avoiding obesity.

sake. What it does mean is making a habit of choosing an active way of approaching a situation rather than a lazy way: walking upstairs rather than taking the elevator; walking to school rather than riding; walking while playing golf rather than riding in a cart; running to get the ball that has rolled away rather than ambling toward it. These choices should be made consistently and not just occasionally if obesity is to be avoided. Those people who naturally enjoy the more active way of doing things are lucky. Those who don't should make an effort to develop new patterns, especially if obesity is a family problem.

Anyone with the type of physical handicap that makes a normal amount of exercise impossible should be especially careful about caloric intake.

Weight Reduction

The treatment of obesity is a complicated problem. In the first place, there is the question of who wants or needs to be treated and how much weight should be lost. Except in unusual situations, anyone who wants to lose weight should be encouraged to do so. Possible exceptions are teen-agers who are not overweight but who want to be as thin as they can possibly be—the boy who is involved in an athletic event such as wrestling, or the girl who has decided she wants to look like a fashion model.

Crash dieting is usually unwise if the goal is to lose too much weight too rapidly and should be undertaken only after consulting a doctor about its advisability. As for adolescents who have become slightly overweight during puberty, they may be ill-advised to try to take off the extra pounds that probably relate to a temporary growth pattern.

Losing Weight
Must Be Self-Motivated

Unless there are compelling medical reasons for not doing so, anyone weighing 20 percent or more over the normal limit for his age and body build should be helped to slim down. It is extremely important, however, for the motivation to come from the person himself rather than from outside pressure.

Unless an overweight person really wants to reduce, he will not succeed in doing so, certainly not permanently, even though he appears to be trying. He must have convinced himself—intellectually and emotionally—that the goal of weight loss is truly worth the effort.

It is very difficult not only for his friends and family but for the person himself to be absolutely sure about the depth of his motivation. A doctor

treating an overweight patient has to assume that the desire to reduce is genuine and will try to reinforce it whenever he can. However, if a patient has made a number of attempts to lose weight over a period of years and has either been unable to reduce to any significant degree, or has become overweight again after reducing, it is probably safe to assume that the emotional desire is absent, or that there are emotional conflicts that stand in the way.

It is very possible that such a person could be harmed psychologically by losing weight, since he

Patent remedies that promise quick and effortless release from obesity have long been on the market; this 1878 ad sells one such product.

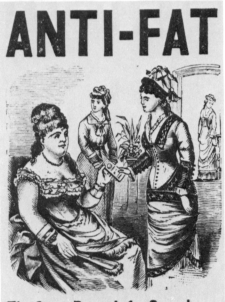

ANTI-FAT

The Great Remedy for Corpulence

ALLAN'S ANTI-FAT

is composed of purely vegetable ingredients, and is perfectly harmless. It acts upon the food in the stomach, preventing its being converted into fat. Taken in accordance with directions, **it will reduce a fat person from two to five pounds per week.**

might need to be overweight for some deep-seated reason. This can be true for both children and adults. Occasionally it is possible for a psychiatrist or psychologist to help the patient remove a psychological block, and then weight reduction can occur if the caloric balance is straightened out.

Effective Planning for Weight Loss

The ultimate key to successful weight reduction is proper eating combined with proper physical activity. This balance is extremely difficult for many people to achieve because it involves a marked change in attitudes and behavior patterns that are generally solidly established and of long duration. Furthermore, once the changes are made, they will have to endure for a lifetime if the weight that has been lost is not to be regained.

It is therefore important that the reducing diet should be somewhat similar to the person's usual eating pattern in terms of style and quality. Ideally, only the caloric content should be changed, and probably the word "dieting" should not be used to describe the process, since most people don't find the idea of permanent dieting congenial.

Similarly, the increased physical activity that must accompany the new eating style should be of a type that the person enjoys. It is virtually impossible for an overweight person to reduce merely by restricting his caloric intake, or merely by increasing his caloric expenditure. The two must go together.

Cutting Down Step by Step

The first thing to determine when planning to lose weight is the number of pounds that have to go. A realistic goal to set is the loss of about one pound a week. This may seem too slow, but remember that at this rate, fifty pounds can be lost in a year.

GETTING STARTED: Start by weighing yourself on arising, and then for two weeks try to eat in your customary manner, but keep a careful record of everything that you eat, the time it is eaten, and the number of calories it contains. During this period, continue to do your usual amount of physical activity.

When the two weeks are over, weigh yourself again at the same time of day as before. If you haven't gained any weight, you are in a basal caloric state. Then check over your food list to see what might be eliminated each day without causing discomfort.

Try to think in terms of eliminating fats and carbohydrates first, because it is essential that you continue to get sufficient vitamins and minerals which are largely found in proteins. The foods described in the chart on page 705 should all continue to be included in your daily food consumption. If you are in the habit of having an occasional drink, remember that there are calories in alcohol but no nutrients, and that most alcoholic beverages stimulate the appetite. See *Low Calorie Diet* sample menus on page 728, and *Nutrients in Common Foods,* pp. **698–716**, for estimating calories in particular foods.

PLANNING MEALS: When you replan your meals, keep in mind that the items you cut down on must add up to between 300 and 400 calories a day if you are going to lose one pound a week.

LOW CALORIE DIET						
Sample Menus						
	800 calories		1,200 calories		1,600 calories	
	Weight grams	Household measure	Weight grams	Household measure	Weight grams	Household measure
Breakfast						
Orange, sliced	125	1 medium	125	1 medium	125	1 medium
Soft cooked egg	50	One	50	One	50	One
Toast	25	1 slice	25	1 slice	25	1 slice
Butter	5	1 teaspoon	5	1 teaspoon	5	1 teaspoon
Coffee or tea	—	As desired	—	As desired	—	As desired
Milk	240	1 cup skim	240	1 cup skim	240	1 cup whole
Luncheon						
Clear broth	—	As desired	—	As desired	—	As desired
Salad (cottage cheese, tomato, plain lettuce leaf)	90	½ cup	90	½ cup	90	½ cup
Egg			50	One	50	One
Green peas					100	½ cup
Baked apple, unsweetened	80	1 small	80	1 small	80	1 small
Bread			25	1 slice	25	1 slice
Butter			5	1 teaspoon	5	1 teaspoon
Milk	240	1 cup skim	240	1 cup skim	240	1 cup whole
Coffee or tea	—	As desired	—	As desired	—	As desired
Dinner						
Roast beef, lean	60	2 ounces	90	3 ounces	120	4 ounces
Carrots, plain	100	½ cup	100	½ cup	100	½ cup
Tossed vegetable salad with vinegar	50	¾ cup	50	¾ cup	50	¾ cup
Pineapple, unsweetened	80	½ cup	80	½ cup	80	½ cup
Bread			25	1 slice	25	1 slice
Butter			5	1 teaspoon	10	2 teaspoons
Coffee or tea	—	As desired	—	As desired	—	As desired
Nourishment						
Peach					100	1 medium

These diets contain approximately 800, 1,200, and 1,600 calories. The 800 calorie diet, even with variations in selections of food, will not meet the recommended daily allowances in iron and thaimine. The approximate composition is as follows:

	800 calories	1,200 calories	1,600 calories
Protein	60 gm.	75 gm.	85 gm.
Fat	30 gm.	50 gm.	80 gm.
Carbohydrate	75 gm.	110 gm.	130 gm.

From the *Clinical Center Diet Manual*, revised edition, prepared by the Nutrition Department, The Clinical Center, National Institutes of Health, Public Health Service, U.S. Department of Health, Education, and Welfare (Public Health Service Publication No. 989), pp. 67–68.

Your total daily food intake should be divided among at least three meals a day, more if you wish. If you need to eat more food or to eat more often, try snacking on low calorie foods such as cabbage, carrots, celery, cucumber, and cauliflower. All of these can be eaten raw between meals.

There is definitely something to be said in favor of having breakfast every morning, or at least most mornings. This may be psychologically difficult, but try to do it, because it will be easier to control your urge to eat too much later in the day.

INCREASING EXERCISE: At the same time that you begin to cut down on your food intake, start to increase your daily exercise in whatever way you find congenial so that the number of calories expended in increased exercise plus the number of calories eliminated from your diet comes to 500 or more. This is your daily caloric loss compared with your so-called basal caloric state.

ACHIEVING YOUR GOAL: You may wish to double your daily caloric loss so that you lose two pounds a week. Do not try to lose any more than that unless you are under close medical supervision.

If you gained weight during your two-week experimental period, you will have to increase your daily caloric loss by 500 for every pound gained per week. Thus, if you gained one pound during the two weeks, you will have to step up your daily caloric loss to 750 to lose a pound a week.

You'll have to keep plugging away to achieve your goal. It will be trying and difficult in many ways. You may get moody and discouraged and be tempted to quit. Don't. You'll probably go on periodic food binges. All this is natural and understandable, so try not to brood about it. Just do the best you can each day. Don't worry about yesterday, and let tomorrow take care of itself.

In many ways it can help, and in some cases it's essential, to have the support and encouragement of family and friends, particularly of those with whom you share meals. You may find it helpful to join a group that has been formed to help its members lose weight and maintain their weight loss. This is good psychological support.

MAINTAINING YOUR WEIGHT LOSS: Once you have achieved your desired weight, you can test yourself to see what happens if you increase your caloric intake. Clearly, anyone who can lose weight in the manner described can't stay in a state of negative caloric imbalance indefinitely. But you will have to be careful, or you'll become overweight again. It's a challenge, but people who stick to a disciplined program can be rewarded by success.

Special Problems

If you do not succeed in losing weight in spite of carrying out the program described above, you may need professional help because of some special problem. A qualified physician may try some special diets, or he may even suggest putting you into a hospital so that he can see to it that you have no caloric food at all for as long as three weeks.

Perhaps the situation is complicated by a metabolic abnormality that can be corrected or helped by medication. Although such conditions are rare, they are not unheard of.

Obesity is almost never caused by a "glandular" problem—which usually means an underactive thyroid. Do not take thyroid pills to reduce unless your thyroid has been found to be underactive on the basis of a specific laboratory test.

The indiscriminate use of pills to reduce, even when prescribed, is never helpful in the long run, although it may appear to be at first. The unsupervised use of amphetamines, for example, can be extremely dangerous. See *Stimulant Drugs*, p. 1362, for further information about the dangers of amphetamine abuse.

Because so many people are eager to reduce, and because losing weight isn't easy, there are many unethical professionals who specialize in the problem. Avoid them. All they are likely to do for you is take your money and make your situation no better—and often worse—than it was to begin with.

Underweight

Weighing too little is a problem which is considerably less common than weighing too much. In fact, in many cases, it isn't accurate to call it a problem at all, at least not a medical one.

There are some times, however, when underweight may indicate the presence of a disease, especially when a person rather suddenly begins and continues to lose weight, even though there has been no change in his eating habits. This is a situation that calls for prompt medical evaluation. Such a person may already be under a doctor's care at the time the weight loss is first noticed.

More often, however, underweight is a chronic condition that is of concern to the person who feels his looks would improve if he could only add some extra pounds. This is especially true in the case of adolescent girls and young women.

What To Do About Weighing Too Little

Chronic underweight is rarely a reflection of underlying disease. It is rather an expression of individual heredity or eating patterns, or a combination of both. Treatment for the condition is the opposite of the treatment for overweight. The achievement of a positive caloric balance comes first; more calories have to be consumed each day than are expended. An underweight person should record his food history over a two-week period in the manner described for an overweight one. Once this has been done, various adjustments can be made.

First of all, he should see that he eats at least three meals a day and that they are eaten in a leisurely way and in a relaxed frame of mind. All of the basic foods should be represented in the daily food intake, with special emphasis on protein. The daily caloric intake should then be gradually increased at each meal and snacks added, so long as the snacks don't reduce the appetite at mealtimes.

Carbohydrate foods are the best ones to emphasize in adding calories. Since the extra food intake may cause a certain amount of discomfort, encouragement and support from family and friends can be extremely helpful. Just as there may be psychological blocks against losing weight, there may well be a complicated underlying resistance to adding it.

Anyone trying to gain weight should remain or become reasonably active physically. Adding a pound or two a month for an adult—and a little more than that for a growing youngster—is an achievable goal until the desired weight is reached. When this happens, there will probably have to be some adjustments in eating and exercise patterns so that a state of caloric balance is achieved.

How Food Relates to Disease

Just as proper food is essential in the prevention of some diseases, it is helpful in the treatment of others. It also plays an important role in protecting and fortifying the general health of a patient while a specific illness is being treated.

The components of therapeutic diets are usually prescribed by the physician in charge, but some general principles will be presented here. Remember that diets designed to treat a given disease must supply the patient's basic nutritional requirements.

Ulcers

Special diet is a major treatment consideration in the case of peptic ulcer, whether located in the stomach (gastric) or in the small intestine (duodenal). A major aim of such a diet is the neutralizing of the acidity of gastric juices by the frequent intake of high protein foods such as milk and eggs. Foods which irritate an ulcer chemically, such as excessive sweets, spices, or salt, or mechanically, such as foods with sharp seeds or tough skins, and foods that are too hot or too cold, should be avoided. It is also advisable to eliminate gravies, coffee, strong tea, carbonated beverages, and alcohol, since all of these stimulate gastric secretion. Such a diet is called a *bland* diet. See *Soft and Bland Soft Diets*, pp. 732–735. A soft diet is recommended for some forms of gastrointestinal distress and for those people who have difficulty chewing. It is often combined with the bland diet recommended for peptic ulcer patients to reduce the likelihood of irritation. See under *Diseases of the Digestive System*, p. 1155, for further information about ulcers.

Diabetes

As the section on diabetes mellitus indicates (see Ch. 31, p. 1220), the major objectives of the special diet are weight control, control of the abnormal carbohydrate metabolism, and as far as possible, psychological adjustment by the patient to his individual circumstances. To some extent, he must calculate his diet mathematically. First, his daily caloric needs have to be determined in terms of his activities:

TYPE OF ACTIVITY	CALORIES PER POUND OF BODY WEIGHT
Sedentary	13.5
Moderate	16
Marked	18

If he is overweight or underweight, the total calories per pound of body weight will have to be adjusted downward or upward by about five calories per pound.

After his total daily caloric needs have been figured out, he can calcu-

SOFT AND BLAND SOFT DIETS
SOFT DIET

Foods allowed on this diet are left whole. The fiber content is modified by using only cooked or canned fruits and vegetables (with skins and seeds removed); refined or finely ground cereals and breads are included. Some restrictions have been placed on highly seasoned and rich foods because of the specific needs for which the soft diet is usually ordered.

BLAND SOFT DIET

If further restrictions on seasonings and food items are necessary, a bland soft diet may be ordered. This diet follows the same pattern as the soft diet outlined below but is modified to eliminate all stimulants, such as meat extractives, spices, condiments (except salt), strongly flavored foods, and beverages that contain caffeine, such as coffee, tea, or cola drinks. The following foods are also omitted: all whole grain breads, rolls, muffins, and cereals; all gravies and salad dressings; pork; broth and soups with a meat base (use only strained cream soups); lettuce. Limit quantities of jelly, sugar, and hard candies. Extremely hot or cold foods are avoided. The foods allowed may be divided into five or six small meals with each feeding containing a good source of protein.

SOFT DIET		
Type of food	Foods included	Foods excluded
Beverages	Coffee, decaffeinated coffee, tea, carbonated beverages, cereal beverages, cocoa, milk.	None
Breads	White; whole wheat, finely ground; rye (without seeds), finely ground; white or whole wheat rolls or muffins, finely ground; plain crackers.	Coarse whole wheat breads; breads, rolls, and muffins with seeds, nuts, raisins, etc.
Cereals	Cooked or prepared cereals, such as corn flakes, strained oatmeal, cream of rice or wheat, farina, hominy grits, cornmeal, puffed rice, other rice cereals.	Cooked or prepared coarse cereals, such as bran, shredded wheat.
Desserts	Plain cake and cookies, sponge cake; custards, plain puddings, rennet desserts; gelatin desserts with allowed fruits; plain ice cream, sherbets (except pineapple), fruit ices.	Pies; pastries; desserts made with coconut, nuts, pineapple, raisins, etc.
Fats	Butter, cream, fortified fats, plain gravies, mayonnaise, cream sauces.	Fried foods; rich highly seasoned sauces and gravies with mushrooms, pimento, etc.

From the *Clinical Center Diet Manual*, revised edition, prepared by the Nutrition Department, The Clinical Center, National Institutes of Health, Public Health Service, U.S. Department of Health, Education, and Welfare (Public Health Service Publication No. 989), pp. 45–52.

SOFT DIET (continued)		
Type of food	Foods included	Foods excluded
Fruits	Raw ripe bananas; canned or cooked fruits without skins or small seeds, such as applesauce, baked apple without skin, apricots, sweet cherries, peaches, pears; fruit juices as desired.	Raw fruits except bananas; canned or cooked fruits with skins, coarse fibers, or seeds, such as figs, raisins, berries, pineapple, etc.
Meat, poultry, fish	Bacon, beef, ham, lamb, pork, veal, poultry, and fish that has been baked, boiled, braised, broiled, or roasted.	Fried meat, poultry, or fish; highly seasoned meats; stews containing celery, onions, etc.; cold cuts, sausages.
Cheese	All except strongly flavored cheeses.	Cheeses with pimento, caraway seeds, etc.; strongly flavored cheeses.
Eggs	Any raw, soft cooked, hard cooked, soft scrambled, poached; omelets made with allowed foods.	Fried eggs, omelets containing mushrooms, etc.
Potato or substitute	Hominy, macaroni, noodles, rice, spaghetti; white or sweet potatoes without skins.	Fried potatoes; potato chips; highly seasoned sauces for spaghetti, macaroni, etc.
Soups	Broth, strained soups; cream soups made with allowed vegetables.	All others
Sweets	Hard candies, simple chocolate candies without nuts or fruit; strained honey, jelly, sugar, syrup.	Candies with whole fruit, coconut, or nuts; jam, marmalade.
Vegetables	Cooked or canned asparagus tips, string beans, wax beans, beets, carrots, chopped spinach, winter squash; tomato puree, tomato juice; raw lettuce leaf as garnish.	Cooked broccoli, brussels sprouts, cabbage, cauliflower, celery, corn, mustard greens, turnip greens, mushrooms, onions, fresh and dried peas, summer squash, whole tomatoes; dried beans, lima beans, lentils. All raw vegetables except lettuce as a garnish.
Miscellaneous	Salt; small amounts of white or black pepper used in cooking; creamy peanut butter.	Hot seasonings, such as chili sauce, red pepper, etc.; coconut, nuts, olives, pickles; spiced fruit.

late the number of grams of carbohydrate he should have each day by dividing his total calories by 10. The number of grams of protein per day as well as the number of grams of fat should be half the number of grams of carbohydrate.

This will mean that 40 percent of his daily calories will come from carbohydrate, 40 percent from fat,

SOFT DIET
Sample Menu

Breakfast
  Orange juice . . . . ½ cup
  Corn flakes . . . . ½ cup
  Poached egg . . . One
  Whole wheat toast . . 1 slice
  Butter or fortified fat . . 1 teaspoon
  Milk, whole . . . . 1 cup
  Coffee or tea . . . . As desired
  Cream . . . . . As desired
  Sugar . . . . . As desired

Luncheon
  Creamed chicken on toast ½ to ¾ cup
  Mashed potato . . . ½ cup
  Buttered carrots . . ½ cup
  Bread, enriched . . 1 slice
  Butter or fortified fat . . 1 teaspoon
  Canned pear halves . . 2 halves
  Milk, whole . . . . 1 cup
  Coffee or tea . . . . As desired
  Cream . . . . . As desired
  Sugar . . . . . As desired

Dinner
  Roast beef, gravy . . . 2 to 3 ounces
  Baked potato . . . . 1 medium
  Buttered asparagus spears 1 serving
  Bread, enriched . . . 1 slice
  Butter or fortified fat . . 1 teaspoon
  Vanilla ice cream . . . ½ cup
  Coffee or tea . . . . As desired
  Cream . . . . . As desired
  Sugar . . . . . . As desired

and 20 percent from protein. One-fifth of the total should be obtained at breakfast and the rest split between lunch and dinner. Snacks that are taken during the day should be subtracted equally from lunch and dinner.

It is important that meals and planned snacks be eaten regularly and that no food servings be added or omitted. Growing children from 1 to 20 years of age who have diabetes will require considerably more daily calories. A rough estimate is 1,000 calories for a one-year-old child and 100 additional calories for each year of age.

Salt-Free Diets

There are a number of chronic diseases which are treated in part by restricting the amount of sodium in the diet. These diseases, which are associated with fluid retention in the body, include congestive heart failure, certain types of kidney and liver diseases, and hypertension or high blood pressure.

BLAND SOFT DIET
Sample Menu *(six small meals)*

Breakfast
Egg, poached .   .   .   .   One
White toast, enriched .   .   1 slice
Butter or fortified fat .   .   1 teaspoon
Hot cocoa .   .   .   .   1 cup

10:00 a.m.
Orange juice .   .   .   .   ½ cup
Corn flakes   .   .   .   ½ cup
Cream   .   .   .   .   ¼ cup
Sugar .   .   .   .   .   2 teaspoons

Luncheon
Creamed chicken on toast   ½ cup
Mashed potato   .   .   .   ½ cup
Buttered carrots .   .   .   ½ cup
Milk .   .   .   .   .   1 cup
Canned pears .   .   .   .   1 half

2:30 p.m.
Milkshake   .   .   .   1 cup
Soda crackers .   .   .   Three

Dinner
Roast beef   .   .   .   2 ounces
Baked potato .   .   .   1 medium
Buttered asparagus   .   .   1 serving
Butter or fortified fat .   .   1 teaspoon
Milk .   .   .   .   .   1 cup
Vanilla ice cream .   .   .   ½ cup

8:30 p.m.
Baked custard   .   .   .   ½ cup
Vanilla wafers   .   .   Two

The restriction of sodium intake helps to reduce or avoid the problem of fluid retention. The normal daily diet contains about seven or more grams of sodium, most of it in the form of sodium chloride or table salt. This amount is either inherent in the food or added during processing, cooking, or at mealtime. Half the weight of salt is sodium.

For people whose physical condition requires only a small restriction of the normal sodium intake, simply not salting food at the table is a sufficient reduction. They may decide to use a salt substitute, but before doing so should discuss the question with their physician.

A greater sodium restriction, for example, to no more than 5 grams a day, requires the avoidance of such high salt content foods as ham, bacon, crackers, catsup, and potato chips, as well as almost entirely eliminating salt in the preparation and serving of meals. Severe restriction—1 gram or less a day—involves special food selection and cooking procedures, as well as the use of distilled water if the local water has more than 20 milligrams of sodium per quart. In restricting sodium to this extent, it is important to make sure that protein and vitamins are not reduced below the minimum daily requirements. See *Sodium Restricted Diets*, pp. 737–740.

Other Diseases Requiring Special Diets

There are several other disorders in which diet is an important consideration: all chronic gastrointestinal disorders, such as ulcerative colitis, enteritis, gall bladder stones, and diverticulitis; a variety of hereditary disorders such as phenylketonuria and galactosemia; atherosclerosis, especially when it is associated with elevated blood levels of cholesterol or triglycerides or both; liver disease such as cirrhosis; many of the endocrine diseases; kidney stones; and sometimes certain neurological diseases such as epilepsy. Diet also plays a special role in convalescence from most illnesses and in post-surgical care. The *Modified Fat Diet* (pp. 741–743) and *Low Fat Diet* (pp. 745–746) are recommended for some diseases of the liver and gall bladder. The *Minimal Residue Diet* (pp. 749–750) is recommended for some digestive troubles and before and after gastrointestinal surgery.

Diet and Individual Differences

Most discussions about food and eating tend to suggest that all normal people have identical gastrointestinal and metabolic systems. This is simply not true. There are many individual differences that explain why one man's meat is another man's poison. A person's intolerance for a given food may be caused by a disorder, such as an allergy or an ulcer, and it is possible that many of these intolerances will ultimately be related to enzyme deficiencies or some other biochemical factor.

More subtle are the negative physical reactions to particular foods as a result of psychological conditioning. In most such cases, the choice is between avoiding the food that causes the discomfort or eating it and suffering the consequences. Of course, compulsive overeating can also cause or contribute to discomfort. Practically no one can eat unlimited quantities of anything without having gastrointestinal discomfort or *dyspepsia*.

The establishment of so-called daily minimum food requirements suggests that every day's intake should be carefully balanced. Although this is beneficial, it is by no means necesary. Freedom from such regimentation can certainly be enjoyed during a holiday, or a trip to another country, or on a prolonged visit to relatives with casual food habits.

Sometimes a change in diet is dictated by a cold or an upset stomach or diarrhea. Liquids containing carbohydrates, such as tea with sugar and light soups, should be emphasized in treating a cold, while at the same time solid food intake should be somewhat reduced. In the case of an upset stomach or diarrhea, the discomfort may be eased by not eating or drinking anything at all for a whole day. This form of treatment may be helpful for an adult, but since children with diarrhea can become dehydrated in a day or so, professional advice is indicated when cutting down liquid intake.

SODIUM RESTRICTED DIETS

DIETS MODERATELY RESTRICTED IN SODIUM

If only a moderate sodium restriction is necessary, a normal diet *without added salt* may be ordered. Such an order is interpreted to mean that the patient will be offered the regular salted food on the general selective menu with the following exceptions:

1. No salt will be served on the tray.
2. Soups that are salted will be omitted.
3. Cured meats (ham, bacon, sausage, corned beef) and all salted cheeses will be omitted.
4. Catsup, chili sauce, mustard, and other salted sauces will be omitted.
5. Salt-free gravies, sauces, and salad dressings will be substituted for the regular salted items.
6. Salted crackers, potato chips, nuts, pickles, olives, popcorn, and pretzels will be omitted.

This diet contains approximately 3 grams of sodium or 7.5 grams of sodium chloride, depending on the type and quantity of the food chosen.

LOW SODIUM DIETS[1]
(1,000 mg. Sodium and 800 mg. Sodium Diets)

Type of food	Foods included	Foods excluded
Beverages	Coffee, tea, carbonated beverages, cereal beverages; milk, cream, or cocoa within stated milk limitations.	All others.
Breads	Any unsalted yeast bread or rolls; quick breads made with "sodium-free" baking powder; unsalted matzoth.	All bread and rolls containing salt, baking powder or baking soda; salted or soda crackers; pretzels.
Cereals	Any cereal that is cooked without salt; puffed rice, puffed wheat; shredded wheat; specially prepared "sodium-free" corn flakes and rice flakes; unsalted popcorn.	All prepared cereals containing salt; hominy grits.

[1]Approximate composition is indicated in the following table. 1,000 milligrams (abbreviated *mg.*) equals 1 gram. The 500, 800, and 1,000 milligram sodium diets meet the recommended nutrient levels of the normal diet.

Nutrient	Unit	500 mg. sodium	800 mg. sodium	1,000 mg. sodium
Sodium	Milligrams	485	775	970
Protein	Grams	70	95	95
Fat	Grams	90	90	90
Carbohydrate	Grams	185	250	250
Calories°		1,830	2,190	2,190

°Calories can be augmented by using additional salt-free fats and oils, white sugar, and pure jellies.

From the *Clinical Center Diet Manual*, revised edition, prepared by the Nutrition Department, The Clinical Center, National Institutes of Health, Public Health Service, U.S. Department of Health, Education, and Welfare (Public Health Service Publication No. 989), pp. 77–86.

LOW SODIUM DIETS *(continued)*		
Type of food	Foods included	Foods excluded
Desserts	Any unsalted dessert; custards and puddings made with allowed milk; puddings made without milk; unflavored gelatin desserts; fruit ices; unsalted fruit pie and fruit whips.	Desserts made with salt, baking powder, or baking soda; flavored gelatin desserts.
Fats	Any unsalted fat or oil, vegetable or animal; unsalted salad dressings.	Salted butter, salted margarine; commercial salad dressings; bacon drippings.
Fruits	Any fresh, canned, or frozen fruit or juice.	Dried fruits prepared with sodium preservatives.
Meat, poultry, fish	Prepared without salt: beef, lamb, fresh pork, veal; poultry; fresh-water fish;[2] liver (limit to one serving per week).	Salted meats; bacon; smoked or canned meats or fish; shellfish; all glandular meats except liver as allowed.
Cheese	Unsalted cottage cheese; specially prepared "sodium-free" yellow cheese.	All other.
Eggs	Limit to one daily, prepared without salt.	Any prepared with salt.
Potato or substitute	Dried beans (navy, pea), macaroni, noodles, potato, rice, spaghetti, sweet potato, all prepared without salt.	Salted potato chips, hominy.
Soups	Unsalted meat broth; cream soups prepared with allowed milk and allowed vegetables.	Bouillon; all soups prepared with salt.
Sweets	Hard candies, honey, jam, jelly, white sugar, syrup.	Commercial candy prepared with sodium salts; brown sugar.
Vegetables, cooked and raw	Two servings (½ cup) of vegetables listed below, fresh, frozen, or canned without salt: asparagus, lima beans,[3] navy beans, snap beans (green or yellow wax), broccoli, brussels sprouts, cabbage, carrots, cauliflower, corn, cucumbers, eggplant, dried lentils, lettuce, mushrooms, okra, onions, parsley, parsnips, black.eyed peas, green peas,[3] green peppers, radishes, rutabaga, squash, tomatoes, turnips, turnip greens.	Beets, beet greens, celery, dandelion greens, kale, frozen lima beans, mustard greens, frozen peas, sauerkraut, spinach, frozen succotash, swiss chard.

[2]Unsalted salt-water fish is usually avoided because of the difficulty of obtaining a consistently unsalted supply.
[3]Use only fresh or canned without salt.

LOW SODIUM DIETS (continued)		
Type of food	Foods included	Foods excluded
Miscella-neous	Herbs and spices, except salt. Unsalted peanut butter.	Salt, celery salt, garlic salt; celery seed, parsley flakes; sauces containing salt, such as catsup, chili sauce, mustard, steak sauces; salted nuts and popcorn; olives, pickles; monosodium glutamate.

Diet and Disease Prevention

Whether or not diet can be helpful in preventing various diseases other than those caused by nutritional deficiency is an unsettled question. Some specialists think that a diet low in cholesterol and saturated fats can help prevent cardiovascular disease caused by atherosclerosis, but the evidence for this point of view is not yet definitive. It has been said for years that vitamin C is helpful in preventing the common cold, and this point of view has recently received a great deal of publicity, but the evidence is not conclusive.

FOOD-BORNE DISEASES: There are several ways in which food can be the *cause* of disease, most commonly when it becomes contaminated with a sufficient amount of harmful bac-

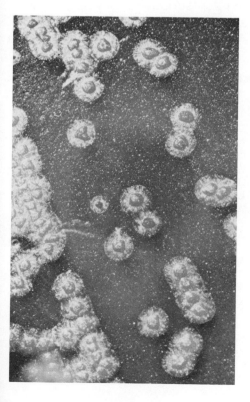

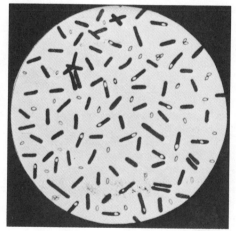

Scientists have isolated the bacterium *Clostridium botulinum* (above), which causes botulism food poisoning. If a seriously ill patient is suspected of having botulism, cultures of his blood and stool are made. The lab technician sees colonies of *C. botulinum* (left) under the microscope, confirming botulism.

LOW SODIUM DIETS (continued)				
Sample Menus				
	500 mg. Sodium		800 mg. Sodium	
	Weight grams	Household measure	Weight grams	Household measure
Breakfast				
Orange, sliced	125	1 medium	125	1 medium
Soft cooked egg	50	One	50	One
Unsalted oatmeal	100	½ cup	100	½ cup
Unsalted toast	25	1 slice	25	1 slice
Unsalted butter	10	2 teaspoons	10	2 teaspoons
Jelly	—	As desired	—	As desired
Milk, low sodium	None		None	
Milk (or cream)	240	1 cup	240	1 cup
Coffee or tea	—	As desired	—	As desired
Sugar	—	As desired	—	As desired
Luncheon				
Unsalted beef patty	60	2 ounces	60	2 ounces
Unsalted fried potatoes	100	½ cup	100	½ cup
Unsalted asparagus	100	½ cup	100	½ cup
Lettuce and tomato salad	100	1 small	100	1 small
Unsalted French dressing	15	1 tablespoon	15	1 tablespoon
Unsalted chocolate cookies	None			1 serving
Canned peaches	100	1 serving	—	As desired
Unsalted bread	25	1 slice	25	1 slice
Unsalted butter	10	2 teaspoons	10	2 teaspoons
Jelly	—	As desired	—	As desired
Milk, low sodium	None		None	
Milk	240	1 cup	240	1 cup
Coffee or tea	—	As desired	—	As desired
Sugar	—	As desired	—	As desired
Dinner				
Unsalted roast chicken	60	2 ounces	90	3 ounces
Unsalted gravy	30	2 tablespoons	30	2 tablespoons
Unsalted mashed potatoes	100	½ cup	100	½ cup
Unsalted green beans	100	½ cup	100	½ cup
Banana salad	100	One	100	One
Unsalted mayonnaise	15	1 tablespoon	15	1 tablespoon
Fresh fruit cup	100	½ cup	100	½ cup
Unsalted bread	25	1 slice	25	1 slice
Unsalted butter	10	2 teaspoons	10	2 teaspoons
Jelly	—	As desired	—	As desired
Milk, low sodium	—	As desired	None	
Milk	None		240	1 cup
Coffee or tea	—	As desired	—	As desired
Sugar	—	As desired	—	As desired
Nourishment				
Orange juice	240	1 cup	—	As desired
Milk	None		240	1 cup

MODIFIED FAT DIET

Type of food	Foods included	Foods excluded
Beverages	Coffee, tea, carbonated beverages, cereal beverages; skimmed milk, nonfat dried milk and buttermilk (made from skimmed milk).	Cream, evaporated milk, whole milk, whole milk beverages.
Breads	Whole wheat, rye, or enriched white bread; plain yeast rolls.	All others, including biscuits, cornbread, French toast, muffins, sweet rolls.
Cereals	Any; whole grain or enriched preferred.	None.
Desserts	Angel food cake; plain puddings made with skimmed milk; gelatin desserts; fruit ices, sherbets; fruit whips; meringues.	Cakes except angel food; cookies; ice cream; pastries; rich desserts.
Fats	Oils: corn, cottonseed, olive, peanut, safflower, soy bean. (If calories permit, 1½ to 3 ounces will be included daily.) Specially prepared margarines.	Bacon drippings, butter, coconut oil, regular fortified fats, salt pork, vegetable shortenings, commerical salad dressings.
Fruits	Any fresh (except avocado), canned, frozen, or dried fruit or juice (one citrus fruit to be included daily).	Avocado.
Meat, fish, poultry, cheese	Limit to 4 ounces daily from Group I or the equivalent from Groups II or III (below). Lean meat trimmed of all visible fat.	Fried meats; fat meats, such as bacon, cold cuts, duck, goose, pork, sausage; fish canned in oil; all other fish except those allowed. All cheese except dry cottage cheese.
Eggs	Egg whites as desired; whole eggs (a maximum of one per day or about 3 per week) poached, soft or hard cooked, fried in allowed oil.	Eggs or egg whites cooked with fat, except those fats allowed.
Group I	7 gms. fat per 30 gms. (1 ounce).	Lean beef, ham, lamb, and pork; tongue; veal; trout.
Group II	3 gms. fat per 30 gms. (1 ounce).	Beef liver, heart, kidney, dried or chipped beef; chicken, turkey; lean fish, such as codfish, haddock, halibut, mackerel, shad, salmon, tuna, whitefish.
Group III	Less than 1 gm. fat per 90 gms. (3 ounces).	Crab, clams, flounder, lobster, oysters, perch, scallops, shrimp.

From the *Clinical Center Diet Manual*, revised edition, prepared by the Nutrition Department, The Clinical Center, National Institutes of Health, Public Health Service, U.S. Department of Health, Education, and Welfare (Public Health Service Publication No. 989), pp. 69–72.

MODIFIED FAT DIET (continued)		
Type of food	Foods included	Foods excluded
Potato or substitute	Hominy, macaroni, noodles, popcorn (prepared with allowed oil), potato, rice, spaghetti.	Potato chips; any of these items fried or creamed unless prepared with allowed fats.
Soups	Bouillon, clear broth, vegetable soup; cream soups made with skimmed milk.	All others.
Sweets	Hard candies, jam, jelly, sugar, syrup; chocolate syrup made only with cocoa, sugar, and water.	All other candies; chocolate.
Vegetables	Any fresh, frozen, or cooked without added fat (one green or yellow vegetable should be included daily).	Buttered, creamed, or fried vegetables unless prepared with allowed fats.
Miscellaneous	Condiments, pickles, salt, spices, vinegar.	Gravies, nuts, olives, peanut butter.

This diet is planned to reduce the intake of fats containing a high degree of either saturated or short-chain fatty acids and to avoid the excessive carbohydrate intake associated with a very low fat diet. This is done through replacement of saturated fat sources with those containing higher quantities of polyunsaturated fatty acids. The fats ordinarily used are corn oil, cottonseed oil, safflower oil, olive oil, peanut oil, and soybean oil. Fats containing large amounts of saturated fatty acids are restricted to approximately 30 grams daily. Carbohydrate and protein are planned to conform to normal levels, with approximately 300–350 grams carbohydrate and approximately 70–80 grams protein. The modified fat diet is planned to meet normal dietary allowances. Calories can be adjusted to fit the needs of the individual. If normal or higher than normal calories are required, fats containing a high percentage of unsaturated fatty acids, such as corn oil, cottonseed oil, etc., may be added.

teria, bacterial toxin, viruses, or other poisonous substances. The gastrointestinal diseases typically accompanied by nausea, vomiting, diarrhea, or stomach cramps that are produced in this way are not, strictly speaking, caused by the foods themselves, and are therefore called food-borne diseases.

Most food-borne illnesses are caused by a toxin in food contaminated by staphylococcal or salmonella bacteria. In general, milk, milk products, raw shellfish, and meats are the foods most apt to be contaminated. This is most likely to happen when such foods are left standing at room temperature for too long between the time they are prepared and the time they are eaten. However, food can also become contaminated at many different points in time and at various stages of processing. Standards enforced by federal and local government agencies provide protection for the consumer for foods bought for the home as well as for use in restaurants, although whether the protection is adequate is a matter of dispute.

MODIFIED FAT DIET (continued)

Sample Menu

	Household measure[1]
Breakfast	
Orange juice	½ cup
Oatmeal	½ cup
Nonfat milk[2]	1 cup
Sugar	2 teaspoons
Poached egg	One
Toast, enriched or whole grain	2 slices
Jelly	1 tablespoon
Coffee or tea	As desired
Luncheon	
Clear broth, fat free	As desired
Lean roast beef	2 ounces
Baked potato	1 medium
Green beans	½ cup
Lettuce and tomato salad, oil dressing	1 serving
Bread, enriched or whole grain	1 slice
Jelly	1 tablespoon
Canned peach halves	2 halves
Nonfat milk[2]	1 cup
Coffee or tea	As desired
Sugar	1 teaspoon
Dinner	
Roast chicken (no skin)	4 ounces
Diced potato	½ cup
Green peas	½ cup
Head lettuce salad, oil dressing	1 serving
Bread, enriched or whole grain	1 slice
Jelly	1 tablespoon
Nonfat milk[2]	1 cup
Fruited gelatin	½ cup
Coffee or tea	As desired
Sugar	1 teaspoon

[1]Household measure is given to indicate the quantity of food necessary to supply 2,200 calories.

[2]As an example of the manner in which oil can be incorporated into the modified fat diet, a recipe for nonfat milk with oil follows:

For one quart of nonfat milk including one and one-half ounces of oil:

Dried powdered skim milk*	3¼ ounces (1⅓ cup)
Corn oil	1½ ounces
Water	to make 1 quart

Blend water with powdered skimmed milk in food blender until thoroughly mixed. Add corn oil and blend at a high speed until fully blended. Fresh skimmed milk may be substituted in the recipe for the powdered skimmed milk and water. The skimmed milk should be served cold, and the addition of flavoring is not recommended.

*Dried skimmed milk powders vary in weight. They may be reliquefied according to the directions on each package.

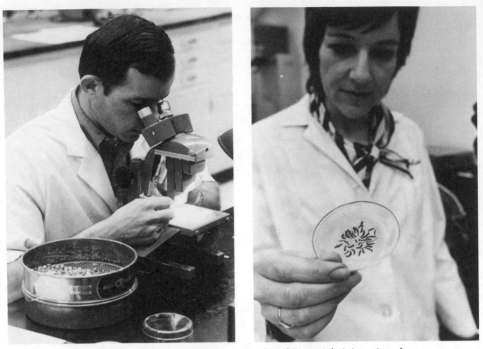

Acting on a consumer complaint, a Food and Drug Administration chemist *(left)* examines popcorn kernels under a microscope for the presence of moth larvae. The picture at right shows the larvae found in the sample.

Food Storage

Food is best protected from contamination when it is stored below 40 degrees Fahrenheit or heated to 145 degrees or more. Cold slows bacterial growth; cooking kills it. Bacteria present in food can double in number every 15 minutes at room temperature.

All food stored in the refrigerator should be covered except ripe fruits and vegetables. Leftover foods cannot be kept indefinitely, nor can frozen foods be stored beyond a certain length of time. Specific information about these time periods for individual items is available from the Agricultural Extension Service in each state.

Commercially processed foods sold in the United States are under government control and generally are safe. However, any food can spoil or become contaminated at any point in time, and the consumer should not buy or serve food whose container (package or can) has been broken, cracked, or appears unusual.

Food Additives

From time to time, concern is expressed about one or another food additive as a hazard to health. Most of these additives are put into foods during processing in order to increase their nutritional value, or to improve their chemical or physical characteristics, such as taste and color. Perhaps as many as 2,000 different substances are used in this way in the United States. Some are natural products such as vanilla, others are chemicals derived from

LOW FAT DIET

Type of food	Foods included	Foods excluded
Beverages	Coffee, tea, carbonated beverages, cereal beverages, skimmed milk or nonfat buttermilk.	Cream, whole milk, whole milk beverages.
Breads	Whole wheat, rye, or enriched white bread; plain yeast rolls.	Muffins, biscuits, sweet rolls, cornbread, pancakes, waffles, french toast.
Cereals	Any: whole grain or enriched preferred.	None.
Desserts	Plain angel food cake; custards and puddings made with skimmed milk and egg allowances; fruit puddings; gelatin desserts; ices; fruit whips made with egg white.	Rich desserts, pastries; sherbets, ice cream; cakes, except angel food.
Fats	None	All fats and oils; salad dressings.
Fruits	Any fresh (except avocado), canned, frozen, or dried fruit or juice (one citrus fruit to be included daily).	Avocado.
Meat, poultry, fish, cheese	Limit to 5 ounces daily: lean meat, such as lean beef, lamb, liver, veal; chicken, turkey, canned salmon or tuna (canned without oil); shellfish, lean whitefish; dry cottage cheese.	Fried meats; fat meats, such as bacon, cold cuts, duck, goose, pork, sausage; fish canned in oil. All cheese except dry cottage cheese.
Eggs	Any poached, soft or hard cooked; limit to one egg daily.	Fried eggs; eggs scrambled with fat.
Potato or substitute	Hominy, macaroni, noodles, potatoes, rice, spaghetti.	Any of these items fried or creamed; potato chips.
Soups	Bouillon, clear broth, vegetable soup; cream soups made with milk.	All others.
Sweets	Hard candies, jam, jelly, sugar, syrup; chocolate syrup made only with cocoa, sugar, and water.	All other candies or chocolate.
Vegetables	Any fresh, frozen or cooked without added fat (one green or yellow vegetable should be included daily).	Buttered, creamed or fried vegetables.
Miscellaneous	Condiments, pickles, salt, spices, vinegar.	Gravies, nuts, olives, peanut butter.

From the *Clinical Center Diet Manual,* revised edition, prepared by the Nutrition Department, The Clinical Center, National Institutes of Health, Public Health Service, U.S. Department of Health, Education, and Welfare (Public Health Service Publication No. 989), pp. 73–75.

LOW FAT DIET (continued)

The low fat diet contains approximately 40 grams of fat. To maintain normal calorie intake with fat restricted, it has a high carbohydrate content. The low fat diet is adequate in all nutrients. Calories can be adjusted to fit the needs of the individual patient. Approximate composition is as follows:

Protein	85 gm.
Fat	40 gm.
Carbohydrate	325 gm.
Calories	2,000

Sample Menu

	Household measure[1]
Breakfast	
Orange juice	½ cup
Oatmeal	½ cup
Skimmed milk	1 cup
Sugar	1 tablespoon
Poached egg	One (limit to one daily)
Toast, enriched or whole grain	2 slices
Jelly	1 tablespoon
Coffee or tea	As desired
Luncheon	
Beef broth, fat free	As desired
Sliced chicken	2 ounces
Baked potato	1 small
Peas	½ cup
Lettuce and tomato salad	1 serving
Lemon ice	½ cup
Bread, enriched or whole grain	1 slice
Jelly	1 tablespoon
Skimmed milk	1 cup
Coffee or tea	As desired
Sugar	1 tablespoon
Nourishment	
Pineapple juice	1 cup
Dinner	
Lean roast beef	3 ounces
Steamed potato	1 small
Carrots	½ cup
Mixed fruit salad	1 serving
Angel food cake	1 serving
Bread, enriched or whole grain	1 slice
Jelly	1 tablespoon
Coffee or tea	As desired
Sugar	1 tablespoon
Nourishment	
Tomato juice	1 cup
Crackers	Five

[1]Household measures are given to indicate the quantity of food necessary to supply 2,000 calories.

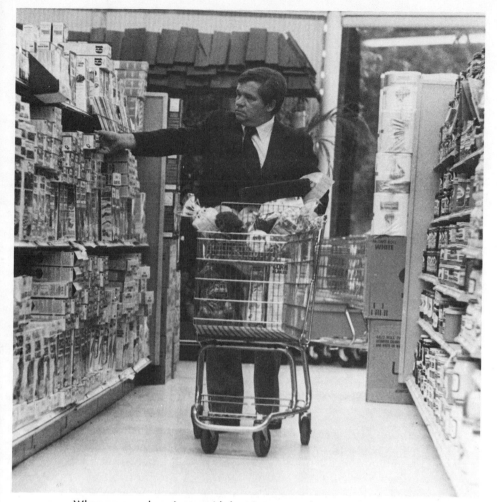

When grocery shopping, avoid choosing any package on which the seal has been broken, or any can that is badly dented or shows signs of rust.

other foods, and a few, like artificial sweeteners, are synthetic. Other additives are referred to as indirect, since they are residues in the food from some stage of growing, processing, or packaging. Although additives are controlled and approved by agencies such as the federal Food and Drug Administration, they continue to be a cause of concern to many people. See under *Food Hazards,* p. 767, for further discussion of food additives.

Organic Foods

Some people feel that industrial methods of food farming and processing introduced during the past century, and more particularly in the last four or five decades, have resulted in foods that are deficient in nutritional value. They have recommended a return to the techniques of food production of an earlier era, in which only organic fertilizers were used. Foods so produced are called *organic foods*. Standard, commercially prepared foods, they feel, lack the health benefits and better tastes of organic foods and may even be damaging to health.

The damage, they believe, is caused because chemical fertilizers, pesticides, and food additives make foods toxic in some way or other. These toxins include female hormones, antibiotics, and an inordinate number of organic and inorganic chemicals. They are thought to cause or contribute to the development of some cancers, arteriosclerosis, and other degenerative diseases, the causes of which really are unknown.

Organic foods are also said to make people less susceptible to viral infections such as common colds, and to tooth decay. All of these claimed health benefits could also be the result of having preserved in organically prepared foods various substances that are eliminated in normal commercial processing.

The organic food philosophy calls for growing your own foods, using only organic fertilizers such as compost or animal (not human) manure, and without using pesticides or herbicides. For those unable to grow their own foods, commercial sources of organic foods are becoming more and more readily available.

Typical Organic Foods

Whole grain cereals such as brown rice, and wheat, beans, vegetables, and fruits are the major sources of organic foods. Unsulfured molasses and natural honey are the primary sweeteners. Sea salt and herbs are used for flavoring. Organic meat is available, but many organic food people are vegetarians. Fertile eggs, cheeses, especially those from raw goat or cow milk, and yogurt also are basic parts of an organic diet. Cold pressed vegetable oils, filtered in a special way, and made from sesame, corn germ, or soy are used regularly; they are not only unsaturated fats and therefore have low cholesterol contents but also contain many natural vitamins. Herb teas, fruit juices, and raw milk are among the preferred liquids. Ideally, all organic foods should be eaten when fresh or in season, since canning or freezing requires the addition of chemicals.

Natural Foods

Several other food styles are associated with organic foods. *Natural foods* are not necessarily grown organically, but are not processed very much. *Macrobiotics* is a special natural food concept, oriental in origin, and based upon the idea of maintaining an equilibrium between foods that make one active *(Yang)* and foods that make one relax *(Yin)*. A proper mixture of grain and vegetables contains an excellent balance of Yin and Yang. Yoga diets center around such natural foods as fruits and nuts.

Psychological Aspects of Food and Meals

Food and meals play an important role in emotional well-being and interpersonal relationships as well as in physical health and appearance.

During Infancy

The infant whose needs are attended to by a loving family develops a general sense of trust and

MINIMAL RESIDUE DIET

Type of food	Foods included	Foods excluded
Beverages	Black coffee, tea, carbonated beverages, cereal beverages.	Milk, milk drinks.
Breads	Salted and soda crackers.	All breads.
Cereals	Cooked rice cereals or refined wheat cereals, made with water.	Whole grain cereals.
Desserts	White angel food cake, arrowroot cookies; ices; clear gelatin dessert.	Custards, puddings; desserts made with milk; ice cream.
Fats	Bacon, butter, fortified fats.	Cream.
Fruits	Strained fruit juices only.	All fruits.
Meat, eggs, poultry, fish, cheese	Beef, lamb, veal; chicken, turkey; white fish; eggs.	Fried meats, poultry, or fish; all cheese.
Potato or substitute	Macaroni, noodles, rice, spaghetti.	Potatoes, hominy.
Soups	Bouillon, broth.	Cream soups.
Sweets	Hard candies without nuts or fruit; honey, jelly, sugar, syrup.	Candies with fruit or nuts; jam, marmalade.
Vegetables	Tomato juice only.	All other vegetables.
Miscellaneous	Salt, small amounts of pepper used in cooking.	All other spices; condiments; nuts, olives, pickles, etc.

Minimal residue diet. The foods included on the minimal residue diet are selected on the basis of the small amount of residue left in the intestines after digestion. Since milk, milk products, fruits, and vegetables are thought to leave a large residue, these foods (except fruit and vegetable juices) have been omitted from the diet. The minimal residue diet is adequate in protein and calories. All other nutrients are below the recommended allowances.

From the *Clinical Center Diet Manual*, revised edition, prepared by the Nutrition Department, The Clinical Center, National Institutes of Health, Public Health Service, U.S. Department of Health, Education, and Welfare (Public Health Service Publication No. 989), pp. 45, 56–57.

security. The major contribution to his emotional contentment is probably made at mealtimes, and perhaps in a special way if he is breast-fed.

For most infants, food comes to be identified with love, pleasure, protection, and the satisfaction of basic needs. If there is an atmosphere of tension accompanying his feeding times, his digestion can be impaired in such a way as to cause vomiting, fretting, or signs of colic. If the ten-

sion and the baby's reaction to it—and inevitably the mother's increasing tension as a consequence—become a chronic condition, the result may be a failure to gain weight normally, and in extreme cases, some degree of mental retardation. Throughout life, good nutrition depends not only on eating properly balanced meals that satisfy the body's physiological requirements, but also on a reasonable de-

MINIMAL RESIDUE DIET *(continued)*	
Sample Menu	

Breakfast

Orange juice	½ cup
Cream of wheat (cooked in water with butter)	½ cup; 1 teaspoon butter
Poached egg	One
Salted crackers	4 to 5
Butter	2 teaspoons
Jelly	1 tablespoon
Coffee or tea	As desired
Sugar	As desired

Luncheon

Roast beef	3 ounces
Buttered noodles	½ cup
Tomato juice	½ cup
Salted crackers	4 to 5
Butter	2 teaspoons
Jelly	1 tablespoon
Plain gelatin dessert	½ cup
Coffee or tea	As desired
Sugar	As desired

Dinner

Grapefruit juice	½ cup
Clear broth	As desired
Baked chicken	4 ounces
Buttered rice	½ cup
Salted crackers	4 to 5
Butter	2 teaspoons
Fruit ice	½ cup
Coffee or tea	As desired
Sugar	As desired

Nourishment

Strained fruit juices	As desired
Plain gelatin desserts	As desired
Fruit ices	As desired

gree of contentment and relaxation while eating.

Everybody develops individual emotional reactions and attitudes about food and its role as a result of conditioning during the years of infancy and childhood. These attitudes relate not only to food itself and to mealtimes in general, but also to other aspects of eating, including the muscle activities of sucking, chewing, and swallowing.

If food symbolized contentment during the early years, it probably will have the same role later on. If it was associated with conflict, then it may be associated throughout life with strife and neurotic eating patterns.

During Childhood

For the preschool child, mealtimes should provide the occasion for the development of interper-

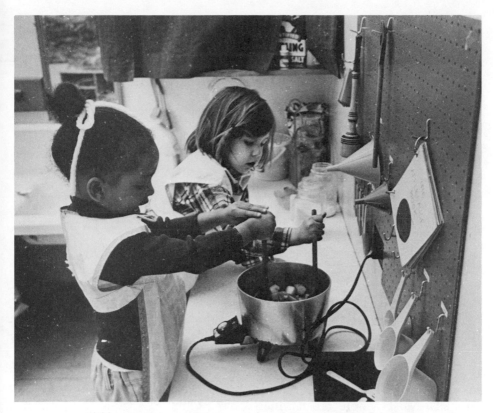

Children assist in preparing a meal at their nursery school, helping them learn about food and nutrition and also the basics of sharing.

sonal relationships, since they are a daily opportunity for both verbal and nonverbal self-expression. The child who eats with enthusiasm and obvious enjoyment is conveying one message; the one who dawdles, picks at food, and challenges his mother with every mouthful is conveying quite a different one.

Meals can become either positive or negative experiences depending in large part on how the adults in the family set the stage. Communication can be encouraged by relaxed conversation and a reasonably leisurely schedule. It can be discouraged by watching television or reading while eating, by not eating together, or by eating and running.

Reasonably firm attitudes about eating a variety of foods in proper quantities at proper times and avoiding excessive catering to individual whims can also help in the development of wholesome eating patterns.

Those who select and prepare the food can transmit special messages of love and affection by serving favorite dishes, by setting the table attractively, and by creating an atmosphere of grace and good humor. Or they can show displeasure and generate hostility by complaining about all the work involved in feeding everyone, or by constant criticism of table manners, or by bringing up touchy subjects likely to cause arguments at the table.

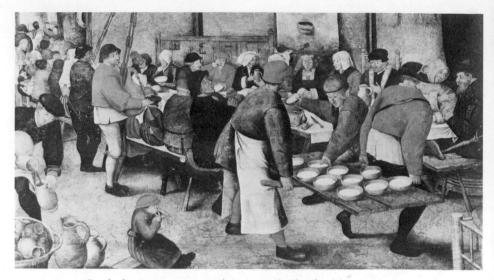

Food plays an important role in many kinds of celebrations, as is portrayed in Pieter Brueghel's painting "Peasant Wedding Feast."

How Food Can Relieve Tension

Food can be instrumental in relieving individual tension as well as in smoothing over minor family conflicts. Most people are familiar with the type of individual who is grumpy before a meal and who visibly brightens when he begins to eat. Sometimes this is due to the condition of *hypoglycemia* in which the blood sugar is too low for comfort. More often, the good spirits come from the psychological uplift brought about by the comradeship of eating.

People often turn to food as a way of relieving tension, thus reverting to a pattern established in childhood. Milk, for example, is often sought in times of stress. The relationship between food and anxiety is a complex one, and if it becomes so distorted that neurosis results, the physical consequences can be extremely unpleasant. Gastrointestinal disorders such as ulcers, bloating, belching, passing gas, diarrhea, and constipation are more often than not emotional rather than purely physical in origin.

The Symbol of Food

Food has many symbolic aspects: it can transmit and reinforce ethnic traditions either regularly or on special holidays. It can be used at lavish dinner parties as an expression of economic success; it can denote worldliness and sophistication in the form of complicated gourmet dishes of obscure origin.

A great deal can be learned about a person by knowing something about his attitudes toward food—not only what, how, when, and where he eats, but also how the groceries are bought, how the refrigerator and pantry shelves are stocked, how the cooking is organized, and how the dishes are cleaned up. In many significant ways, all of us are not only *what* we eat; we truly express who we are by *how* we eat.

CHAPTER 14

The Environment and Health

"Ecology . . . pollution . . . deterioration of the environment . . . the quality of life. . . ."

These words are with us constantly, in the news, political speeches, informed conversation. Heated controversy flairs over just how contaminated the globe is, the extent of the danger, the cost of cleaning up the mess, and whether any solution is realistically possible.

One thing is clear and incontestable: the quality of the environment is crucial to health, perhaps more important than any individual personal health measures you can employ. According to the federal Task Force on Research Planning in Environmental Health Science: ". . . the environment plays a predominant role in man's health; . . . rapid technologic change, increased population, and greater concentration of people into urban centers are compounding the problems of maintaining the environment at a healthful level."

Kinds of Pollution

Harmful ingredients in the environment are often the result of pollution; however, natural components—ultraviolet radiation in sunlight, for example—can also be contributing factors. These pollutants and the occasional natural counterparts can damage health in a variety of ways; even though there is as yet no scientific proof linking some of these pollutants with a specific malady, the statistical or circumstantial evidence is impressive. Most health experts believe, for example, that there is a direct connection between air pollution and various forms of respiratory illness.

Excessive noise, sometimes referred to as the "third pollution," after air and water pollution, is known to cause temporary and permanent hearing loss, anxiety, tension, and insomnia; it is strongly suspected of contributing to cardiovascular disease.

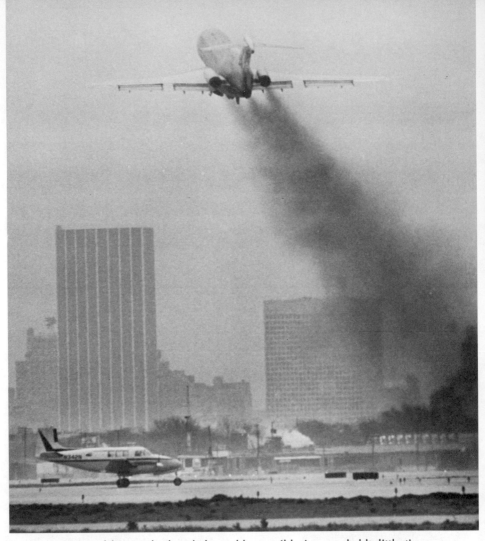

Jet travel has made the whole world accessible in remarkably little time, but it has also contributed to the problems of air and noise pollution.

Many of the products of the technological age are toxic. Quantities of them find their way into the air, water, and food. Apart from outright poisoning, some of these contaminants are implicated in the development of cancer. Others are thought to cause mutations in the consumer, resulting in abnormal and sometimes nonviable offspring.

OCCUPATIONAL DISEASE: Because of our jobs, some of us are vastly more exposed to these dangerous contaminants than others. Occupational disease linked to specific pollutants has a long and unpleasant history. Chimney sweeps in 18th-century London developed cancer of the scrotum from long exposure to coal soot, which contained potent cancer-producing agents (*carcinogens*). The malady was called "soot-wart." The Mad Hatter in Lewis Carroll's *Alice in Wonderland* represents a well-known type, a victim of "hatter's disease"—chronic mercury poisoning. (Mercury was used in the preparation of felt for hats.) During the latter part of the 19th century, skin cancer was a frequent hazard of work in the coal tar, paraffin, oil, and lignite tar industries. Bladder cancer began to appear among workers in the new aniline dye industry; it wasn't until 1938 that the carcinogen responsible was identified.

Today, miners contract *black lung disease* and *silicosis* from inhaling coal and other dusts. Cotton workers suffer chest-tightening *byssinosis* ("white lung disease") from inhaling cotton dust. Asbestos workers have seven times more lung cancer than the general population, and risk several other lung diseases, among them silicosis. Recently, some clothing workers were exposed to similar risks when they unknowingly manufactured 100,000 women's coats from a cloth containing eight percent asbestos fiber. One authority advised any woman in possession of such a coat to "bury

it." Merely rubbing or brushing the coat would produce asbestos levels in the air 10,000 times higher than normal. See also *Lung Disease*, p. 1196.

Added to all these and other traditional occupational hazards are those from a bewildering new profusion of synthetic chemicals whose dangerous properties may become known only long after they are in production.

RADIATION: Finally, there is a category of contaminants about which so little is known that they are provoking raging debate: ionizing radiation (such as that from nuclear reactors and other radioactive sources), microwave radiation (such as that from microwave ovens), and laser radiation. The Task Force quoted earlier points out with some asperity that the United States allows a level of microwave radiation for occupational exposure that is 1,000 times

A protest against nuclear power plants invokes memories of the major accident at the Three Mile Island plant near Harrisburg, Pa., in 1979.

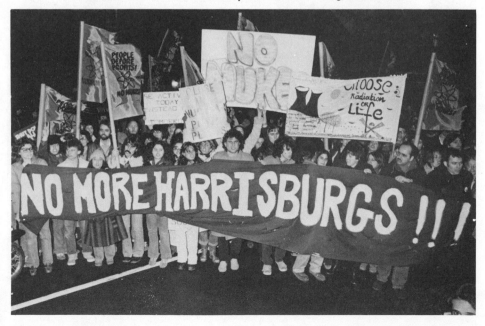

higher than the maximum set by Soviet Russia and other Eastern European countries. Microwaves, similar to radio waves and used in communications as well as ovens, are measurable in the environment of one-half the U.S. population.

Air Pollution

Most air pollution results from the incomplete burning of fuels and other materials, such as garbage. There are hundreds of different pollutants; some are visible as the yellowish brown haze that hangs over most large cities, but most are invisible. There is some debate over the precise relation between these various contaminants and the level of respiratory disease among the general population, although many experts think that the evidence now linking them with asthma, emphysema, and bronchitis is very strong.

Inversions

No one can doubt that high concentrations of air pollution are deadly. Modern history has seen some appalling examples. They usually

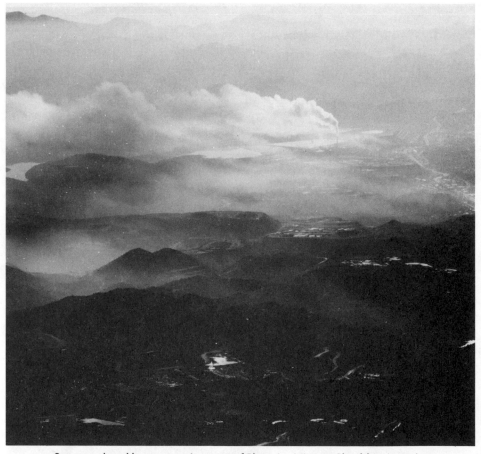

Smog produced by copper mines east of Phoenix, Arizona. Should an inversion trap such concentrated pollution, the health hazards can be enormous.

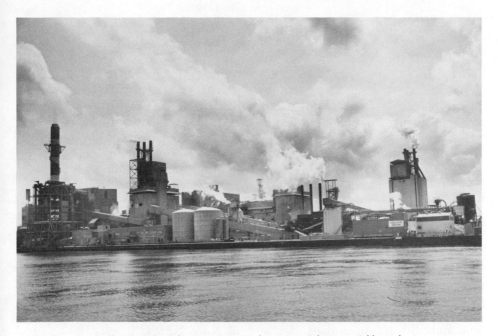

Sulfur dioxide in factory emissions becomes air-borne quickly and is a major source of air pollution over large areas of the U.S.

occur in a region that is subject to a freak weather condition called an *inversion,* during which a mass of warm air sits like a lid on top of cool air, trapping it and preventing the pollutants that are produced daily from being ventilated. The pollutants accumulate in this stagnant air until they sometimes reach high concentrations, with lethal results.

The Meuse valley in Belgium, a center of heavy industry with many coal-burning factories, experienced an inversion in 1930 that trapped the smoke for five days. Some 60 people died as a result and 6,000 were sickened.

A killer smog brought a new menace to London's notorious pea-soupers in December, 1952. For five days an impenetrable, smoky fog paralyzed the city. Hospitals were jammed with people gasping for breath. When the smog finally lifted, medical statisticians calcu-

lated that 4,000 deaths during and immediately after the siege could be attributed to the smog.

The United States has known its share of such tragedies. Perhaps the worst and most famous was the inversion that hit Donora, Pennsylvania, in October, 1948, in a valley similar in topography and in pollution-creating industry to the Meuse. The inversion lasted six days—six days of ever more unhealthy air. At its peak, more than half of the valley's 14,000 persons had been stricken; at least 20 deaths were blamed on the pollution. Many more persons suffered irreversible damage to their health, according to a U.S. Public Health Service study.

Sulfur Dioxide

Today, numbers of cities still report unsatisfactory or unhealthy air conditions with some frequency, but at least local and national officials are aware of the seriousness of the problem. New York City officials have stated that between 1,000 and 2,000 deaths a year there probably result from sulfur dioxide—the main toxic component of killer smogs—and other particles suspended in the air. Sulfur dioxide is spewed into the air—more than 23 million tons in the country, and 380,000 tons in New York City alone—when heavy fuel oil and coal are burned to provide heat, generate electricity, and provide industrial power. These fuels are generally rich in sulfur. Recently, some localities have passed legislation requiring the use of low-sulfur coal and oil for certain uses.

No one knows exactly how sulfur dioxide affects the respiratory tract. The likelihood is that it irritates the lungs and contributes to a reduction of the lungs' oxygen-handling capacity. Persons especially vulnerable to smogs are those suffering from bronchial asthma, chronic bronchitis (some studies show 13 percent of U.S. men have the disease) and emphysema, because their respiratory capacity is already defective. In emphysema, for example, the elasticity of the air sacs in the lungs has progressively broken down, usually after prolonged infection or repeated bronchial irritation (such as is produced by cigarette smoking). Deaths from emphysema are twice as high in cities as in rural areas.

Other Contaminants

Other major contaminants that have been identified as dangerous are nitrogen oxides, lead, carbon monoxide, hydrocarbons, and soot—the visible particles of carbon suspended in the air.

Dust may be harmful by transporting corrosive chemicals or other irritants to the lungs. Ordinarily, particles in the air are trapped in the nasal passages, but very small ones can slip past into the lungs. These tiny motes are called submicron particles—less than one twenty-five-thousandth of an inch in size.

Auto Exhausts

The major contributor of these harmful agents is the automobile. Auto exhausts contribute more than one-half the total of all atmospheric contaminants; in large cities, the figure is much higher. For example, in New York City cars, buses, and trucks contribute an estimated 77% by weight of all air pollution.

How can these substances affect your health? Nitrogen oxides irritate the eyes and the respiratory tract. Moreover, when nitrogen oxide and hydrocarbons mix in the presence of sunlight, they form other noxious substances in what is called a photochemical smog that has a typical yellowish cast. The new ingredients produced include ozone—a poisonous form of oxygen—and peroxyacetyl nitrate (PAN), which is intensely irritating to the eyes. Los Angeles was the first city to experience these smogs; they now occur in many other cities as well.

Auto exhaust hydrocarbons include varieties that are suspected of being carcinogens, that is, of contributing to the development of cancer in susceptible individuals. This link so far has been proven only in animals. Dr. Ernest Wynder of the Sloan-Kettering Institute for Cancer Research, however, got

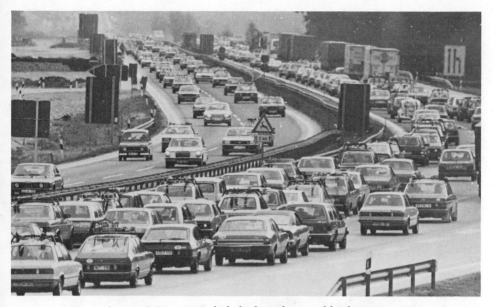

Auto emissions, particularly hydrocarbons and lead, are a major source of air pollution in industrialized countries.

some provocative results by painting the skin of laboratory mice with the residues collected from filters exposed to New York air. The mice developed cancer.

Carbon monoxide is an odorless, colorless gas that is lethal even in very small concentrations because it combines with hemoglobin readily and thus replaces oxygen in the blood. In concentrations that have been measured in heavy city traffic, it can make you tired, headachy, drowsy, and careless.

LEAD POISONING: Lead is an extremely poisonous substance. Acute cases of lead poisoning produce headache, nausea, cramps, anemia, numbness, loss of control of wrist and ankle, and finally, coma and death. The symptoms of chronic lead poisoning are much more subtle and harder to pinpoint. Test animals that have consumed lead in amounts comparable to those ingested by men over long periods

have had their life spans reduced by 20 percent, experienced increased infant mortality rates, sterility, and birth defects. Testifying before the Senate Subcommittee on Energy, Natural Resources and the Environment, Carl L. Klein, an assistant Secretary of the Interior, said that "there can be little doubt that exposure of mothers to lead has a damaging effect upon fertility, the course of pregnancy, and the development of the fetus."

One expert estimated that auto exhausts were releasing 300,000 tons of lead annually into the air, some of which winds up in the water supply. Industrial users also vent large quantities of lead into lakes and rivers.

Experts are now debating exactly how much airborne lead can be tolerated. But a strange phenomenon is occurring in big cities such as New York. The tragedy of slum children developing lead poisoning has been explained readily because it is known that they nibble lead-bearing paint peeling from their walls. Yet a number of instances of high lead levels in the blood of middle-class children have been discovered. Those children live in dwellings painted with modern house paints containing no lead. Some doctors have concluded that the children have been poisoned by auto exhausts. Lead levels in high traffic areas of New York are sometimes 25 times higher than the legal limit in California.

The outlook for any drastic improvements in the air pollution scene is not good. The federal government has extended the deadline for auto manufacturers to reduce

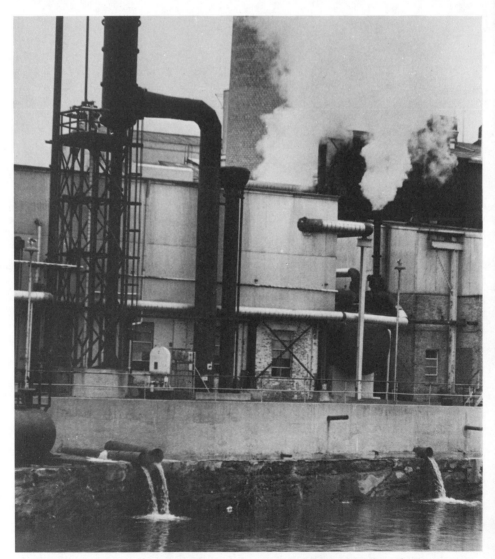

Lead is an extremely poisonous substance. Industries often dump large quantities of waste products containing lead into nearby waterways.

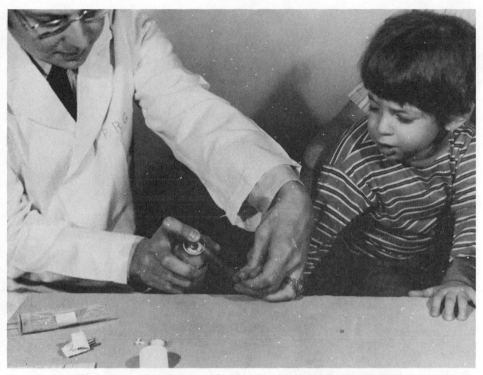

After taking a few drops of blood to test for lead poisoning, a technician sprays the finger with collodion, a coating agent for wounds.

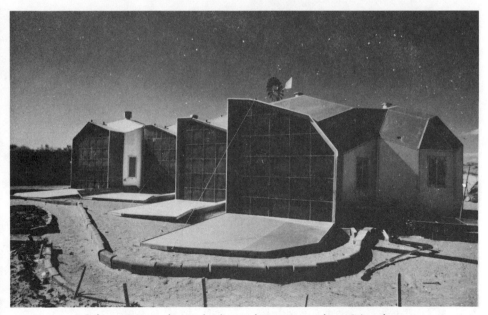

Solar energy can be used to heat a home, as seen here. It is a clean source of energy, but it is not yet practicable on a large scale.

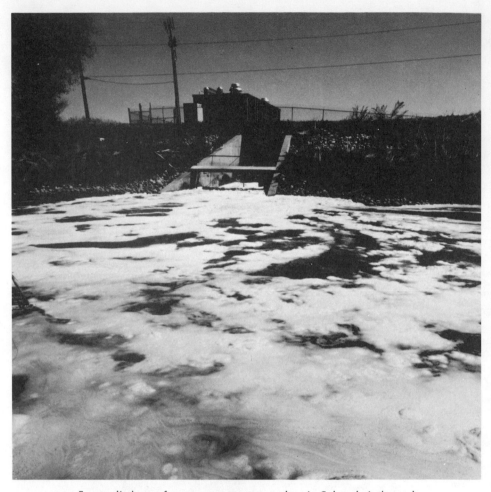

Foamy discharge from a water treatment plant in Colorado is the end product of a water supply that has been infiltrated with detergents.

exhaust emissions until 1979. In any event, the pollution contribution of older cars will continue into the '80s.

Energy production, the other major air polluter, also offers little hope for immediate improvement, because it will be many years before we can rely heavily on other than fossil fuels such as coal and oil. Supplies of nonpolluting natural gas are in too short supply to do us much good. There is still a good deal of controversy over the safety of nuclear power plants, and it will

be some time before solar energy can make a dent in the energy crisis. See under *Lung Disease*, p. 1196, for additional information about the effects of air pollution on health.

Water Pollution

The quality of water is intimately tied to our physical well-being, and we have, therefore, come to expect high standards of cleanliness and purity in the water we drink and bathe in. Public health authorities are increasingly concerned, however, at the progressive deterioration of this country's water supply. This deterioration results from years of abuse in which natural waterways were inundated with quantities of raw sewage, waste products of industrial and chemical plants and slaughterhouses, petroleum residues, poisonous herbicides and insecticides—the list is almost endless, but our water supply is not. In 1970, the Division of Water Hygiene, part of the federal Environmental Protection Agency, concluded that some 969 of the nation's individual water supplies were substandard.

Many householders do not need to be told that their water is less than sparkling and delicious. Bad tastes and odors, off colors and cloudiness plague many regions and make water drinking distasteful, even if it is not yet dangerous. In Suffolk County on New York's Long Island, for example, water in the region's wells had become so infiltrated with detergents that a glass of water was likely to have a head of detergent foam. After much controversy, the County banned the sale of all laundry products containing detergents.

The problem is that some synthetic detergents are not *biodegradable*—they are not broken down by microorganisms in the soil and water, and thus become water pollutants. Even biodegradable synthetic detergents may add another pollutant—phosphates—to water. Phosphates overstimulate the growth of the primitive water plants called algae, which overrun lakes and streams; the algae consume vast quantities of oxygen, thereby choking out other life, such as game and food fish.

Oil Spills

With the increasing reliance on supertankers to carry industrial and heating oil from abroad, the danger

Volunteers use straw to absorb oil spilled on a California beach, but even prompt cleanup efforts do not prevent damage from a spill.

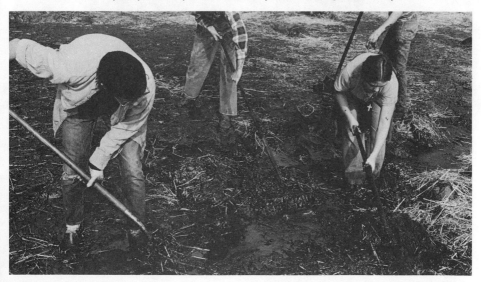

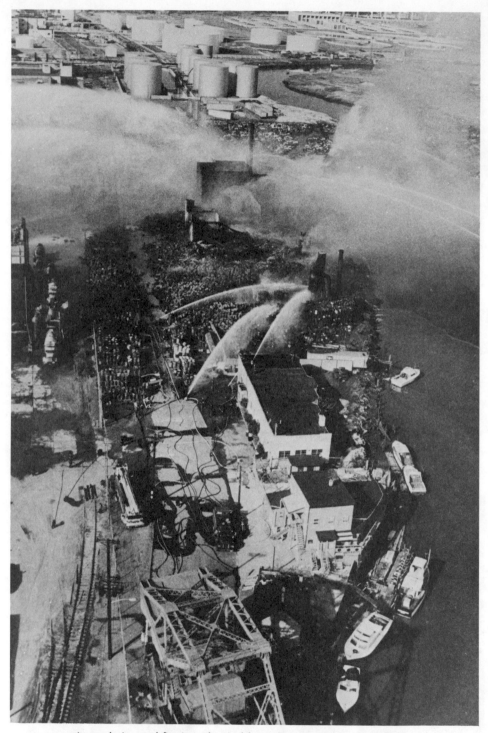

An explosion and fire in a chemicals' warehouse sent toxic fumes into the atmosphere rapidly—a common type of industrial accident.

of major oil spills occurring near a coastal area is becoming ever greater. Several of these huge ships have been grounded and broken apart by the seas, their vast cargoes spilling out heavy oil into the ocean, where currents can carry it many miles before it disperses and gradually sinks to the ocean floor. Sometimes, of course, the currents carry the oil toward land, where it fouls beaches and kills water birds. Other accidents have involved smaller tankers plying the inland waterways; their oil cargoes have polluted rivers and lakes, killing fishes and despoiling recreational areas.

Microbes in Sewage

The risk to health from drinking contaminated water depends on the contaminant. It is fairly rare in this country for cases of typhoid, for example, caused by a pathogenic bacillus, to be contracted through an impure water supply. But you may risk gastrointestinal upsets caused by other organisms if you swim at a beach that is posted "Polluted Waters," as so many beaches now are. The cause is generally the dumping of raw sewage nearby, or of sludge, the solid mass that is left after some kinds of sewage treatment. In New York Harbor there is a dead sea 21 miles square where nothing can live.

Chemical Contamination

In addition to the danger of infection from viral and microbial agents in polluted water, there is mounting danger from chemical contamination. Literally hundreds of chemical compounds find their way into the water supply, some of them in potentially dangerous quantities. At-

tention has focused most recently on the heavy metals and especially mercury. In a recent study, the U.S. Geological Survey reported that small amounts of seven toxic metals were present in many of the country's lakes and streams, with dangerous concentrations seemingly rare. The metals are mercury, arsenic, cadmium, chromium, cobalt, lead, and zinc. Aside from being generally poisonous, some of these metals are implicated in specific health problems. Cadmium, for example, has been linked to hypertension due to kidney malfunction. In Taiwan, skin cancer has been proved to rise with the quantity of arsenic in well water.

The Dangers of Mercury

Mercury represents a special case. For years, experts thought that since mercury was heavier than water and couldn't dissolve in it, it was therefore safe to dump large quantities of the metal into the waterways on the assumption that it would lie harmlessly on the bottom. They were, however, wrong. Bacteria can convert some of the metallic form of the element into a water-soluble form, which enters the food chain and eventually winds up, concentrated, in fish. When dangerous levels of this form of mercury were found in some waters and in food fish, the boom was lowered. There was a scare over canned tuna (the government later said that 97 percent of the canned tuna on the market was safe to eat) and swordfish. Lakes and rivers across the country were closed to commercial and sport fishing, and some remain closed.

The reason is not hard to understand. Mercury is an exceedingly

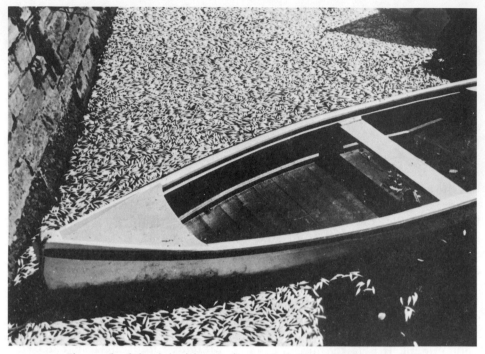

Thousands of dead shad float in the Anacostia River, Washington, D.C. The oxygen content of the water was decreased by industrial pollution.

toxic substance. The U.S. Food and Drug Administration has established the safe limit of mercury in food at half a part per million, comparable to a thimbleful in an Olympic-sized swimming pool. Even infinitesimal amounts absorbed by the body over a period of time can produce blindness, paralysis, and brain damage.

SWORDFISH: In an extremely unusual action, the Food and Drug Administration in 1971 advised the public to stop eating swordfish. The FDA had no power to ban the fish legally, but the move curtailed the consumption of swordfish in this country for some time. FDA investigators had discovered that only 42 of 853 samples of the fish contained acceptable levels of mercury. The average level of the remaining samples was twice the permissible amount. Soon after the announcement, doctors disclosed the first death in this country attributable to eating mercury-contaminated swordfish—that of a woman who had been eating large quantities of the fish on a weight-reducing diet.

The population of Minimata, a Japanese coastal town, was afflicted in 1953 by a strange malady that killed 40, crippled 70. The Minimatans had eaten the local fish and shellfish, which had absorbed mercury discharged into the water in a water soluble form by a nearby plastics factory. Similar cases of mass mercury poisoning have occurred in Italy, Guatemala, and Pakistan.

Pollution experts are particularly worried about mercury because even if we stopped producing mercury compounds and discharging mercury wastes into the country's waters today, the problem would continue to worsen. The enormous store of metallic mercury already discharged and sitting on river and lake bottoms continues to be converted slowly into soluble forms. One chemist has estimated that in the St. Clair River system alone (between Detroit and southwestern Ontario), about 200,000 pounds of metallic mercury have been discharged in the last 20 years.

Recently, high amounts of selenium, an element considered more toxic than mercury, have been found in microscopic animal life in Lake Michigan downwind from Chicago and Milwaukee.

PCBs: Among the chief water pollutants today are the *polychlorinated biphenyls* (PCBs), highly toxic chemicals used industrially in carbonless copying paper and as an additive in lubricants, paints, and other products. PCBs, which require many years for the process of being altered chemically (biodegraded) to take place, have been found in unusually large quantities in waterways downstream from manufacturing plants. In January, 1977, the federal Environmental Protection Agency banned the direct discharge of PCBs into any U.S. waterway. Tests had shown that fish in some rivers, such as the Hudson River, had levels of PCB far higher than the permissible level. PCBs, which are related chemically to DDT— banned in 1972—are found in major bodies of water throughout the world because of their many industrial uses. No one knows what the long-term effects of ingesting small quantities of PCB's will be.

Food Hazards

Contaminants found in water often make their way into food products in the cooking and packaging processes, so that many of the comments on water apply here. Some dilute water pollutants become highly concentrated as they pass up the food chain and end in fish or other foods for man. Mercury was cited earlier as one example. Contamination of food with harmful microorganisms is an everpresent concern wherever standards of cleanliness and sanitation are low.

Additives

Food entails a whole new set of problems because of the thousands of new ingredients that have been added to it, directly and indirectly, in recent years. These substances include many that have been deemed necessary because of the revolution in food technology—the rise of packaged convenience foods of all kinds. Labels on today's convenience foods list preservatives, thickeners, mold inhibitors, fillers, emulsifiers, and artificial colors and flavors. The trouble with food additives is that we have had little time to learn about their effect on the body, especially over a long period of time. The Food and Drug Administration does set standards in this area; but in the opinion of many experts, these safeguards are inadequate. According to Bess Myerson, then Commissioner of New York City's Department of Consumer Affairs, "The food that we eat is becoming as polluted as the air we breathe. Inadequate federal regulations allow manufacturers of prepared foods to ignore potential health hazards. No reasonable person would knowingly drink a glass full of the chemicals he unwittingly consumes in his daily diet."

What are some of these chemicals, and how could they be dangerous? One that was imbibed freely by large numbers of Americans and in great quantities was sodium cyclamate, the artificial sweetener used in diet drinks and foods. It was eventually withdrawn after it was linked to cancer and chromosome damage in experimental animals. The controversy continues, however, and some accused the government of acting precipitately in this case. Cyclamates are still recommended for diabetics and dieters.

Nitrates and nitrites are used in enormous quantities as preservatives in food. Recently, Food and Drug Administration chemists found that these chemicals had apparently given rise to substances called nitrosamines in samples of fish. Nitrosamines are powerful carcinogenic agents, even in small amounts. The amounts found in the fish were minuscule, up to 26 parts per billion. These chemicals are also thought to be capable of producing genetic and birth defects.

Recently, a red dye used to color maraschino cherries and other food substances was ordered withdrawn from the market because it was implicated in certain studies as having potentially carcinogenic properties.

In Sweden, a geneticist and microbiologist named Dr. Bjorn Gillsberg has warned that unless we start to screen potentially mutagenic (causing changes in the genes) substances from our food we face an

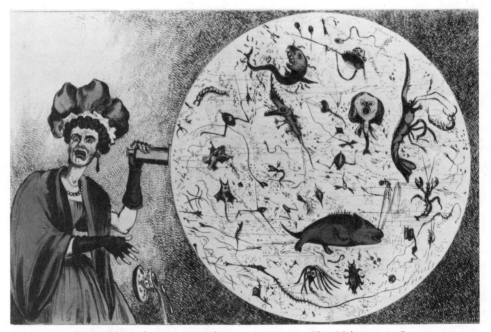

The problem of contaminated water is not new. This 19th-century English etching shows a horrified citizen with a cup of drinking water enormously magnified according to the artist's imaginative conception.

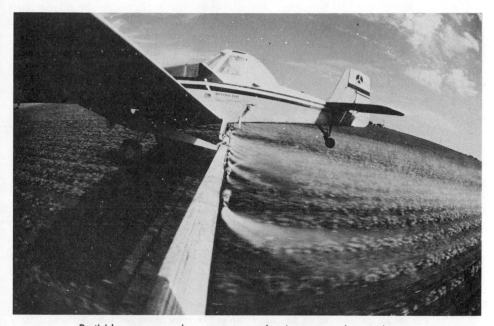

Pesticides are sprayed on crops to combat insect pests, but residues of chemical pesticides contaminate the crops and the soil, too.

epidemic of birth defects, loss of fertility, and other genetic damage. He cited sodium bisulphate, a chemical used to prevent peeled potatoes from darkening, as a potentially dangerous additive.

The federal Task Force on Research Planning in Environmental Health Science estimates there are some 10,000 of these chemicals—additives and residues—to be found in our foods, and it holds that "only a portion . . . have been studied thoroughly enough to meet exacting, present-day standards."

Pesticide Residues

Every year until recently, synthetic organic pesticides have drenched the territory of the United States in an amount equivalent to 220 pounds for every square mile. American mother's milk now contains four times the level of DDT that is permitted in cow's milk. We know that DDT and similar compounds have had devastating effects on many forms of wildlife, especially fish and birds. Some scientists fear the genetic and other effects of these compounds on human beings. As the result of widespread clamor, the use of DDT and related pesticides is on the wane in many parts of the world.

Noise Pollution

Most people are aware that their health may be threatened by the contamination of the air they breathe or the water they drink or swim in. Some know that dangerous substances may pollute the food they eat. But few realize that we are all adversely affected by a pollutant so common it tends to be overlooked—noise.

Noise is generally defined as any unwanted sound. It is the most widespread form of pollution in the United States. Who has not been driven to distraction by the wail of sirens, the din of construction noise, cars, trucks, and buses? The old joke about city-dwellers being so used to noise that they were kept awake by the silence of a vacation retreat in the country is an expression of just how much noise most of us have accepted as inevitable.

The joke has a new twist now, because rural and suburban areas are plagued by their own varieties of noise. Farms have become increasingly more mechanized, and agricultural machinery contributes its ear-splitting toll. The once-inviolate stillness of snow-blanketed wilderness is now ruptured by the buzz of snowmobiles. Suburban homes are filled with the sound of electric dishwashers, garbage disposals, air conditioners, vacuum cleaners, and power tools—all potent noise makers—while from their backyards comes the insistent roar of power lawn mowers.

Worst of all is the situation of some workers, who, in addition to all this domestic noise, must suffer high noise levels on the job. Boilermakers and jackhammer operators are obvious examples, but cab

Noise pollution is on the rise. These jackhammer operators will suffer a hearing loss from their continual exposure to loud noise.

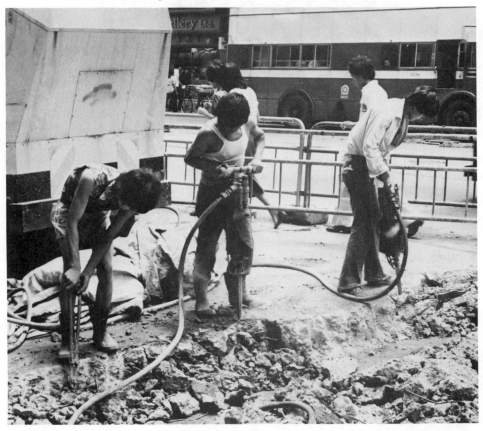

drivers, bookkeeping machine operators, and parents of young children are all subject to special, if less conspicuous, hazards.

For noise is not just annoying, it is potentially dangerous, both physically and mentally. Dr. Vern Knudsen, a specialist in sound and chancellor emeritus at UCLA, has said, "Noise, like smog, is a slow agent of death. If it continues to increase for the next 30 years as it has for the last 30, it could become lethal."

Effect of Sound on the Eardrum

How can mere sound have such dire effects? Sound is a form of energy, and energy can be destructive as well as constructive. Sound is caused by anything that moves back and forth—vibrates. For us to hear sound over a distance, the energy of this vibrating motion must be transmitted to our ears over a distance, via sound waves. A sound wave in air is a succession of regions of compressed air and partial vacuums, or areas of high and low air pressure. (Sound waves can also travel through liquids and solids.) We hear sound because our eardrums are moved back and forth by these changes in air pressure. The eardrum, or *tympanic membrane,* can be incredibly delicate, perceiving a sound that moves it only one billionth of a centimeter—the threshold of hearing—equivalent, perhaps, to the rustle of one blade of grass against another. If the intensity of sound pressure becomes too great, at something like a billion billion times the energy at the threshold of hearing, we experience pain, and the eardrum or the delicate structures inside the ear may be damaged.

The intensity of sounds is often measured in units called *decibels,* or *db*. These units are logarithmic— that is, 10 db is ten times as powerful as 1 db, 20 db is 100 times as powerful, 30 db is 1,000 times as powerful, and so on. On this scale, 0 db is at the threshold of hearing; rustling leaves, 20 db; a quiet office, about 50 db; conversation, 60 db; heavy traffic, 90 db; a pneumatic jackhammer six feet away, 100 db; a jet aircraft 500 feet overhead, 115 db; a Saturn rocket's takeoff, 180 db.

For most people, the pain threshold is about 120 db; deafening ear damage will result at 150 db. But damage of various kinds can come from much lower exposures. Temporary hearing impairment can result from sounds over 85 db now found in modern kitchens with all appliances going. If the ears don't get a chance to recover, the impairment will become permanent.

Damage to the Inner Ear

Although very loud noise can damage the eardrum, most physiological damage from noise occurs in the snail-shaped, liquid-filled cochlea, or inner ear. Sound transmitted to the cochlea produces waves in the liquid, which in turn move delicate and minute structures called hair cells or *cilia* in that part of the cochlea known as the organ of Corti. The motion of the cilia is transformed into electrical impulses that conduct the sensation of sound to the brain.

The cilia can easily be fatigued by noise, causing a temporary loss of hearing, or a shift in the threshold of hearing. If they are not given a chance to recuperate, they will be permanently damaged, and irreversible hearing loss will result. There

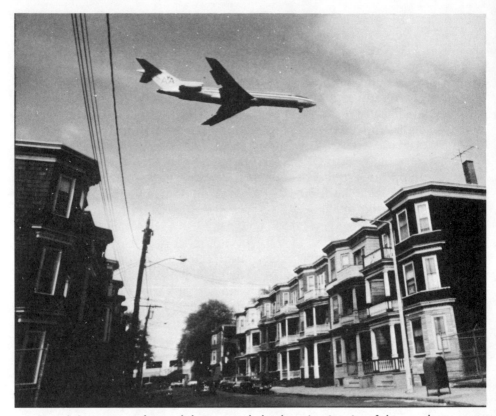

It is easy to understand the protests lodged against jet aircraft by people who endure the hearing hazards posed by living near a major airport.

are some 23,000 cilia in the average cochlea; different sets of cilia respond to different frequency bands. The cilia responding to sound frequencies of 4,000 to 6,000 cps (cyles per second) are especially vulnerable to damage. The region of 85–95 db is generally regarded as the beginning of dangerous sound intensities. In general, the louder the noise, the longer it lasts, the higher it is, and the purer in frequency, the more dangerous it is. Thus, jet engines and powerful sirens are particularly hazardous.

Noise and Mental Illness

Moreover, noise has a definite effect on mental well-being. No one knows exactly how, but noise can produce irritability, tension, and nervous strain. Extreme noise conditions can cause, or at least contribute to, mental illness. British medical authorities have reported a significantly higher incidence of mental illness among people exposed to aircraft noise.

Dr. Jack C. Westman, Director of the Child Psychiatry Division of the University of Wisconsin Medical School, thinks that unwanted noise in the home is contributing to divorce and the generation gap:

We scapegoat, take out our tensions in other ways. Mothers yell at the youngsters, and parents bicker and fight between themselves. The average kitchen is like a boiler room, and what we thought was our friendly dishwasher is adding to the unhealthy surroundings by contributing to the noise.

A Growing Problem

Unfortunately, the noise problem seems to be getting worse. The U. S. Surgeon General states that as many as 16 million citizens are now losing their hearing from on-job noise. The U. S. Department of Commerce's Panel on Noise Abatement recently observed that noise pollution in the United States is reaching a serious level—a conclusion that most authorities had reached some time ago. Noise experts generally agree that the overall sound level in this country is rising at the rate of 1 db per year—or doubling every decade. There is every reason to believe that the rate of increase will rise in the coming years. Some scientists predict that even at the current rate, everyone in America will be deaf by the year 2000. Measurements conducted in average American towns show that noise levels have boomed four times higher than 1956 values and 32 times those in 1938. A New York City task force on noise control found that noise had reached a level "intense, continuous and persistent enough to threaten basic community life." The Federal Council for Science and Technology reckons that this major health hazard costs the nation $4 billion a year in decreased efficiency and lost compensation.

Some experts have linked the rise in diseases of the cardiovascular system to this steady increase in noise pollution. Noise elevates blood pressure and raises the amount of cholesterol in the blood.

A group of Africans living in the hushed environment of the Southeast Sudan retain acute hearing and youthful arteries into advanced old age. But when they move to their noisy capital, their hearing deteriorates, and their rate of heart disease goes up.

Protection Against Noise

What can you do to protect yourself and your family from the effects of noise pollution? You can't do much to control some forms of noise—such as traffic noise—directly. But you can support local, state, and federal legislation that seeks to control or eliminate some forms of noise. For example, many communities have laws that forbid blowing car horns except in emergencies; regrettably, such laws are poorly enforced, and the noise contribution from impatient drivers in our metropolitan areas is staggering.

You have at your constant command two effective noise-control instruments—your hands. Cupping your ears with them during noise of extraordinary pitch and intensity may help preserve your hearing. If you regularly encounter loud or irritating noise on your job or travels, buy a pair of ear protectors and wear them. This solution is no more far-fetched than wearing sunglasses on dazzling days at the beach.

If you're responsible for the running of an office or plant, seek professional sound engineers' advice to make sure that you've taken advantage of the latest techniques and materials to cut noise to a minimum.

One of the most important things you can do is to stay clear of avoidable dangerous noise. A prevalent

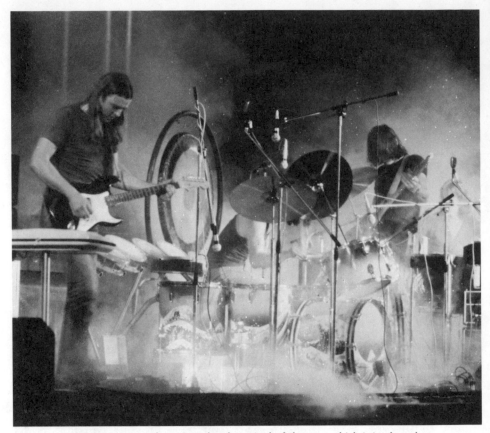

Listening to rock music at levels typical of those at which it is played
or reproduced may blow not only one's mind but one's hearing as well.

source of this kind of sound is rock music played or reproduced at damaging levels. If you or your children pooh-pooh this threat, here are the facts: listening to this music at levels typical of those now current may not only your mind, but your hearing, too.

Dr. Ralph R. Rupp, head of the audiology division of the speech clinic of the University of Michigan, together with his assistant, Larry J. Koch, measured sound levels produced by a rock combo. In the rehearsal room, these averaged 120–130 db during loud passages. All members of the combo reported ringing in their ears or other uncom-

fortable symptoms for from eight hours to several days after their get-togethers—signs of temporary or permanent hearing damage. Dr. Rupp says that people who either play or listen to music at such high levels may pay an enormous price in terms of eventual hearing loss. He suggests that rock musicians wear ear protectors that could reduce the sound levels at the ear by 20 or 30 db. He also proposes that local governments set safe maximum allowable noise limits for electronic amplification in clubs and discothèques.

In another test, Dr. Kenneth Pollock of the University of Florida found that the sound levels at a swinging teen club dropped to a safe 90 db only when he moved his equipment 40 feet outside the club. Ten teen-agers suffered hearing losses after dancing for three hours near the bandstand, where the din averaged 120 db. Listening to music via earphones offers a particularly effective means of going deaf—all it takes is a twist of the dial and you are instantly assaulted with sound levels that are practically unbearable. Dr. David M. Lipscomb of the University of Tennessee says, "We are apparently reaching the point where young people are losing sufficient hearing to jeopardize their occupational potential."

Yet another form of noise introduced to our novelty-hungry society is that from snowmobiles—those off-road vehicles that have enjoyed an amazing boom in recent years.

Some ranch hands, foresters, and Arctic Indians and Eskimos have found the snowmobile literally a lifesaver in their harsh, snowbound winters, but most snowmobiles are used for recreational purposes. If you ride a snowmobile for any reason, you should know that its snarl is a definite hazard to your hearing, and wear special ear protectors. John G. Bollinger, a professor of mechanical engineering at the University of Wisconsin, measured snowmobile noise in a project to determine how they might be quietened. He recorded levels of about 110 db at a point six inches in front of the driver's head. Noise of this intensity can cause temporary hearing loss for an occasional rider, and permanent hearing loss for someone who spends several hours a day on the snowmobile.

CHAPTER 15

Skin and Hair

Not many people have perfectly proportioned faces and bodies, but practically anyone, at any age, can present an attractive appearance if skin is healthy-looking and glowing and hair is clean and shining. Healthy skin and hair can be achieved through good health habits, cleanliness, and personal grooming. Expensive skin-and-hair products may boost self-confidence, but they are a poor substitute for proper diet, exercise, enough sleep, and soap and water or cleansing creams.

The condition of skin and hair reflects a person's physical and emotional health. Of course, general appearance is determined not only by what is going on inside the body, but by outward circumstances, such as extremes of temperature or the use of harsh soaps. Appearance can also be altered temporarily by cosmetics and permanently by surgery.

THE SKIN

The skin is one of the most important organs of the body. It serves as protection against infection by germs and shields delicate underlying tissue against injury. Approximately one-third of the bloodstream flows through the skin, and as the blood vessels contract or relax in response to heat and cold, the skin acts as a thermostat that helps control body temperature. The two million sweat glands in the skin also regulate body temperature through the evaporation of perspiration. The

ANATOMY OF THE SKIN

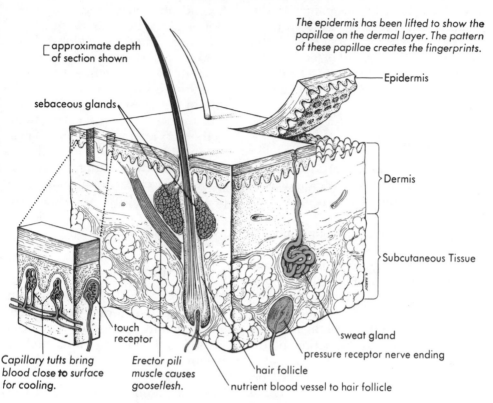

The epidermis has been lifted to show the papillae on the dermal layer. The pattern of these papillae creates the fingerprints.

approximate depth of section shown

sebaceous glands

Epidermis

Dermis

Subcutaneous Tissue

touch receptor

sweat gland

pressure receptor nerve ending

Capillary tufts bring blood close to surface for cooling.

Erector pili muscle causes gooseflesh.

hair follicle

nutrient blood vessel to hair follicle

many delicate nerve endings in the skin make it a sense organ responsive not only to heat and cold, but to pleasure, pain, and pressure.

Certain cells in the skin produce a protective pigmentation that determines its color and guards against overexposure to the ultraviolet rays of the sun. By absorption and elimination, the skin helps regulate the body's chemical and fluid balance. One of the miracles of the skin is that it constantly renews itself.

Structure of the Skin

The skin is made up of two layers. The outer layer or *epidermis* has a surface of horny, nonliving cells that form the body's protective en-velope. These cells are constantly being shed and replaced by new ones which are made in the lower or inner layer of the epidermis.

Underneath the epidermis is the *dermis*, the thicker part of the skin. It contains blood vessels, nerves, and connective tissue. The sweat glands are located in the dermis, and they collect fluid containing water, salt, and waste products from the blood. This fluid is sent through tiny canals that end in pores on the skin's surface.

The oil or *sebaceous* glands that secrete the oil which lubricates the surface of the skin and hair are also located in the dermis. They are most often associated with hair *follicles*. Hair follicles and oil glands are found over most of the body, with the exception of the palms of the hands and the soles of the feet.

The layer of fatty tissue below the dermis, called *subcutaneous* tissue, acts as an insulator against heat and cold and as a shock absorber against injury.

Skin Color

The basic skin color of each person is determined at birth, and is a part of his heritage that cannot be changed.

MELANIN: There are four pigments in the normal skin that affect its color: melanin, oxygenated hemoglobin, reduced hemoglobin, and various carotenes. Of these, *melanin* is the most powerful. The cells that produce it are the same in all races, but there is wide variation in the amount produced, and wide variation in its color, which ranges from black to light tan. Every adult has about 60,000 melanin-producing cells in each square inch of skin.

Melanin cells also affect eye color. When the cells are deep in the eye, the color produced is blue or green. When they are close to the surface, the eye is brown. An *albino*, a person with no melanin, has eyes that appear pink because the stronger pigment that ordinarily masks the blood vessels is lacking.

HEMOGLOBIN: The pigment that gives blood its color, called hemoglobin, has the next greatest effect on skin color. When it is combined with oxygen, a bright red is the result, and this in turn produces the rosy complexion associated with good health in light-skinned people. When such people suffer from reduced hemoglobin due to anemia,

they appear to be excessively pale. A concentration of reduced hemoglobin gives the skin a bluish appearance. Since hemoglobin has a weaker coloring effect than the melanin that determines basic skin color, these variations are more visible in lighter-skinned individuals.

CAROTENES: The weakest pigments in the skin are the *carotenes*. These produce a yellowish tone that is increased by eating excessive amounts of carrots and oranges. In people with black or brown skin, excess carotene is usually masked by the melanin pigment.

Aging Skin

Skin appearance is affected by both internal and external factors. The silken quality of a baby's skin is due mainly to the fact that it has not yet begun to show the effects of continued exposure to sun and wind. The skin problems associated with adolescence reflect the many glandular changes that occur during the transition to adulthood. As the years pass, the skin becomes the most obvious indicator of aging.

Heredity, general health, and exposure to the elements are some of the factors that contribute to aging skin. Because people with darker skin have built-in protection against the ravages of the sun, their skin usually has a younger appearance than that of lighter-skinned people of comparable age.

In general, the skin of an older person is characterized by wrinkles and shininess. It feels thinner when pinched because it has lost its elasticity and part of the underlying fat that gives firmness to a younger skin.

Constant exposure to sunlight is now thought to play a more important role in the visible aging of skin than the aging process itself. Such exposure also appears to be directly related to the greater frequency of skin cancer among farmers, sailors, and others who spend most of their working hours out-of-doors.

Care of the Skin

Healthy, normal skin should be washed regularly with mild soap and warm water to remove grease, perspiration, and accumulated dirt. For those with a limited water supply or inadequate bath and shower facilities, sponge baths are a good

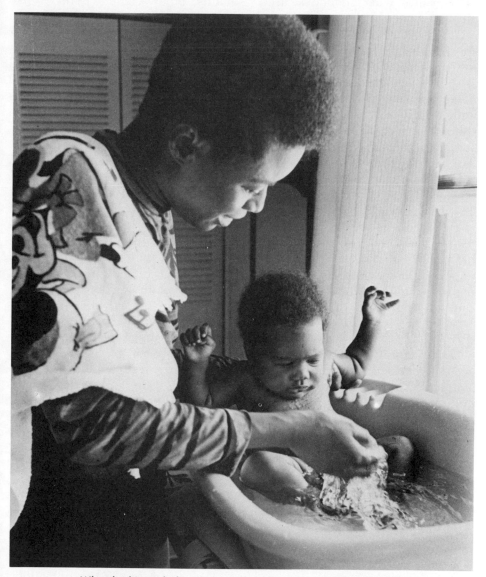

When bathing a baby, care must be taken to see that soap is thoroughly rinsed off after washing, since it can act as a skin irritant.

substitute if the sponge or wash-cloth is thoroughly rinsed as various parts of the body are washed. Many people feel that a shower is a much more efficient way of getting clean than a bath, since the bath water becomes the receptacle for the dirt washed from the body, instead of its being rinsed away.

No matter what method is used, all soap should be thoroughly rinsed off the skin after washing. Unless specifically prescribed by a doctor, medicated or germicidal soaps should not be used, since they may be an irritant. Skin should be dried with a fluffy towel, and bath towels should never be shared. Hands should be washed several times a day, and fingernails kept clean.

Facial skin requires special care because of its constant exposure. The face should be cleaned in the morning and before bedtime. Some women may prefer to use a cleansing cream rather than soap and water. Everyone should avoid massaging soap into the skin, since this may cause drying.

Dry and Oily Skin

Both heredity and environment account for the wide variation in the amount of oil and perspiration secreted by the glands of different people. Also, the same person's skin may be oily in one part of the body and dry in another.

DRY SKIN: This condition is the result of loss of water from the outer surface of the epidermis and its insufficient replacement from the tissues below. Some causes of the moisture loss are too frequent use of soap and detergents, and constant exposure to dry air. Anyone spending a great deal of time in air-conditioned surroundings in which the humidity has been greatly lowered is likely to suffer from dry skin.

To correct the condition, the use of soap and water should be kept to a minimum for those parts of the body where the skin is dry. Cleansing creams or lotions containing lanolin should be used on the face, hands, elbows, and wherever else necessary. If tub baths are taken, a bath oil can be used in the water or applied to the skin after drying. Baby oil is just as effective and much cheaper than glamorously packaged and overadvertised products. Baby oil or a protective lotion should also be used on any parts of the body exposed to direct sunlight for any extended length of time. Applying oil to the skin will not, however, prevent wrinkles.

OILY SKIN: The amount of oil that comes to the surface of the skin through the sebaceous glands is the result not only of heredity, but also of temperature and emotional state. In warm weather, when the skin perspires more freely, the oil spreads like a film on the surface moisture. Non-oily foundation lotions can be helpful in keeping the oil spread to a minimum, and so can frequent washing with soap and water. When washing is inconvenient during the day, cleansing pads packaged to fit in pocket or purse are a quick and efficient solution for both men and women.

Too much friction from complexion brushes, rough washcloths, or harsh soaps may irritate rather than improve an oily skin condition.

Deodorants and Antiperspirants

Sweat glands are present almost everywhere in the skin except for the lips and a few other areas. Most of them give off the extremely dilute salt water known as sweat, or perspiration. Their purpose is to cool the body by evaporation of water. Body odors are not produced by perspiration itself, but by the bacterial activity that takes place in the perspiration. The activity is most intense in warm, moist parts of the body from which perspiration cannot evaporate quickly, such as the underarm area.

DEODORANTS: The basic means of keeping this type of bacterial growth under control is through personal cleanliness of both skin and clothing. Deodorant soaps containing antiseptic chemicals are now available. Though they do not kill bacteria, they do reduce the speed with which they multiply.

Underarm deodorants also help to eliminate the odor. They are not meant to stop the flow of perspiration, but rather to slow down bacterial growth and mask body odors with their own scent. Such deodorants should be applied immediately after bathing. They are usually more effective if the underarm area is shaved, since the hair in this unexposed area collects perspiration and encourages bacterial growth.

ANTIPERSPIRANTS: Antiperspirants differ from deodorants in that they not only affect the rate of bacterial growth, but also reduce the amount of perspiration that reaches the skin surface. Since the action of the chemical salts they contain is cumulative, they seem to be more effective with repeated use. Antiperspirants come under the category of drugs, and their contents must be printed on the container. Deodorants are considered cosmetics, and may or may not name their contents on the package.

No matter what the nature of the advertising claim, neither type of product completely stops the flow of perspiration, nor would it be desirable to do so. Effectiveness of the various brands differs from one person to another. Some may produce a mild allergic reaction; others might be too weak to do a good job. It is practical to experiment with a few different brands, using them under similar conditions, to find the type that works best for you.

Creams and Cosmetics

The bewildering number of creams and cosmetics on the market and the exaggerated claims of some of their advertising can be reduced to a few simple facts. In most cases, the higher price of such products is an indication of the amount of money spent on advertising and packaging rather than on the ingredients themselves. Beauty preparations should be judged by the user on their merits rather than on their claims.

COLD CREAMS AND CLEANSING CREAMS: These two products are essentially the same. They are designed to remove accumulated skin secretions, dirt, and grime, and should be promptly removed from the skin with a soft towel or tissue.

LUBRICATING CREAMS AND LOTIONS: Also called night creams, moisturizing creams, and conditioning creams, these products are supposed to prevent the loss of moisture from the skin and promote its smoothness. They are usually left on overnight or for an extended length of time. Anyone with dry skin will find it helpful to apply

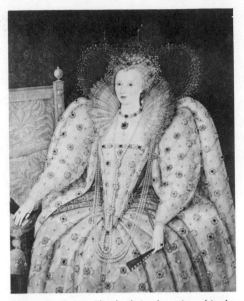

England's Queen Elizabeth I, who reigned in the 1500s, is usually portrayed as very pale. An amateur cosmetician, she almost always wore white-lead powder.

a moisturizer under foundation cream. This will help keep the skin from drying out even further, and protect it against the effects of air conditioning.

VANISHING CREAMS AND FOUNDATION CREAMS: These products also serve the purpose of providing the skin with moisture, but are meant to be applied immediately before putting on makeup.

REJUVENATING CREAMS: There is no scientific proof that any of the "royal jelly," "secret formula," or "hormone" creams produce a marked improvement on aging skin. They cannot eliminate wrinkles, nor can they regenerate skin tissue.

MEDICATED CREAMS AND LOTIONS: These products should not be used except on the advice of a doctor since they may cause or aggravate skin disorders of various kinds.

LIPSTICKS: Lipsticks contain lanolin, a mixture of oil and wax, a coloring dye, and pigment, as well as perfume. Any of these substances can cause an allergic reaction in individual cases, but such reactions are uncommon. Sometimes the reaction is caused by the staining dye, in which case a "nonpermanent" lipstick should be used.

COSMETICS AND THE SENSITIVE SKIN: Anyone with a cosmetic problem due to sensitive skin should consult a *dermatologist*, a physician specializing in the skin and its diseases. Cosmetic companies will inform a physician of the ingredients in their products, and he can then recommend a brand that will agree with the patient's specific skin problems. He may also recommend a special nonallergenic preparation.

EYE MAKEUP: Eye-liner and mascara brushes and pencils—and lipsticks for that matter—can carry infection and should never be borrowed or lent. *Hypoallergenic* makeup, which is specially made for those who get allergic reactions to regular eye makeup, is available and should be used by anyone so affected.

SUNTANNING LOTIONS: See under *Aches, Pains, Nuisances, Worries,* p. 837, for a discussion of sunburn.

HAIR

Hair originates in tiny sacs or follicles deep in the dermis layer of skin tissue. The part of the hair below the skin surface is the root; the part above is the shaft. Hair follicles are closely connected to the sebaceous glands which secrete oil to the scalp and give hair its natural sheen.

Hair grows from the root outward, pushing the shaft farther from the scalp. Depending on its color, there may be as many as 125,000 hairs on an adult's head. The palms of the hands, the soles of the feet, and the lips are the only completely hairless parts of the surface of the body.

Texture

Each individual hair is made up of nonliving cells that contain a tough protein called *keratin*. Hair texture differs from one part of the body to another. In some areas, it may be soft and downy; in others, tough and bristly. Hair texture also differs between the sexes, among individuals,

A hairdresser uses rollers to curl a client's hair. Hair styles, including length and degree of curling, are a matter of fashion.

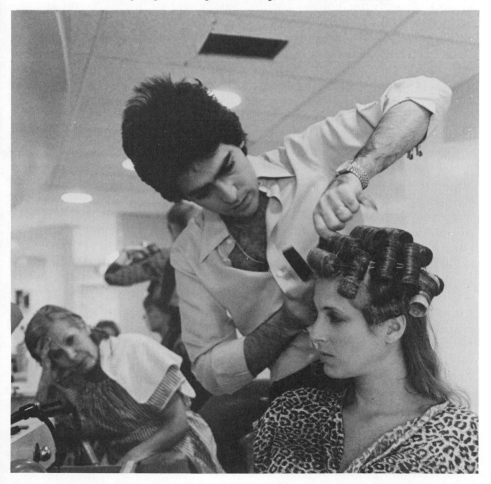

and among the different races.

If an individual hair is oval in cross-section, it is curly along its length. If the cross-section is round, the hair is straight. Thick, wiry hair is usually triangular or kidney-shaped. The fineness or coarseness of hair texture is related to its natural color.

CURLING: Anyone using a home permanent preparation should read and follow instructions with great care. If a new brand is tried, the instructions should be read all over again, since they may be quite different from the accustomed ones.

Electric curling irons are not safe because they may cause pinpoint burns in the scalp which are hardly noticeable at the time but may lead to permanent small areas of baldness. The danger can be minimized, however, if instructions for use are followed exactly and the recommended moisturizing lotions are used. It is especially important that the iron not be hot enough to singe the hair. The results, even if there is no damage, are not long lasting and are adversely affected by dampness. Setting lotions used with rollers or clips have a tendency to dull the hair unless they are completely brushed out.

STRAIGHTENING: The least harmful as well as the least effective way of straightening the hair temporarily is the use of pomades. They are usually considered unsatisfactory by women because they are too greasy, but are often used by men with short unruly hair. Heat-pressing the hair with a metal comb is longer-lasting but can cause substantial damage by burning the scalp. When this method is used, humidity or scalp perspiration will cause the hair to revert to its natural curl. The practice of ironing the hair should be discouraged since it causes dryness and brittleness, with resultant breakage. Chemical straighteners should be used with great care since they may cause serious burns. Special efforts must be made to protect the eyes from contact with these products.

Hair Color

In the same way that melanin colors the skin, it also determines hair color. The less melanin, the lighter the hair. As each hair loses its melanin pigment, it gradually turns gray, then white. It is assumed that the age at which hair begins to gray is an inherited characteristic and therefore can't be postponed or prevented by eating special foods, by taking vitamins, or by the external application of creams. The only way to recolor gray hair is by the use of a chemical dye.

DYES AND TINTS: Anyone wishing to make a radical change in hair color should consult a trained and reliable hairdresser. Trying to turn black hair bright red or dark red hair to blonde with a home preparation can sometimes end up with unwanted purplish or greenish results. When tints or dyes are used at home to lighten or darken the hair color by one or two shades, instructions accompanying the product must be followed carefully. Anyone with a tendency to contract contact dermatitis (see page 792) should make a patch test on the skin to check on possible allergic reactions. Hair should be tinted or dyed no more often than once a month.

DYE STRIPPING: The only safe way to get rid of an unwanted dye color that has been used on the hair is to let

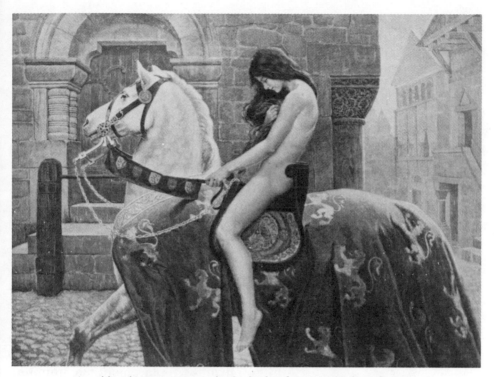

An old etching portrays Lady Godiva's infamous ride through the streets of Coventry, England, clad only in her long, beautiful hair.

it grow out. The technique known as stripping takes all color from the hair and reduces it to a dangerously weak mass. It is then redyed its natural color. Such a procedure should never be undertaken by anyone except a trained beautician, if at all.

BLEACHING: Hydrogen peroxide is mixed with a hair-lightener to pre-bleach hair before applying blond tints. Bleaching with peroxide alone can cause more damage to the hair than dyeing or tinting it with a reliable commercial preparation, because it causes dryness, brittlenesss, and breakage.

General Hair Care

Properly cared for hair usually looks clean, shiny, and alive. Unfortunately, too many people mask the natural good looks of their hair with unnecessary sprays and "beauty" preparations.

WASHING THE HAIR: Hair should be washed about once a week—more often if it tends to be oily. The claims made by shampoo manufacturers need not always be taken too seriously, since most shampoos contain nothing more than soap or detergent and a perfuming agent. No shampoo can restore the natural oils to the hair at the same time that it washes it. A castile shampoo is good for dry hair, and one containing tincture of green soap is good for oily hair.

Thorough rinsing is essential to eliminate any soap deposit. If the local water is hard, a detergent shampoo can be rinsed off more easily than one containing soap.

DRYING THE HAIR: Drying the

hair in sunlight or under a heat-controlled dryer is more satisfactory than trying to rub it dry with a towel. Gentle brushing during drying reactivates the natural oils that give hair its shine. Brushing in general is excellent for the appearance of the hair. Be sure to wash both brush and comb as often as the hair is washed.

Hair pomades should be avoided or used sparingly, since they are sometimes so heavy that they clog the pores of the scalp. A little bit of olive oil or baby oil can be rubbed into dry hair after shampooing. This is also good for babies' hair.

There is no scientific evidence that creme rinses, protein rinses, or beer rinses accomplish anything for the hair other than making it somewhat more manageable if it is naturally fine and flyaway.

Dandruff

Simple dandruff is a condition in which the scalp begins to itch and flake a few days after the hair has been washed. There is no evidence that the problem is related to germ infection.

Oiliness and persistent dandruff may appear not only on the scalp, but also on the sides of the nose or the chest. In such cases, a dermatologist should be consulted. Both light and serious cases often respond well to prescription medicines containing tars. These preparations control the dandruff, but there is no known cure for it.

Nits

Head lice sometimes infect adults as well as children. These tiny parasites usually live on the part of the scalp near the nape of the neck, and when they bite, they cause itching.

They attach their eggs, which are called *nits*, to the shaft of the hair, and when they are plentiful, they can be seen by a trained eye as tiny, silvery-white ovals. This condition is highly contagious and can be passed from one head to another by way of combs, brushes, hats, head scarfs, and towels. A doctor can be consulted for information on effective ways of eliminating nits—usually by the application of chemicals and the use of a fine-toothed comb.

Baldness

Under the normal circumstances of combing, brushing, and shampooing, a person loses anywhere from 25 to 100 hairs a day. Because new hairs start growing each day, the loss and replacement usually balance each other. When the loss rate is greater than the replacement rate, thinning and baldness are the result.

ALOPECIA: The medical name for baldness is *alopecia,* the most common form of which is *male pattern baldness.* Dr. Eugene Van Scott, Professor of Dermatology of Temple University's Health Sciences Center, sums up the opinion of medical authorities on the three factors responsible for this type of baldness: sex, age, and heredity. Unfortunately, these are three factors over which medical science has no control.

OTHER CAUSES OF BALDNESS: Other forms of baldness may be the result of bacterial or fungus infections, allergic reactions to particular medicines, radiation, or continual friction. It has also been suggested that constant stress from hair curlers or tightly pulled ponytails can cause loss of hair. These forms of baldness usually disappear when the cause is

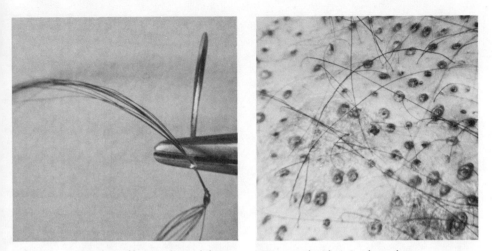

Synthetic fibers, (*above, left*) are sometimes used as hair implants, but scalp tissue can be badly infected (*above, right*) by the operation.

eliminated.

Although diet has very little to do with baldness, poor nutrition can result in hair that is dry, dull, and brittle enough to break easily. Any serious illness can lead to hair loss as well. It is thought that vitamin A taken in grossly excessive amounts can contribute to hair loss.

Women ordinarily lose some of their hair at the end of pregnancy, after delivery, and during the menopause, but regrowth can be expected in a few months.

It is now possible for anyone suffering from temporary baldness or from male pattern baldness to choose from a wide variety of attractively styled wigs and hairpieces.

A surgical procedure for treating male pattern baldness and baldness in women is called hair transplantation; it is discussed under *Surgery*, p. 900.

Hair Removal

Over the centuries and around the world, fashions in whiskers and beards come and go, but the average American male still subjects at least part of his face to daily shaving. Although feminine shaving practices are a more recent phenomenon, most American women now consider it part of good grooming to remove underarm and leg hair with a razor as often as twice a week. Shaving removes not only the dead skin cells that make up the protective layer of the body's surface, but also some of the living skin underneath. Instead of being harmful, this appears to stimulate rather than damage new skin growth.

Male Shaving

The average beard grows about two-tenths of an inch a day. However, the density of male face hair varies a great deal depending on skin and hair color. In all races, the concentration is usually greatest on the chin and in the area between the nose and upper lip.

There is no proof that an electric razor is safer or better for all types of skin than a safety razor. Both types

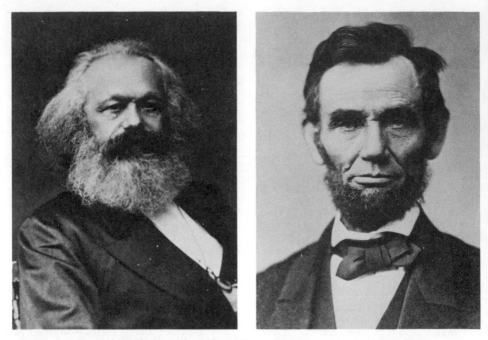

Beards were fashionable in the 1800s, and we are accustomed to seeing portraits of Karl Marx (*above, left*) and Abraham Lincoln with beards.

result in nicks and cuts of the living skin tissue, depending on the closeness of the shave.

Twice as many men prefer wet shaving to dry because the use of soap and hot water softens the hair stubble and makes it easier to remove. Shaving authorities point out that thorough soaking is one of the essentials of easy and safe shaving. Leaving the shaving lather on the face for at least two minutes will also soften whiskers a good deal.

The razor should be moistened with hot water throughout the process, and the chin and upper lip left for last so that the heavier hair concentration in these areas has the longest contact with moisture and lather.

OILY SKIN: Men with oily skin should use an aerosol shaving preparation or a lather type applied with a brush. These are really soaps and are more effective in eliminating the oils that coat the face hair, thus making it easier to shave.

DRY SKIN: A brushless cream is advisable for dry skin since it lubricates the skin rather than further depriving it of oil.

INGROWN HAIRS: One of the chief problems connected with shaving is that it often causes ingrown hairs, which can lead to pore-clogging and infection. Hair is more likely to turn back into the skin if it is shaved against the grain, or if the cutting edge of the blade is dull and rough rather than smooth. Men with coarse, wiry, curly hair may find that whisker ends are more likely to become ingrown than men with fine hair. The problem is best handled by shaving with the grain, using a sharp blade, and avoiding too close a shave, particularly in the area around the neck.

SHAVING AND SKIN PROBLEMS: For men with acne or a tendency to skin problems, the following advice is offered by Dr. Howard T. Behrman, Director of Dermatological Research, New York Medical College:

• Shave as seldom as possible, perhaps only once or twice a week, and always with the grain.

• If wet shaving is preferred, use a new blade each time, and shave as lightly as possible to avoid nicking pimples.

• Wash face carefully with plenty of soap and hot water to make the beard easy to manage, and after shaving, rinse with hot water followed by cold.

• Use an antiseptic astringent face lotion.

• Instead of plucking out ingrown hairs, loosen them gently so that the ends do not grow back into the skin.

• Although some people with skin problems find an electric shaver less irritating, in most cases, a wet shave seems best.

Female Shaving

Millions of American women regularly shave underarm and leg hair, and most of them do so with a blade razor. In recent years, various types of shavers have been designed with blade exposure more suited to women's needs than the standard type used by men. To make shaving easier and safer, the following procedures are recommended:

• Since wet hair is much easier to cut, the most effective time to shave is during or immediately following a bath or shower.

• Shaving cream or soap lather keeps the water from evaporating, and is preferred to dry shaving.

• Underarm shaving is easier with a contoured razor designed for this purpose. If a deodorant or antiperspirant causes stinging or irritation after shaving, allow a short time to elapse before applying it.

• Light bleeding from nicks or scrapes can be stopped by applying pressure to a sterile pad placed on the injured area.

Unwanted Hair

The technical word for excess or unwanted hair on the face, chest, arms, and legs is *hirsutism*. The condition varies greatly among different ethnic strains, and so does the attitude toward it. Women of southern European ancestry are generally hairier than those with Nordic or Anglo-Saxon ancestors. Caucasoid peoples are hairier than Negroid peoples. The sparsest amount of body hair is found among the Mongolian races and American Indians.

Although heredity is the chief factor in hirsutism, hormones also influence hair growth. If there is a sudden appearance of coarse hair on the body of a young boy or girl or a woman with no such former tendency, a glandular disturbance should be suspected and investigated by a doctor.

A normal amount of unwanted hair on the legs and under the arms is usually removed by shaving. When the problem involves the arms, face, chest, and abdomen, other methods of removal are available.

Temporary Methods of Hair Removal

BLEACHING: Unwanted dark fuzz on the upper lip and arms can be lightened almost to invisibility with a commercially prepared bleach or with a homemade paste consisting of baking soda, hydrogen peroxide (bleaching strength), and a few drops of ammonia. Soap chips can be used instead of baking soda. The paste should be left on the skin for a few minutes and then washed off. It is harmless to the skin, and if applied repeatedly, the hair will tend to break off as a result of constant bleaching.

CHEMICAL DEPILATORIES: These products contain alkaline agents that cause hair to detach easily at the skin surface. They can be used on and under the arms, and on the legs and chest. However, they should not be used on the face unless the label says it is safe to do so. Timing instructions should be followed carefully. If skin irritation results, this type of depilatory should be discontinued in favor of some other method.

ABRASIVES: Devices which remove hair from the skin surface by rubbing are cheap but time-consuming. However, if an abrasive such as pumice is used regularly, the offending hairs will be shorter with each application. A cream or lotion should be applied to the skin after using an abrasive.

WAXING: The technique of applying melted wax to the skin for removal of excess facial hair is best handled by an experienced cosmetician. The process involves pouring hot wax onto the skin and allowing it to cool. The hairs become embedded in the wax, and are plucked out from below the skin surface when the wax is stripped off. Since this method is painful and often causes irritation, it is not very popular, although the results are comparatively long-lasting.

PLUCKING: The use of tweezers for removing scattered hairs from the eyebrows, face, and chest is slightly painful but otherwise harmless. It is not a practical method for getting rid of dense hair growth, however, since it takes too much time.

Permanent Hair Removal by Electrolysis

The only permanent and safe method of removing unwanted hair is by *electrolysis*. This technique destroys each individual hair root by transmitting electric current through fine wire needles into the opening of the hair follicle. The hair thus loosened is then plucked out with a tweezer. The older type of electrolysis machine uses galvanic current. The newer type, sometimes called an electrocoagulation machine, uses modified high frequency current. In either case, the efficiency and safety of the technique depends less on the machine than on the care and skill of the operator.

Since the process of treating each hair root is expensive, time-consuming, and uncomfortable, it is not recommended for areas of dense hair growth such as the arms or legs. Before undertaking electrolysis either at a beauty salon or at home, it would be wise to consult a dermatologist about individual skin reaction.

Nails

Fingernails and toenails are an extension of the epidermis or outer layer of the skin. They are made of elastic tissue formed from keratin, the substance that gives hair its strength and flexibility.

Some of the problems associated with fingernails are the result of too much manicuring. White spots, for example, are often caused by too much pressure at the base of the nail when trying to expose the "moon"

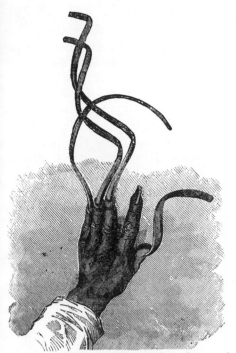

An old engraving portrays the long fingernails supposedly in vogue among the upper classes in ancient China.

—the white portion which contains tissue not yet as tough as the rest of the nail.

To ensure the health of toenails, feet should be bathed once a day and the nails cleaned with a brush dipped in soapy water. Shoes should fit properly so that the toenails are not subjected to pressure and distortion. In order to avoid ingrown toenails, trimming should be done straight across rather than by rounding or tapering the corners.

SPLITTING: Infection or injury of the tissue at the base of a fingernail may cause its surface to be rigid or split. Inflammation of the finger joints connected with arthritis will also cause nail deformity. For ordinary problems of splitting and peeling, the nails should be kept short enough so that they don't catch and tear easily. For practical purposes, the top of the nail should not be visible when the palm is held about six inches from the eye. As the nails grow stronger, they can be grown longer without splitting.

BRITTLENESS: This condition seems to be caused by external factors such as the chemicals in polish removers, soaps, and detergents. It is also a natural consequence of aging. Commercial nail-hardening preparations that contain formaldehyde are not recommended, since they are known to cause discoloration, loosening, or even loss of nails in some cases.

Nail damage can be reduced by wearing rubber gloves while doing household chores. Hand cream massaged into the skin around the nails will counteract dryness and lessen the possibility of hangnails. Although nail polish provides a shield against damage, it should not be worn all the time, particularly if the nail is polished right down to the base, since this prevents live tissue from "breathing."

DISORDERS OF THE SKIN

The skin is subject to a large number of disorders, most of which are not serious even though they may be temporarily uncomfortable. A disorder may be caused by one or another type of allergy; by excessive heat or cold; or by infection from fungi, bacteria, viruses, or parasites. There are also many skin ailments that are caused or aggravated by emotional disturbances.

The symptoms and treatment of the more common disorders are discussed in the following pages. Any persistent change in skin condition should be brought to the attention of a doctor.

Allergies and Itching

Itching and inflammation of the skin may be caused by an allergic reaction, by exposure to poisonous plants, or by a generalized infection.

Dermatitis

Dermatitis is the term used for an inflammation of the skin. The term for allergic reactions of the skin resulting from surface contact with outside agents is *contact dermatitis*. This condition is characterized by a rash and may be brought on by sensitivity to cosmetics, plants, cleaning materials, metal, wool, and so on. Other forms of dermatitis can be caused by excesses of heat or cold, by friction, or by sensitivity to various medicines. Dermatitis is usually accompanied by itching at the site of the rash.

Poison Ivy

This common plant, unknown in Europe, but widespread every-where in the United States except in California and Nevada, produces an allergic reaction on the skin accompanied by a painful rash and blisters. Some people are so sensitive to it that they are affected by contact not only with the plant itself, but with animal fur or clothing that might have picked up the sap weeks before.

A mild attack of poison ivy produces a rash and small watery blisters that get progressively larger. The affected area of the skin becomes crusty and dry, and after a few weeks, all symptoms vanish. If the exposed area is thoroughly washed with laundry soap immediately after contact, the poison may not penetrate the skin.

If the symptoms do develop, they can be relieved with Burow's solution—one part solution to fifteen parts of cool water—or with the application of calomine lotion. If the symptoms are severe, and espe-

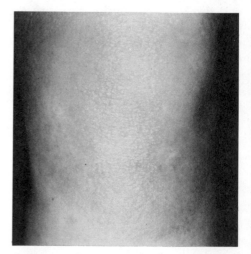

A close-up of contact dermatitis of the knee, an allergic skin reaction caused by surface contact with a substance such as wool.

cially if the area around the eyes is involved, a doctor should be consulted. He may prescribe an application or an injection of cortisone.

The best way to avoid the unpleasantness of a poison ivy attack is to learn to recognize the plant and stay away from it. Children especially should be warned against putting the leaves and berries in their mouths.

Poison oak and poison sumac produce somewhat the same symptoms and should also be avoided.

Under no circumstances should these plants be burned in order to eliminate them, since the inhaling of the contaminated smoke even from a distance can cause a serious case of poisoning. The application

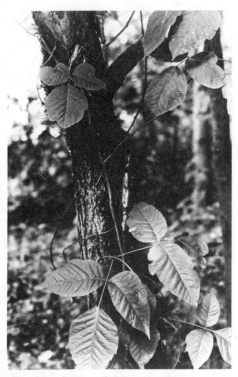

The glossy leaves of the poison ivy plant are arranged in clusters of three, and often have irregularly-shaped notches.

of special sprays, if the instructions are followed carefully, will get rid of the plants without affecting people or the neighborhood greenery.

Hives

These are large, irregularly shaped swellings on the skin that burn and itch. The cause is unknown, but allergic reactions to certain foods and medicine or to insect bites have been suggested as possible causes. The swellings of hives usually disappear within a day or so, but they can be very uncomfortable while they last. The itching and burning can often be relieved by applying cold water and a calomine solution. However, some people are sensitive to cold and develop wheals when subjected to intense cold. Commercial preparations containing surface anesthetics are seldom effective and may cause allergic reactions.

If the outbreak of hives can be traced to a specific food such as shellfish or strawberries, the food should be eliminated from the diet. If a medicine such as penicillin or a sulfa drug is the cause, the doctor should be told about the reaction.

Eczema

This condition is an allergic reaction that produces itching, swelling, blistering, oozing, and scaling of the skin. It is more common among children than among adults and may sometimes cover the entire body, although the rash is usually limited to the face, neck, and the folds of the knees and elbows. Unlike contact dermatitis, it is likely to be caused by an allergy to a food or a pollen or dust. Advertised cures for eczema cannot control the cause and sometimes make the condition worse. A doctor should be consulted if the symptoms are severe, particularly if the patient is an infant or very young child.

Itching

The technical name for the localized or general sensation on the skin which can be relieved by scratching is *pruritus*. Itching may be caused by many skin disorders, by infections, by serious diseases such as nephritis or leukemia, by medicines, or by psychological factors such as tension. A doctor should always be consulted to find the cause of persistent itching, since it may be the symptom of a basic disorder. Repeated scratching may provide some relief, but it can also lead to infection.

Anal Pruritus

If itching in the anal area is so severe that only painful scratching will relieve it, the condition is probably *anal pruritus*. It is often accompanied by excessive rectal mucus that keeps the skin irritated and moist. This disorder is most commonly associated with hemorrhoids, but many other conditions, such as reactions to drugs, can cause it. Anxiety or tension can also contribute to it. Sitz baths with warm water are usually recommended. Every effort should be made to reduce scratching and to keep the anal skin clean and dry. Cortisone cream may be prescribed in persistent cases.

Skin Irritations and Weather

Extremes of weather produce local inflammations and other skin problems for many people.

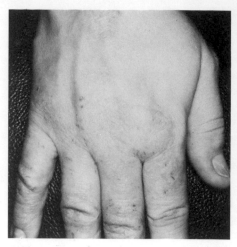

Unlike contact dermatitis, eczema (or *atopic dermatitis*) is caused by an allergic reaction to a food or an airborne substance such as pollen.

Chapping

In cold weather, the sebaceous glands slow down the secretions that lubricate the skin, causing it to become dry. When dry skin is exposed to wintry weather, it becomes irritated and is likely to crack, particularly around the lips. Chapped skin is especially sensitive to harsh soaps. During such periods of exposure, the skin can be protected with a mild cream or lotion. A lubricating ointment should be used on the lips to prevent them from cracking. Children who lick their lips constantly no matter what the weather can benefit from this extra protection. Chapped hands caused by daily use of strong soaps and detergents can be helped by the use of a lubricating cream and rubber gloves during housework.

Frostbite

Exposure to extreme cold for a prolonged period may cause freezing of the nose, fingers, toes, or ears, thus cutting off the circulation to the affected areas. Frostbitten areas are of a paler color than normal and are numb. They should not be rubbed with snow or exposed to intense heat. Areas should be thawed gradually, and a doctor should be consulted for aftercare in extreme cases.

Chilblain

A localized inflammation of the skin, called *chilblain,* is common among people who are particularly sensitive to cold because of poor circulation. Chilblains may occur in the ears, hands, feet, and face, causing itching, swelling, and discoloration of the skin. Anyone prone to chilblain should dress protectively during the cold weather and use an electric pad or blanket at night. Affected parts should not be rubbed or massaged, nor should ice or extreme heat be applied directly, since these measures may cause additional damage. Persistent or extreme attacks of chilblain should be discussed with a doctor.

Chafing

This condition is an inflammation of two opposing skin surfaces caused by the warmth, moisture, and friction of their rubbing together. Diabetics, overweight people, and those who perspire heavily are particularly prone to chafing. Chafing is accompanied by itching and burning, and sometimes infection can set in if the superficial skin is broken. Parts of the body subject to chafing are the inner surfaces of the thighs, the anal region, the area under the breasts, and the inner surfaces between fingers and toes.

To reduce the possibility of chafing, cool clothing should be worn and strenuous exercise avoided during hot weather. Vaseline or a Vitamin A and D ointment may be applied to reduce friction. In general, the treatment is the same as that for diaper rash in infants. If the condition becomes acute, a doctor can prescribe more effective remedies.

Prickly Heat

This skin rash is usually accompanied by itching and burning. It is caused by an obstruction of the sweat ducts so that perspiration does not reach the surface of the skin, but backs up and causes pimples the size of a pinhead. If the obstruction is superficial, the pimples are white; if it is deeper, they are red. The condition can be brought on by other minor skin irritations, by continued exposure to moist heat such as a compress, or by exercise in humid weather. Infants and people who are overweight are especially prone to prickly heat.

The discomfort can be eased by wearing lightweight, loose-fitting clothing, especially at night, and keeping room temperature low. Alcoholic beverages, which tend to dehydrate the body, should be avoided. Tepid baths and the application of cornstarch to the affected skin areas will usually relieve itching. If the rash remains for several days, a doctor should be consulted to make sure it does not arise from some other cause.

Calluses and Corns

As a result of continued friction or pressure in a particular area, the skin forms a tough, hard, self-protecting layer known as a *callus.* Calluses are common on the soles of the feet, the palms of the hands, and, among guitarists and string players, on the tips of the fingers. A heavy callus which presses against a bone in the foot because of poorly fitted shoes can be very painful. The hard surface can be reduced somewhat by the use of pumice, or by gently paring it with a razor blade that has been washed in alcohol.

Corns are a form of callus that appear on or between the toes. They usually have a hard inner core that causes pain when pressed against underlying tissue by badly fitted shoes. A hard corn that appears on the surface of the little toe can be removed by soaking for about ten minutes and applying a few drops of ten percent salicylic acid in collodion. The surface should be covered with a corn pad to reduce pressure, and the corn lifted off when it is loose enough to be released from the skin. Anyone suffering from a circulatory disease and particularly from diabetes should avoid home treatment of foot disturbances. Those with a tendency to callus and corn formations should be especially careful about the proper fit of shoes and hose. A *chiropodist* or *podiatrist* is a trained specialist in foot care who can be visited on a regular basis to provide greater foot comfort.

Fungus Infections

Fungi are plantlike parasitic growths found in the air, in water, and in the soil. They comprise a large family that includes mushrooms, and are responsible for mildew and mold. Only a small number cause disease.

Ringworm

This condition is not caused by a worm, but by a group of fungi that live on the body's dead skin cells in those areas that are warm and damp because of accumulated perspiration. One form of ringworm attacks the scalp, arms, and legs, especially of children, and is often spread by similarly affected pets. It appears as reddish patches that scale and blister and frequently feel sore and itchy. Ringworm is highly contagious and can be passed from person to person by contaminated objects such as combs and towels. It should therefore be treated promptly by a doctor. Ringworm can best be prevented by strict attention to personal cleanliness.

Athlete's Foot

Another form of ringworm, *athlete's foot,* usually attacks the skin between the toes and under the toenails. If not treated promptly, it can cause an itching rash on other parts of the body. Athlete's foot causes the skin to itch, blister, and crack, and as a result, leaves it vulnerable to more serious infection from other organisms. The disorder

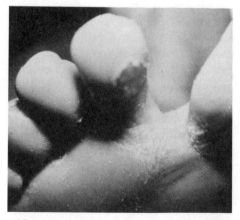

Athlete's foot, a form of ringworm, is marked by a cracking of the skin between the toes or under the toenails. Itching and soreness are usual symptoms.

can be treated at home by gently removing the damaged skin, and, after soaking the feet, thoroughly drying and dusting between the toes with a medicated foot powder. Some of the powder should be sprinkled into shoes. If the condition continues, a fungicidal ointment can be applied in the morning and at night. Persistent cases require the attention of a doctor.

Scabies

An insectlike parasite causes the skin irritation called *scabies*, otherwise known as "the itch." The female itch mite burrows a hole in the skin, usually in the groin or between the fingers or toes, and stays hidden long enough to build a tunnel in which to deposit her eggs. The newly hatched mites then work their way to the skin surface and begin the cycle all over again. There is little discomfort in the early period of infestation, but in about a week, a rash appears accompanied by extreme itching, which is usually most severe at night. Constant scratching during sleep can lead to skin lesions that invite bacterial infection.

Scabies is very contagious and can spread rapidly through a family or through a community, such as a summer camp or army barracks. It can also be communicated by venereal contact.

Treatment by a doctor involves the identification of the characteristic tunnels from which sample mites can be removed for examination. Hot baths and thorough scrubbing will expose the burrows, and medical applications as directed by the doctor usually clear up the condition in about a week.

Bacterial Infections

The skin is susceptible to infection from a variety of bacteria. Poor diet and careless hygiene can lower the body's resistance to these infectious agents.

Boils

These abscesses of the skin are caused by bacterial infection of a hair follicle or a sebaceous gland. The pus that accumulates in a boil is the result of the encounter between the bacteria and the white blood cells that fight them. Sometimes a boil subsides by itself and disappears. Sometimes the pressure of pus against the skin surface may bring the boil to a head; it will then break, drain, and heal if washed with an antiseptic and covered with a sterile pad. Warm water compresses can be applied for ten minutes every hour to relieve the pain and to encourage the boil to break and drain. A fresh dry pad should be applied after each period of soaking.

Anyone with a serious or chronic illness who develops a boil should consult a doctor. Since the bacteria can enter the bloodstream and cause a general infection with fever, a doctor should also be consulted for a boil on the nose, scalp, upper lip, or in the ear, groin, or armpit.

Carbuncles

This infection is a group of connected boils and is likely to be more painful and less responsive to home treatment. Carbuncles may occur as the result of poor skin care. They tend to occur in the back of the neck where the skin is thick, and the abscess tends to burrow into deeper tissues. A doctor usually lances and drains a deep-seated carbuncle, or he may prescribe an antibiotic remedy.

Impetigo

This skin infection is caused by staphylococcal or streptococcal bacteria, and is characterized by blisters that break and form yellow crusted areas. It is spread from one person to another and from one part of the body to another by the discharge from the sores. Impetigo occurs most frequently on the scalp, face, and arms and legs. The infection often is picked up in barber shops, swimming pools, or from body contact with other infected people or household pets.

Special care must be taken, especially with children, to control the spread of the infection by keeping the fingers away from infected parts. Bed linens should be changed daily, and disposable paper towels as well as paper plates and cups should be used during treatment. A doctor should be consulted for proper medication and procedures to deal with the infection.

Barber's Itch

Sycosis, commonly called *barber's itch,* is a bacterial infection of the hair follicles of the beard, accompanied by inflammation, itching, and the formation of pus-filled pimples. People with stiff, curly hair are prone to this type of chronic infection, since their hair is more likely to curve back and reenter the skin. The infection should be treated promptly to prevent scarring and the destruction of the hair root. In some cases, doctors recommend antibiotics. If these are not effective, it may be nec-

essary to drain the abscesses and remove the hairs from the inflamed follicles. During treatment, it is best to avoid shaving, if possible. If one must shave, the sterilization of all shaving equipment and the use of a brushless shaving cream are recommended.

Erysipelas

An acute streptococcal infection of the skin, *erysipelas* can be fatal, particularly to the very young or very old, if not treated promptly. One of its symptoms is the bright redness of the affected areas of the skin. These red patches enlarge and spread, making the skin tender and painful. Blisters may appear nearby. The patient usually has a headache, fever, chills, and nausea. Erysipelas responds well to promptly administered antibiotics, particularly penicillin. The patient is usually advised to drink large amounts of fluid and to eat a nourishing, easily digested diet.

Viral Infections

The most common skin conditions caused by viruses are cold sores, shingles, and warts, discussed below.

Cold Sores

Also called fever blisters, *cold sores* are technically known as *herpes simplex.* They are small blisters that appear most frequently in the corners of the mouth, and sometimes around the eyes and on the genitals. The presumed cause is a virus that lies dormant in the skin until it is activated by infection or by excessive exposure to sun or wind. There is no specific cure for cold sores, but the irritation can be eased by applying drying or cooling agents such as camphor ice or cold water compresses. Recurrent cold sores, especially in infants, should be called to a doctor's attention.

Recent studies have shown that a variety of the herpes simplex virus called HSV-2 (for Herpes simplex virus-Type 2) can be a serious danger to the fetus of a pregnant woman. For a discussion of this condition, see Ch. 21, p. 997. The variety that causes cold sores is called Type 1.

Shingles

The virus infection of a sensory nerve, accompanied by small, painful blisters that appear on the skin along the path of the nerve—usually on one side of the chest or abdomen—is called *shingles.* The medical name for the disorder, which is caused by the chicken pox virus, is *herpes zoster,* Latin for "girdle of blisters." When a cranial nerve is involved, the blisters appear on the face near the eye. The preliminary symptom is neuritis with severe pain and, sometimes, fever. The blisters may take from two to four weeks to dry up and disappear. Although there is no specific cure, the pain can be alleviated by aspirin. In severe cases, or if the area near the eye is involved, a doctor should be seen.

Warts

These growths are caused by a virus infection of the epidermis. They never become cancerous, but can be painful when found on the soles of the feet. In this location, they are known as *plantar warts,* and they cause discomfort because

constant pressure makes them grow inward. Plantar warts are most likely to be picked up by children because they are barefooted so much of the time, and by adults when their feet are moist and they are walking around in showers, near swimming pools, and in locker rooms. Warts can be spread by scratching, by shaving, and by brushing the hair. They are often transmitted from one member of the family to another. Since warts can spread to painful areas, such as the area around or under the fingernails, and since they may become disfiguring, it is best to consult a doctor whenever they appear.

In many ways, warts behave rather mysteriously. About half of them go away without any treatment at all. Sometimes, when warts on one part of the body are being treated, those in another area will disappear. The folklore about "witching" and "charming" warts away has its foundation in fact, since apparently having faith in the cure, no matter how ridiculous it sounds, sometimes brings success. This form of suggestion therapy is especially successful with children.

There are several more conventional ways of treating warts. Depending on their size and the area involved, electric current, dry ice, or various chemicals may be employed. A doctor should be consulted promptly when warts develop in the area of the beard or on the scalp, since they spread quickly in these parts of the body and thus become more difficult to eliminate.

Sebaceous Cysts

When a sebaceous gland duct is blocked, the oil which the gland secretes cannot get to the surface of the skin. Instead, it accumulates into a hard, round, movable mass contained in a sac. This mass is known as a *sebaceous cyst.* Such cysts may appear on the face, back, ears, or in the genital area. A sebaceous cyst that forms on the scalp is called a *wen,* and may become as large as a billiard ball. The skin in this area will become bald, because the cyst interferes with the blood supply to the hair roots.

Some sebaceous cysts just disappear without treatment. However, those that do not are a likely focus for secondary infection by bacteria, and they may become abscessed and inflamed. It is therefore advisable to have cysts examined by a doctor for possible removal. If such a cyst is superficial, it can be punctured and drained. One that is deeper is usually removed by simple surgical procedure in the doctor's office.

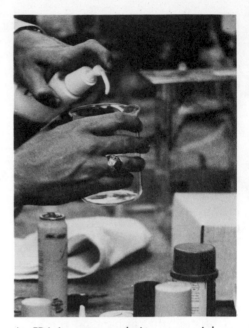

An FDA inspector analyzing commercial cosmetics. The use of such products should be discontinued if they cause irritation.

Acne

About 80 percent of all teen-agers suffer from the skin disturbance called *acne.* It is also fairly common among women in their twenties. Acne is a condition in which the skin of the face, and often of the neck, shoulders, chest, and back, is covered to a greater or lesser extent with pimples, blackheads, whiteheads, and boils.

The typical onset of acne in adolescence is related to the increased activity of the glands, including the sebaceous glands. Most of the oil that they secrete gets to the surface of the skin through ducts that lead into the pores. When the surface pores are clogged with sebaceous gland secretions and keratin, or when so much extra oil is being secreted that it backs up into the ducts, the result is the formation of the skin blemishes characteristic of acne. Dirt or make-up does not cause acne.

The blackheads are dark not because they are dirty, but because the fatty material in the clogged pore is oxidized and discolored by the air that reaches it. When this substance is infected by bacteria, it turns into a pimple. Under no circumstances should such pimples be picked at or squeezed, since the pressure can rupture the surrounding membrane and spread the infection further.

Although a mild case of acne usually clears up by itself, it is often helpful to get the advice of a doctor so that it does not get any worse.

CLEANLINESS: Although surface dirt does not cause acne, it can contribute to its spread. Therefore, the affected areas should be cleansed with a medicated soap and hot water twice a day. Hair should be shampooed frequently and brushed away from the face. Boys who are shaving should soften the beard with soap and hot water. The blade should be sharp and should skim the skin as lightly as possible to avoid nicking pimples.

CREAMS AND COSMETICS: Nonprescription medicated creams and lotions may be effective in reducing some blemishes, but if used too often, they make the skin dry. They should be applied according to the manufacturer's instructions and should be discontinued if they cause additional irritation. If makeup is used, it should have a non-oily base and be completely removed before going to bed.

FORBIDDEN FOODS: Although acne is not caused by any particular food, it can be made worse by a diet overloaded with candy, rich pastries, and fats. Chocolate and cola drinks must be eliminated entirely in some cases.

PROFESSIONAL TREATMENT: A serious case of acne, or even a mild one that is causing serious emotional problems, should receive the attention of a doctor. He may prescribe antibiotics, usually considered the most effective treatment, or recommend sunlamp treatments. He can also be helpful in dealing with the psychological aspects of acne that are so disturbing to teen-agers.

Psoriasis

Psoriasis is a noncontagious chronic condition in which the skin on various parts of the body is marked by bright red patches covered with silvery scales. The areas most often affected are the knees, elbows, scalp, and trunk, and less frequently, the areas under the arms and around the genitals.

The specific cause of psoriasis has not yet been discovered, but it is thought to be an inherited abnormality in which the formation of new

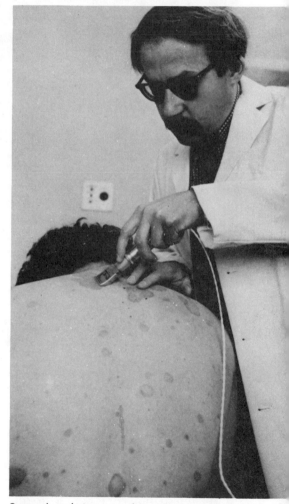

Research techniques involving the removal of tissue from a psoriatic back for study hold out hope for a cure.

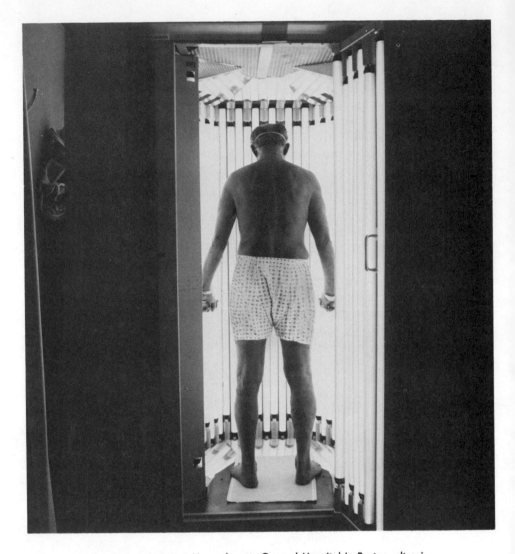

In an experiment at Massachusetts General Hospital in Boston, ultraviolet light is used to activate drugs taken orally by a psoriasis patient.

skin cells is too rapid and disorderly. In its mild form, psoriasis responds well to a variety of long-term treatments. When it is acute, the entire skin surface may be painfully red, and large sections of it may scale off. In such cases, prompt hospitalization and intensive care are recommended.

CONDITIONS THAT CAN BRING ON AN OUTBREAK: It has been observed that the onset or aggravation of psoriasis can be triggered by some of the following factors:

• Bruises, burns, scratches, and overexposure to the sun

• Sudden drops in temperature—a mild, stable climate is most beneficial

• Sudden illness from another source, or unusual physical or emotional stress

• Infections of the upper respiratory tract, especially bacterial throat infections and the medicines used to cure them.

TREATMENT: Although there is no specific cure for psoriasis, these are some of the recommended treatments:

• Controlled exposure to sunlight or an ultraviolet lamp

• Creams or lotions of crude coal tar or tar distillates, used alone or in combination with ultraviolet light

• Psoralen and ultraviolet light (PUVA), a combined systemic-external therapy in which a psoralen drug is taken orally before exposure to ultraviolet light

• Systemic drugs, such as methotrexate, which can be taken orally

• Steroid hormone medications applied to the skin surface under dressings.

Pigment Disorders and Birthmarks

The mechanism which controls skin coloration is described above under *Skin Color.* Abnormalities in the creation and distribution of melanin result in the following disorders, some of which are negligible.

Freckles

These are small spots of brown pigment which frequently occur when fair-skinned people are exposed to the sun or to ultraviolet light. For those whose skin gets red rather than tan during such exposure, freckles are a protective device. In most cases, they recede in cold weather. A heavy freckle formation that is permanent can be covered somewhat by cosmetic preparations. No attempt should be made to remove freckles with commercial creams or solutions unless supervised by a doctor.

Liver Spots

Flat, smooth, irregularly placed markings on the skin, called *liver spots,* often appear among older people, and result from an increase in pigmentation. They have nothing to do with the liver and are completely harmless. Brownish markings of similar appearance sometimes show up during pregnancy or as a result of irritation or infection. They usually disappear when the underlying cause is eliminated.

Liver spots are permanent, and the principal cause is not aging, but the accumulated years of exposure to sun and wind. They can be disguised and treated in the same way as freckles. A liver spot that becomes hard and thick should be called to the doctor's attention.

Moles

Clusters of melanin cells, called *moles,* may appear singly or in groups at any place on the body. They range in color from light tan to dark brown; they may be raised and hairy or flat and smooth. Many moles are present at birth, and most make their appearance before the age of twenty. They rarely turn into malignancies, and require medical attention only if they become painful, if they itch, or if they suddenly change in size, shape, or color.

There are several ways of removing moles if they are annoying or particularly unattractive. They can be destroyed by the application of an electric needle, by cauterizing, and by surgery. A mole that has been removed is not likely to reappear. The hairs sometimes found in moles can be clipped close to the surface of the skin, or they can be permanently removed. Hair removal often causes the mole to get smaller.

Vitiligo

The condition called *vitiligo* stems from a loss of pigment in sharply defined areas of the skin. There is no known cause for this abnormality of melanin distribution. It may affect any part of the body and may appear any time up to middle age. It is particularly conspicuous when it occurs among blacks, or when a lighter skinned person becomes tanned except around the paler patches. There is no cure for vitiligo, but cosmetic treatment with pastes and lotions can diminish the contrast between affected areas and the rest of the skin.

Birthmarks

About one-third of all infants are born with the type of birthmark called a *hemangioma,* also known as a vascular birthmark. These are caused by a clustering of small blood vessels near the surface of the skin. The mark, which is flat, irregularly shaped, and either pink, red, or purplish, is usually referred to as "port wine stain." There is no known way to remove it, but with cosmetic covering creams, it can usually be successfully masked.

The type of hemangioma which is raised and bright red—called a strawberry mark—spontaneously disappears with no treatment in most cases during early childhood. If a strawberry mark begins to grow rather than fade, or if it begins to ulcerate, a physician should be promptly consulted.

See under *Cancer,* p. 1273, for a discussion of skin cancer; see under *Puberty and Growth,* p. 542, for a discussion of adolescent skin problems, see under *Aches, Pains, Nuisances, Worries,* p. 839, for further discussion of minor skin problems.

CHAPTER 16

The Teeth and Gums

Although a human baby is born without teeth, a complete set of 20 *deciduous,* or baby teeth (also called *primary teeth*) already has formed within the gums of the offspring while it still is within the mother's womb. The buds of the permanent or secondary teeth are developing even before the first baby tooth appears at around the age of six months. The baby teeth obviously are formed from foods eaten by the mother. Generally, if the mother follows a good diet during pregnancy, no special food items are required to insure an adequate set of deciduous teeth in the baby.

It takes about two years for the full set of deciduous teeth to appear in the baby's mouth. The first, usually a central incisor at the front of the lower jaw, may erupt any time between the ages of three and nine months. The last probably will be a second molar at the back of the upper jaw. Like walking, talking, and other characteristics of infants, there is no set timetable for the eruption of baby teeth. One child may get his first tooth at three months while another must wait until nine months, but both would be considered within a normal range of tooth development.

The permanent teeth are never far behind the deciduous set. The first permanent tooth usually appears around the age of six years, about four years after the last of the baby teeth has erupted. But the last of the permanent molars, the third molars or *wisdom teeth,* may not break through the gum line until the offspring is an adult.

Types of Teeth

The permanent teeth number thirty-two. In advancing from deciduous to permanent teeth, the human gains six teeth in the lower

805

jaw, or *mandible,* and six in the upper jaw, or *maxilla,* of the mouth. The primary set of teeth includes the following:

UPPER JAW	LOWER JAW
2 central incisors	2 central incisors
2 lateral incisors	2 lateral incisors
2 cuspids	2 cuspids
2 first molars	2 first molars
2 second molars	2 second molars

The permanent set of teeth has an equivalent combination of incisors, cuspids, and first and second molars. But it also includes:

2 first bicuspids	2 first bicuspids
2 second bicuspids	2 second bicuspids
2 third molars	2 third molars

An *incisor* is designed to cut off particles of food, which is then pushed by muscles of the tongue and cheeks to teeth farther back in the mouth for grinding. The front teeth, one on each side, upper and lower, are central incisors. Next to each central incisor is a lateral incisor.

A *cuspid* is so named because it has a spear-shaped crown, or *cusp.* It is designed for tearing as well as cutting. Cuspids sometimes are called *canine teeth* or *eye teeth; canine teeth* owe their name to the use of these teeth by carnivorous animals such as dogs for tearing pieces of meat. There are four cuspids in the mouth, one on the outer side of each lateral incisor in the upper and lower jaws.

Bicuspids sometimes are identified as *premolars.* The term bicuspid suggests two cusps, but a bicuspid may in fact have three cusps. The function of the bicuspids is to crush food passed back from the incisors and cuspids. The permanent set of teeth includes a total of eight bicuspids.

The *molars,* which also number eight and are the last teeth at the back of the mouth, are the largest and strongest teeth, with the job of grinding food. The third molars, or wisdom teeth, are smaller, weaker, and less functional than the first and second molars.

Structure of the Tooth

The variety of shapes of teeth make them specialized for the various functions in preparing food for digestion—biting, chewing, and grinding. All varieties, however, have the same basic structure.

Enamel

The outer covering of the part of the tooth that is exposed above the gum line is *enamel,* the hardest substance in the human body. Enamel is about 97 percent mineral and is as tough as some gemstones. It varies in thickness, with the greatest thickness on the surfaces that are likely to get the most wear and tear.

Enamel begins to form on the first tooth buds of an embryo at the age of about 15 weeks, depending upon substances in the food eaten by the mother for proper development. Once the tooth has formed and erupted through the gum line, there is nothing further that can be done by natural means to improve the condition of the enamel. The enamel

THE STRUCTURE OF A TOOTH

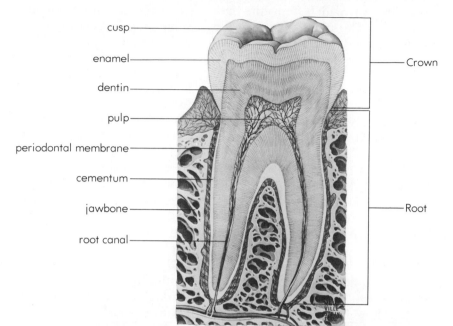

cusp
enamel
dentin
pulp
periodontal membrane
cementum
jawbone
root canal

Crown

Root

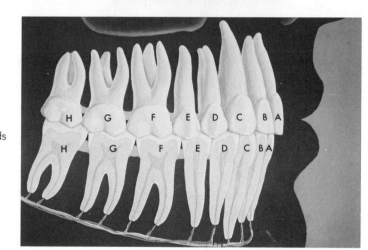

THE ADULT
TEETH

A. central incisors
B. lateral incisors
C. cuspids
D. first bicuspids
E. second bicuspids
F. first molars
G. second molars
H. third molars
X. artery, vein,
   and nerve

has no blood supply, and any changes in the tooth surface will be the result of wearing, decay, or injury.

While the health and diet of the mother can affect the development of tooth enamel in the deciduous teeth, certain health factors in the early life of a child can result in defective enamel formation of teeth that have not yet erupted. Some infectious or metabolic disorders, for example, may result in enamel pitting.

Dentin

Beneath the enamel surface of a tooth is a layer of hard material—

though not as hard as enamel—called *dentin,* which forms the bulk of a tooth. The dentin forms at the same time that enamel is laid down on the surface of a developing tooth, and the portion beneath the crown of the tooth probably is completed at the same time as the enamel. However, the dentin, which is composed of calcified material, is not as dense as the enamel; it is formed as myriad tubules that extend downward into the pulp at the center of the tooth. There is some evidence that dentin formation may continue slowly during the life of the tooth.

Cementum

The *cementum* is a bonelike substance that covers the root of the tooth. Though harder than regular bone, it is softer than dentin. It contains attachments for fibers of a periodontal ligament that holds the tooth in its socket. The periodontal ligament serves as a kind of hammock of fibers that surround and support the tooth at the cementum surface, radiating outward to the jawbone. This arrangement allows the tooth to move a little while still attached to the jaw. For example, when the teeth of the upper and lower jaws are brought together in chewing, the periodontal ligament allows the teeth to sink into their sockets. When the teeth of the two jaws are separated, the hammocklike ligament permits the teeth to float outward again.

Pulp

The cavity within the dentin contains the *pulp.* There is a wide pulp chamber under the crown of the tooth and a pulp canal that extends from the chamber down through the root or roots. Some teeth, such as the molars, may contain as many as three roots, and each of the roots contains a pulp canal.

The pulp of a tooth contains the blood vessels supplying the tooth and the lymphatic system. Although the blood supply arrangement is not the same for every tooth, a typical pattern includes a dental artery entering through each passageway, or *foramen,* leading into the root of a tooth. The artery branches into numerous capillaries within the root canal. A similar system of veins drains the blood from the tooth through each foramen. A lymphatic network and nerve system also enter the tooth through a foramen and spreads through the pulp, as branches from a central distribution link within the jawbone. The nerve fibers have free endings in the tooth, making them sensitive to pain stimuli.

Supporting Structures

The soft, pink gum tissue that surrounds the tooth is called the *gingiva,* and the bone of the jaw that forms the tooth socket is known as *alveolar bone.* The gingiva, alveolar bone, and periodontal ligaments sometimes are grouped into a structural category identified as the *periodontium.* Thus, when a dentist speaks of periodontal disease he is referring to a disorder of these supporting tissues of the teeth. The ailment known as *gingivitis* is an inflammation of the gingiva or gum tissue around the teeth.

Care of the Teeth and Gums

Years ago, loss of teeth really was unavoidable. Today, thanks to modern practices of preventive dentistry,

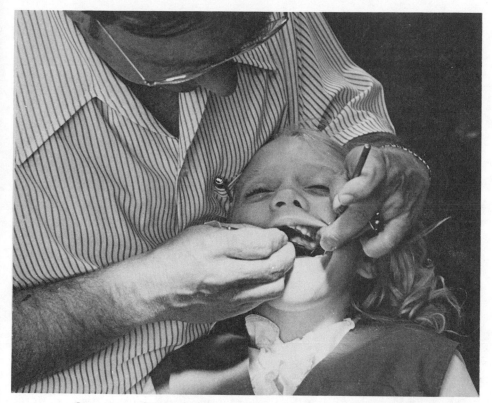

Preventive medicine is the best medicine involving teeth. Dentists recommend regular checkups for everyone, but especially for children.

it is possible for nearly everyone to enjoy the benefits of natural teeth for a lifetime. But natural teeth can be preserved only by daily oral-hygiene habits and regular dental checkups.

The Dental Examination

During the teen years, careful supervision by the dentist and cooperation from the teen-ager are especially necessary. The poor eating habits of many youngsters are reflected in high cavity rates, which may be greater during adolescence than in later life. Neglect of proper dental care also occurs in the middle years when an often-used excuse is that eventual loss of teeth is inevitable. After the permanent teeth are established, the dentist should be visited every six months, or at whatever intervals he recommends for an individual patient who may need more or less care than the typical patient.

The dentist, like the family doctor, usually maintains a general health history of each patient, in addition to a dental health history. He examines each tooth, the gums and other oral tissues, and the *occlusion*, or bite. A complete set of X-ray pictures may be taken on the first visit and again at intervals of perhaps five to seven years. During routine visits, the dentist may take only a couple of X-ray pictures of teeth on either side of the mouth; a complete set of X rays may result in a file of 18 or 20 pictures covering every tooth in the mouth.

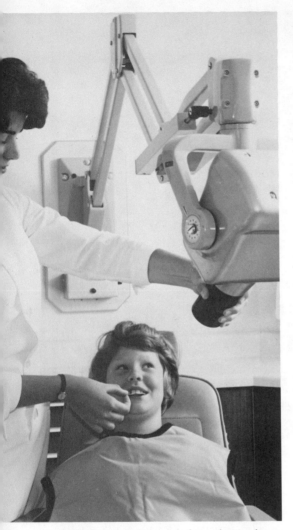

A complete set of X rays helps a dentist determine whether a child's teeth are growing in correct alignment.

X rays constitute a vital part of the dental examination. Without them the dentist cannot examine the surfaces between the teeth or the portion of the tooth beneath the gum, a part that represents about 60 percent of the total length of the tooth. The X rays will reveal the condition of the enamel, dentin, and pulp, as well as any impacted wisdom teeth and the alveolar bone, or tooth sockets. Caps, fillings, abscessed roots, and bone loss due to gum disease also are clearly visible on a set of X rays.

Other diagnositc tests may be made, such as a test of nerve response. Sometimes the dentist will make an impression of the teeth, an accurate and detailed reverse reproduction, in plaster of Paris, plastic impression compound, or other material. Models made from these impressions are used to study the way the teeth meet. Such knowledge is often crucial in deciding the selection of treatment and materials.

After the examination, the dentist will present and explain any proposed treatment. After oral restoration is completed, he will ask the patient to return at regular intervals for a checkup and *prophylaxis,* which includes cleaning and polishing the teeth. Regular checkups and prophylaxis help prevent periodontal diseases affecting the gum tissue and underlying bone. Professional cleaning removes hard deposits that trap bacteria, especially at the gum line, and polishing removes stains and soft deposits.

Dental Care in Middle Age

Although periodontal (gum) disease and cavities—called *dental caries* by dentists—continue to threaten oral health, two other problems may assume prominence for people of middle age: replacing worn-out restorations, or fillings, and replacing missing teeth. No filling material will last forever. The whitish restorations in front teeth eventually wear away. Silver restorations tend to crack and chip with age because they contract and expand slightly when cold or hot food and drinks come in contact with them.

Even gold restorations, the most permanent kind, are subject to decay around the edges, and the decay may spread underneath.

If a needed restoration is not made or a worn-out restoration is not replaced, a deep cavity may result. When the decay reaches the inner layer of the tooth—the dentin—temporary warning twinges of pain may occur. If the tooth still is not restored, the decay will spread into the pulp that fills the inner chamber of the tooth. A toothache can result from inflammation of the pulp, and although the pain may eventually subside, the pulp tissue dies and an abscess can form at the root of the tooth.

Dental Care During Pregnancy

It may be advisable for a pregnant woman to arrange for extra dental checkups. Many changes take place during pregnancy, among them increased hormone production. Some pregnant women develop gingivitis (inflammation of the gums) as an indirect consequence of hormonal changes. A checkup by the dentist during the first three months of pregnancy is needed to assess the oral effects of such changes, and to make sure all dental problems are examined and corrected. Pregnant women should take special care to brush and floss their teeth to minimize these problems.

Dental X rays are important for adults, too, because they permit the dentist to see the state of your fillings, tooth roots, and gums.

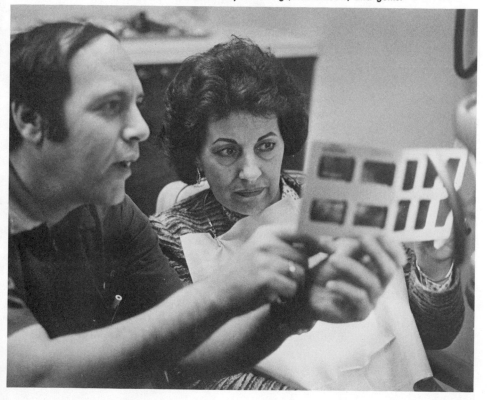

INFECTION: To avoid the problem of toxic substances or poisons circulating in the mother's bloodstream, all sources of infection must be removed. Some of these sources can be in the mouth. An abscessed tooth, for example, may not be severe enough to signal its presence with pain, but because it is directly connected to the bloodstream it can send toxic substances and bacteria through the mother's body with possible harmful effects to the embryo.

It is during pregnancy that tooth buds for both the deciduous and permanent teeth begin to form in the unborn child. If the mother neglects her diet or general health care during this period, the effects may be seen in the teeth of her child.

What You Can Do: Observing Good Oral Hygiene

FLUORIDATION: Among general rules to follow between dental checkups are using fluorides, maintaining a proper diet, and removing debris from the teeth by brushing and by the use of dental floss. Fluorides are particularly important for strengthening the enamel of teeth in persons under the age of 15. Many communities add fluorides to the water supply, but if the substance is not available in the drinking water, the dentist can advise the patient about other ways of adding fluoride to water or other fluids consumed each day. Studies show that children who drink fluoridated water from birth have up to 65 percent fewer cavities than those who do not drink fluoridated water. However, using excessive amounts of fluoride in the drinking water can result in mottled enamel.

DIET: Although a good diet for total health should provide all of the elements needed for dental health, several precautions on sugars and starches should be added. Hard or sticky sweets should be avoided. Such highly refined sweets as soft drinks, candies, cakes, cookies, pies, syrups, jams, jellies, and pastries should be limited, especially between meals. One's intake of starchy foods, such as bread, potatoes, and pastas, should also be controlled. Natural sugars contained in fresh fruits can provide sweet flavors with less risk of contributing to decay if the teeth are brushed regularly after eating such foods. Regular chewing gum may help remove food particles after eating, but it deposits sugar; if you chew gum, use sugarless gum.

Since decay is promoted each time sugars and other refined carbohydrates are eaten, between-meals snacks of sweets should be curtailed in order to lessen the chances of new or additional caries. Snack foods can be raw vegetables, such as carrots or celery, apples, cheese, peanuts, or other items that are not likely to introduce refined carbohydrates into the mouth between meals.

BRUSHING: Brushing the teeth is an essential of personal oral hygiene. Such brushing rids the mouth of most of the food debris that encourages bacterial growth, which is most intense twenty minutes after eating. Therefore, the teeth should be cleaned as soon as possible after a meal.

There is no one kind of toothbrush that is best for every person. Most dentists, however, recommend a soft toothbrush with a straight handle and flat brushing surface that can clean the gums without irritating

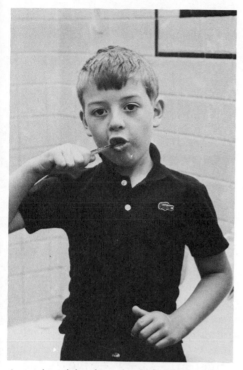

A good tooth-brushing should hit the top, front, and inside of each and every tooth and should also include the area where the gums meet the teeth.

brushed first, before moisture has softened the brush. The cheek and tongue surfaces of the lower teeth are brushed next. Hold the brush parallel to the teeth with the bristle edges angled against and touching the gums. Using short strokes, move the brush back and forth several times before proceeding to the next one or two teeth. Use the same technique on all the inner surfaces of your teeth as well. For the hard-to-brush inner surfaces of the front teeth, hold the handle of the brush out in front of the mouth and apply the tip in an up-and-down motion. For all brushing, a scrubbing motion —but without too much pressure— should be used.

Some people prefer electric toothbrushes, which require less effort to use than ordinary toothbrushes. These are available with two basic motions—up-and-down and back-and-forth. Your dentist may advise which kind best serves an individual needs and proper use of equipment. Some dentists point out that back-and-forth brushing applied with too much pressure can have an abrasive effect on tooth enamel because it works against the grain of the mineral deposits. The American Dental Association also evaluates electric toothbrushes and issues reports on the safety and effectiveness of various types.

REMOVING DEBRIS WITH DENTAL FLOSS: Brushing often does not clean debris from between the teeth. But plaque and food particles that stick between the teeth usually can be removed with dental floss. A generous length of floss, about 18 inches, is needed to do an effective job. The ends can be wrapped several times around the first joint of the middle

them. As for claims about whether toothbrushes should have bristles with square corners or rounded shapes, a dentist may point out that there are both curved and straight surfaces in the mouth so what one design offers in advantages may be offset by equivalent disadvantages. There also are special brushes for reaching surfaces of crooked teeth or cleaning missing-tooth areas of the mouth.

Although several different methods may be used effectively, the following is the technique most often recommended. Brush the biting surfaces, or tops, of the back upper and lower teeth. The lines and grooves on these surfaces make them prone to decay. They should be

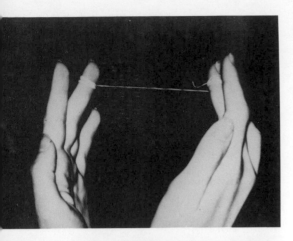

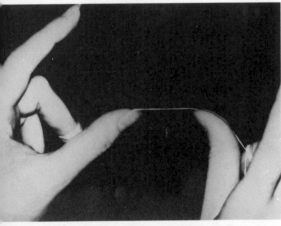

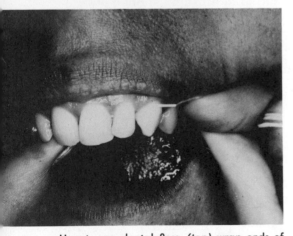

How to use dental floss: *(top)* wrap ends of floss several times around middle fingers; *(middle)* hold center part of floss between thumbs; *(bottom)* insert floss between teeth and work back and forth gently.

finger of each hand. Using the thumbs or index fingers, the floss is inserted between the teeth with a gentle, sawing, back-and-forth motion. Then it is slid gently around part of a tooth in the space at the gum line and gently pulled out; snapping the floss in and out may irritate the gums. After brushing and flossing, the mouth should be rinsed with water. A mouthwash is unnecessary, but it may be used for the good taste it leaves in the mouth.

The dentist may recommend the use of an oral irrigating device as part of dental home care. These units produce a pulsating stream of water that flushes food debris from between teeth. They are particularly useful for patients wearing orthodontic braces or for those who have had recession of the gums, creating larger spaces between the teeth.

The person who wants to see the areas of plaque on his teeth can chew a *disclosing tablet,* available at most pharmacies, which leaves a harmless temporary stain on plaque surfaces. Some dentists recommend the use of disclosing tablets about once a week so that patients can check on the effectiveness of their tooth cleaning techniques.

TOOTH DECAY

In addition to wear, tear, and injury, the major threat to the health of a tooth is bacteria. Bacteria can cause tooth decay, and the human mouth is a tremendous reservoir of bacteria because the mouth is warm, dark, moist, and usually contains tiny particles of food which help nourish the organisms. The bacteria found in the mouth are of two kinds, *aerobic* and *anaerobic*. Aerobic bacteria need oxygen to survive; anaerobic bacteria do not. Anaerobic bacteria can find their way through cracks and crevices into areas of the mouth or teeth where there is little or no oxygen and continue their *cariogenic*, or decay, activity.

Saliva

Saliva offers some protection against the decay germs, for reasons not well understood, but there are crevices and deep pockets around the teeth and gums where saliva does not penetrate. Paradoxically, saliva itself contains millions of different bacterial organisms. Dental scientists have calculated that one ounce of saliva may contain as many as 22 billion bacteria. Even a presumably healthy mouth may contain more than ten varieties of bacteria, plus protozoa and yeast cells. The yeast cells and at least three of the different kinds of bacteria are capable of producing acids that erode the tough enamel surface of a tooth.

Bacterial Acids and Plaque

The acids produced by decay bacteria actually are waste products of the organisms' digestive processes; bacteria, like other living creatures, eventually excrete waste products after a meal. As unpleasant as the thought may be, tooth decay can be the result of feeding a colony of germs in the mouth. Bacterial growth—hence the production of harmful acids—is encouraged by the consumption of too many foods composed of refined sugars. The sugars of candies, cakes, soft drinks, and the like are easier for the bacteria to eat and digest than those of fruits, vegetables, and other less thoroughly processed foods. Even a tiny bit of food remaining in the mouth after a meal may be enough to support many millions of bacteria for 24 hours or more.

An additional contributing factor to tooth decay is *plaque* formation. Plaque is a sticky, transparent substance that forms a film over the surface of the teeth. Plaque forms every day, which is the reason that the teeth must be brushed every day. Plaque frequently begins with deposits of soft food debris along the gum line after a meal; it consists mainly of bacteria and its products. When mixed with mucus, molds, tissue cells from the membranes lining the mouth, and mineral salts, it takes the form of a white, cheesy substance called *materia alba*. If not removed regularly by brushing and the use of dental floss, this substance becomes a thick, sticky mass which has been compared to epoxy cement. Then it becomes a rough-surfaced hard substance with the texture of stone, otherwise known as *dental calculus*, or *tartar*.

Other Causes of Decay

Bacterial acid is not the only way in which the tooth enamel may be damaged to permit the entry of decay bacteria. Certain high acid foods and improper dental care can erode the molecules of enamel. Temperature extremes also can produce cracks and other damage to the enamel; some dental scientists have suggested that repeated exposure to rapid temperature fluctuations of 50°F., as in eating alternately hot and cold foods or beverages, can cause the enamel to develop cracks.

Complications of Tooth Decay

Once decay activity breaks through the hard enamel surface, the bacteria can attack the dentin. Since the dentin is about 30 percent organic material, compared to 5 percent in the enamel layer, the decay process can advance more rapidly there. If the tooth decay is not stopped at the dentin layer, the disease organisms can enter the pulp chamber where they will multiply quickly, producing an acute inflammation and, if unchecked, spread through the blood vessels to other parts of the body. Osteomyelitis, an infection of the membrane covering the skeletal bones, and endocarditis, an extremely dangerous heart ailment, are among diseases in other parts of the body that can begin with untreated tooth decay.

Periodontal disease, described below, is another possible complication of tooth decay.

Treatment of Tooth Decay

The portion of a tooth invaded by decay is called a *cavity;* it may be compared to an ulcer that develops because of disease in soft tissues. In treating the decay process, the dentist tries to prevent further destruction of the tooth tissue. The dentist also tries to restore as much as possible the original shape and function of the diseased tooth. The procedure used depends on many factors, including the surfaces affected (enamel, dentin, etc.) and the tooth face and angle involved as well as whether the cavity is on a smooth area or in a pit or fissure of the tooth surface.

The decayed portions of the tooth are removed with various kinds of carbide burrs and other drill tips as well as with hand instruments. The dentist may also use a caries removal system that reduces or eliminates drilling. In this system two solutions are combined in one liquid and squirted in a pulsating stream onto the decayed area. The stream does not harm gums or healthy teeth; rather, it softens the caries so that it can easily be scraped away. Used, generally, in conjunction with rotary or hand instruments, the "squirt" system may make anesthesia unnecessary.

In other cases an anesthetic may be injected for the comfort of the patient. The dentist usually asks whether the patient prefers to have an anesthetic before work commences. In the cleaning process, an effort is made to remove all traces of diseased enamel or dentin, but no more of the tooth material than is necessary.

The cleaned cavity is generally filled in a layering procedure. The layers of liners and bases used before insertion of the filling are determined by the depth of the cavity and other factors. If pulp is exposed, special materials may be applied to help the pulp recover from the irritation of the procedure and to form a firm base for the amalgam, inlay, or other restorative substance that becomes the filling.

In the 1980s, new ceramic materials came into use for fillings. Many dentists believed that ceramics could provide more natural-looking restorations. With ceramics, also, teeth would be less sensitive to changes of temperature—a problem with some more traditional materials.

Tooth Extraction

When it becomes necessary to remove a diseased, damaged, or malpositioned tooth, the procedure is handled as a form of minor surgery, usually with administration of a local anesthetic to the nerves supplying the tooth area. However, there is no standard routine for extraction of a tooth because of the numerous individual variations associated with each case. The dentist usually has a medical history of the patient available, showing such information as allergies to drugs, and medications used by the patient which might react with those employed in oral surgery. Because the mouth contains many millions of bacteria, all possible precautions are taken to prevent entry of the germs into the tooth socket.

The condition of the patient is checked during and immediately after tooth extraction, in the event that some complication develops. The patient is provided with analgesic (pain-killing) and other needed medications along with instructions regarding control of any postoperative pain or bleeding. The dentist also may offer special diet information with suggested meals for the recovery period, which usually is quite brief.

DRY SOCKET: Severe pain may develop several days after a tooth has been extracted if a blood clot that forms in the socket becomes dis-

"The Transplanting of Teeth," an early painting, portrays the shambles of a dentist's office before licensing requirements were introduced.

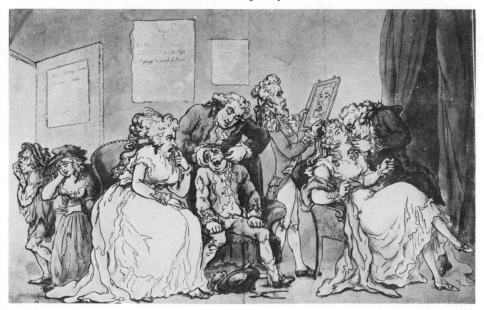

lodged. The condition, commonly called *dry socket,* can involve infection of the alveolar bone that normally surrounds the roots of the tooth; loss of the clot can expose the bone tissue to the environment and organisms that produce *osteitis,* or inflammation of the bone tissue. Dry socket may be treated by irrigating the socket with warm salt water and packing it with strips of medicated gauze. The patient also is given analgesics, sedatives, and other medications as needed to control the pain and infection.

General anesthetics are sometimes necessary for complicated oral surgery. In such cases, there are available dental offices or clinics that are as well equipped and staffed as hospital operating rooms.

Endodontic Therapy

Tooth extraction because of caries is less common today than in previous years, although an estimated 25 million Americans have had all of their teeth removed. Modern preventive dentistry techniques of *endodontics* now make it possible to save many teeth that would have been extracted in past decades after the spread of decay into the pulp canal. The procedures include *root canal therapy, pulp capping,* and *pulpotomy.*

ROOT CANAL THERAPY: Once the tooth has fully developed in the jaw, the nerve is not needed, so if the pulp is infected the nerve as well as the pulp can be removed. Only minor effects are noticeable in the tooth structure after the pulp is removed, and the dentist compensates for these in filling the tooth after root canal therapy.

Briefly, the procedure of root canal work begins by examination and testing of the pulp viability. The pulp may be tested by heat, cold, or by an electrical device called a *vitalometer,* which measure the degree of sensation the patient feels in a tooth. If the pulp is dead, the patient will feel no sensation, even at the highest output of current.

After the degree of vitality in the pulp has been determined, a local anesthetic is injected and the dentist begins removing the pulp, using rotary drills and hand instruments. By means of X-ray pictures, the dentist measures the length of the root, which may be about one and a half times the length of the crown. Stops or other markers are placed on the root excavation tools to show the dentist when the instrument has reached the end of the root. The canal is then sterilized and filled with gutta-percha—a tough plastic substance—silver, or a combination of the two, and a cap is added.

PULP CAPPING: Pulp capping consists of building a cap over the exposed pulp with layers of calcium hydroxide paste, which is covered by zinc oxide and topped with a firm cement.

PULPOTOMY: A pulpotomy procedure involves removal of the pulp in the pulp chamber within the crown of the tooth, while leaving the root-canal pulp in place. The amputated pulp ends are treated and a pulp capping procedure is used to restore the crown of the tooth.

PERIODONTAL DISEASE

It is important in the middle years of life and later to continue good oral-hygiene habits and the practice of having regular dental checkups. Studies have found that after the age of 50 more than half the people in America have periodontal disease. At the age of 65, nearly everybody has this disease.

The Course of the Disease

The combination of bacterial action described above and the roughness of the resulting calculus injures the surrounding gum tissue and makes it susceptible to infection and recession. The irritation causes swelling, inflammation, and bleed-ing into the crevices between the teeth and gums, which is one of the early signs of impaired tissue health.

The inflammation of the gums, known as *gingivitis,* can spread to the roots of the teeth if not treated. The gums separate from the teeth, forming pockets that fill up with more food particles and colonies of bacteria. As the disease progresses, the bone support for the teeth is weakened and the affected teeth begin to loosen and drift from their normal position. Finally, unless the disease is treated in time, the teeth may be lost.

Periodontal disease is sometimes called *pyorrhea,* a Greek word

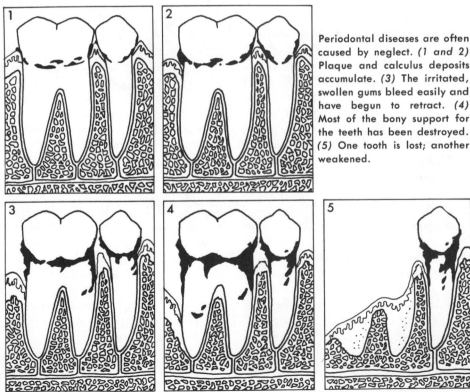

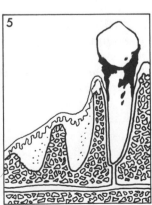

Periodontal diseases are often caused by neglect. *(1 and 2)* Plaque and calculus deposits accumulate. *(3)* The irritated, swollen gums bleed easily and have begun to retract. *(4)* Most of the bony support for the teeth has been destroyed. *(5)* One tooth is lost; another weakened.

meaning a discharge of pus. But pyorrhea is a somewhat misleading term because it identifies only one manifestation of the disease, an abscess that usually forms along the side of an affected tooth. In some cases, a membrane forms around the abscess, creating a pus-filled cyst in the tooth socket.

Other Signs and Complications

Another manifestation of periodontal disease is periodontal atrophy, or recession of the gingiva, or gum tissue, and the underlying bone away from the outer layer of the tooth that joins it to its socket. Recession tends to expose the dentin below the gum line, which is not protected by a layer of enamel. The exposed dentin may be hypersensitive to hot or cold foods or beverages, air, and sweet or sour food flavors.

Inflammation of the gingival tissue in periodontal disease may be increased in intensity by toxic chemicals from tobacco smoke, bacterial infections, vitamin deficiencies, and defective dental restorations. The normal pink color of the gingival tissue may be altered by periodontal disease to a bright red or a darker coloration ranging to bluish purple.

The inflamed gingival tissue may lead to a complication called *periodontitis* in which the bone under the gum tissue is gradually destroyed, widening the crevice between the tooth and surrounding tissues. Pregnant women seem particularly vulnerable to periodontitis and gingivitis if they have been experiencing periodontal disorders, because the temporary hormonal imbalance of the pregnancy tends to exaggerate the effects of this condition.

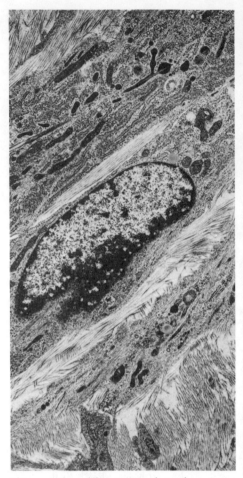

The periodontal ligaments, shown here in an electron micrograph, anchor the teeth in the sockets, allowing a slight amount of movement.

One kind of gingivitis that involves projections of gum tissue between the teeth is sometimes referred to as *trench mouth*, because it was not an uncommon form of periodontal disease affecting soldiers during World War I. The infection is associated with poor oral hygiene along with nutritional deficiencies and general depressed condition of health.

Causes

At one time it was assumed that

periodontal diseases were associated with the life styles of persons living in more technologically advanced societies, where soft, rich foods are eaten regularly, providing materials toward the formation of plaque and support of bacteria in the plaque. But recent investigations show that people living in the less developed nations, who are relatively free of tooth decay, eventually develop periodontal disease. However, this does not alter the fact that the accumulation of plaque and harmful bacteria are the chief cause of periodontal disease as well as of tooth decay.

Although periodontal disease generally becomes troublesome in middle age, there is some evidence that early symptoms of gingival disorders occur during childhood or adolescence. Also, because more people live longer today, periodontal disease has become more common than in the past.

BRUXISM: *Bruxism*—the nervous habit, often unconsciously done, of clenching and grinding the teeth— can contribute to the development of periodontal disease. Bruxism frequently occurs during sleep.

MALOCCLUSION: Another contributing cause to periodontal disease is repeated shock or undue pressure on a tooth because of *malocclusion,* or an improper bite. This effect accelerates damage to the tooth and gum structure during such simple activities as biting and chewing.

Treatment

Periodontal treatment may include a variety of techniques ranging from plaque removal to oral surgery to form new contours on the alveolar bone surrounding the tooth. If treatment is not begun until periodontal disease is well advanced, it may be difficult to fit replacement teeth, or *dentures,* as substitutes for lost teeth. Dentures fit over the ridges of the jaws, and if the top edge of the ridge has been destroyed by periodontal disease, the procedure for holding the denture firmly in place will be complicated.

DENTURES

If it becomes necessary to have some teeth removed, they should be replaced as soon as possible with a *bridge*—a mounting for false teeth anchored to natural teeth on either side—or a partial or full denture.

Why Missing Teeth Must Be Replaced

Chewing ability and clarity of speech may be impaired if missing teeth are not replaced. Also, each tooth functions to hold the teeth on either side and opposite it in place. If a tooth is lost, the tooth opposite may erupt further and the teeth on either side shift in their positions because there is no counterforce to keep them in place. Food particles lodge in the spaces created by the shifting teeth, plaque forms, and periodontal disease develops, causing the loss of additional teeth. This loss may take years if the movement of intact teeth is slow, but if they tilt and shift rapidly into the empty spaces, the remaining teeth may be lost in a much shorter time.

The loss of a few teeth can also alter a person's appearance. The cheeks may become puckered and the lips drawn together, making the individual look older than he is.

Fitting of Dentures

Modern techniques and materials of construction and the skill of modern dentists should assure well-fitting, natural-looking dentures. The dentist selects the tooth shade and shape that are best for an individual's face size, contours, and coloring. No one, however, has perfectly arranged, perfectly white natural teeth. Tooth coloring depends upon genetic factors and changes as one grows older. These factors must be considered in designing dentures.

Bridges and Partial Dentures

Several different types of dental appliances may be constructed to fill empty spaces. Some, such as dental bridges, may be attached to the remaining natural teeth by cementing them. Others, such as complete sets of dentures, are removable.

A bridge may be made entirely of gold, a combination of gold and porcelain, or combinations of gold and porcelain and other materials. If there is a sound natural tooth on either side of the space, a *pontic*, or suitable substitute for the missing tooth, may be fused to the metal bridge. The crown retainer on either side of the pontic may then be cemented to the crowns of the neighboring natural teeth.

If there are no natural teeth near the space created by an extracted tooth, a partial denture may be constructed to replace the missing teeth. This appliance usually fastens by a clasp onto the last tooth on each side of the space. A bar on the inside of the front teeth provides stability for the partial denture.

A "Maryland bridge," a fixed partial denture developed by the University of Maryland's Baltimore College of Dental Surgery, eliminates the need for crowns to anchor false teeth. With the Maryland bridge, hidden metal "wings" are used to anchor the partial denture. The wings are bonded to the backs of neighboring teeth. Because it eliminates the need for drilling, the Maryland bridge saves healthy teeth, makes anesthesia unnecessary, and reduces costs considerably.

New materials have brought bonding into more common use as an alternative to crowning and for cosmetically restoring chipped, malformed, stained, or widely spaced teeth. In the bonding process the dentist isolates a tooth with a rubber dam, cleans and dries the tooth, and applies a phosphoric acid solution that produces microscopic pores in the enamel. The etched area is then filled in with a liquid plastic. To that base the dentist applies thin layers of tooth-colored plastics known as composite resins. The layers can be sculpted, hardened with a beam of light or by some other method, contoured, and polished.

A removable partial denture should be taken out and cleaned whenever the natural teeth are brushed. A special brush, usually cone-shaped to fit into the clasp, is available as a cleaning tool. The pontic, or tooth substitute of a bridge, remains in place permanently and is brushed like a natural tooth.

A bridge or partial denture helps prevent further deterioration of the mouth if it is kept clean and in good condition. But a dentist should check bridges and partial dentures periodically to make sure they have not become loosened. A loose clasp of a partial denture can rock the teeth to which the device is attached, causing damage and possible loss.

Complete Dentures

Before a full set of removable dentures is constructed, the dentist will take Xrays to determine whether there are any abnormalities in the gum ridges, such as cysts or tooth root tips that may have to be removed. If the gums are in poor condition, treatments may be needed to improve the surfaces of the ridges on which the dentures will be fitted. The dentist may also have to reconstruct the bone underlying the gums —the alveolar ridge. Human bone "harvested" from another part of the patient's body has for decades been used in such reconstruction, but is today giving way to ceramic materials.

Two ceramic materials used in such surgery are hydroxylapatite and beta tricalcium phosphate. Oral surgeons have reported good results with both. The new materials are said to be safer and simpler to use and less expensive than human bone. They also eliminate the need for preliminary surgery to obtain transplants of the patient's bone.

With preliminary work done, the dentist makes an impression of the patient's mouth. Tooth and shade choices are discussed. Several other appointments may be arranged before the new dentures are delivered to the patient. Appointments may be needed for "try-ins" of dentures as they are being constructed and for adjustments after completion of the set.

Although dentures do not change with age, the mouth does. Therefore, it is necessary for the denture-wearer to have occasional dental checkups. At denture checkup appointments, the dentist examines oral tissues for irritation and determines how the dentures fit with respect to possible changing conditions of the mouth. If the dentures no longer fit properly, a replacement may be recommended. The dentist also seeks to correct any irritations of the oral tissues of the mouth and polishes the dentures, making them smooth and easier to keep clean between checkups. If any of the teeth in the dentures has become damaged, the dentist can repair or replace the denture tooth.

Care of Dentures

Dentures should be cleaned daily with a denture brush and toothpaste; once a week they should be soaked for seven or eight hours in a denture cleaner. To avoid breaking them during the brushing process, fill a wash basin with water and place it under the dentures while they are being cleaned; if they are dropped, the dentures will be cushioned by the water. A harsh abrasive that could scratch the denture surface should not be used. Scratches allow stains to penetrate the surface of the dentures, creating permanent discoloration.

The use of adhesives and powders is only a temporary solution to ill-fitting dentures. In time, the dentist may rebuild the gum side of the denture to conform with the shape of the patient's gum ridge. The patient should never try to make his own changes in the fit of dentures. Rebuilding the gum side of the dentures, or *relining,* as it is called, usually begins with a soft temporary material if the patient's gums are in poor condition, and requires several appointments over a period of two or three weeks while the gum tissues are being restored to good health.

Most patients show some concern over the replacement of natural teeth with dentures, even when a set of complete dentures is needed to replace an earlier set. Some people associate the loss of teeth with old age in the same way that others resist the advice that they should wear eyeglasses or a hearing aid. The fact is that many millions of persons of all ages have found they can improve their eating, speaking, and physical appearance by obtaining attractive and well-fitted dentures.

ORTHODONTICS

Orthodontics is a term derived from the Greek words for straight, or normal, teeth. Straight teeth are easier to keep clean and they make chewing food more efficient. There also is a cosmetic benefit in being able to display a smile with a set of straight teeth, although many dentists consider the cosmetic aspect of orthodontics as secondary to achieving proper occlusion, or bite.

Causes of Improper Bite

The causes of orthodontic problems can be hereditary or due to an infectious or other kind of disease, to the premature loss of primary teeth, to the medications used in treatment, or to individual factors such as injury or loss of permanent teeth. A person may have congenitally missing teeth resulting in spaces that permit drifting of neighboring teeth or collapse of the dental arch. Or he may develop extra (supernumerary) teeth due to an inherited factor. The supernumerary teeth may develop during the early years of life while the deciduous teeth are in use. A supernumerary tooth may force permanent teeth into unnatural positions.

Nutritional disorders can also affect the development of jaws and teeth, while certain medications can cause abnormal growth of gingival, or gum, tissues, resulting in increased spaces between the teeth.

Teeth that erupt too early or too late, primary teeth that are too late in

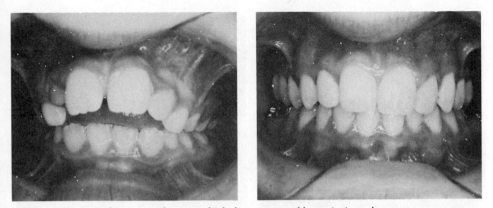

(Left) An open bite, in which the upper and lower incisors do not meet. *(Right)* The same patient after orthodontic correction.

falling out when permanent teeth have developed, and habits such as grinding of the teeth, thumb-sucking, or pushing the tongue against the teeth are among other factors that can result in *malocclusion,* or improper bite, and the need for orthodontic treatment.

Diagnosis of Orthodontic Problems

Each child should visit a dentist before the eruption of his permanent teeth for an examination that may determine the need for orthodontic treatment. Since there are many genetic and other influences that help shape the facial contours and occlusion of each individual, there are no standard orthodontic procedures that apply to any or all children. The dentist may recommend what treatment, if any, would be needed to produce normal occlusion and when it should begin; some dentists advise only that necessary procedures for correcting malocclusion be started before the permanent set of teeth (excluding wisdom teeth) has become established, or around the age of 12 or 13. However, there are few age limits for orthodontic care, and an increasing number of adults are receiving treatment today for malocclusion problems that were neglected during childhood.

In the normal or ideal occlusion positions of the teeth, the first and second permanent upper molars fit just slightly behind the same molars of the lower jaw; all of the teeth of the upper jaw are in contact with their counterparts of the lower jaw. In this pattern of occlusion, all of the biting surfaces are aligned for optimum use of their intended functions of cutting, tearing, or grinding.

There are numerous variations of malocclusion but generally, in simple deformities, the teeth of the upper jaw are in contact with lower jaw teeth once removed from normal positions. Other variations include an *open bite,* in which the upper and lower incisors do not contact each other, or *closed bite,* in which there is an abnormal degree of overlapping *(overbite)* of the front teeth.

Diagnosis is made with the help of X-ray pictures, photographs of the face and mouth, medical histories, and plaster models of the patient's teeth and jaws. The plaster models are particularly important because the dentist can use them to make ex-

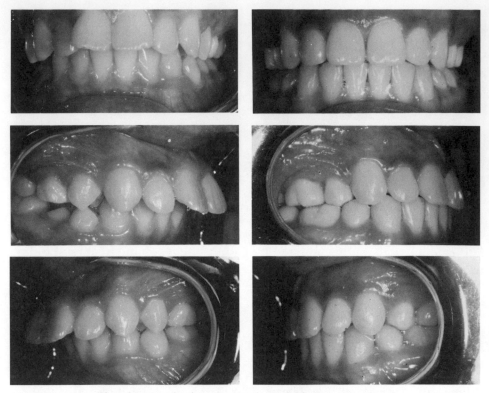

The photographs demonstrate the orthodontic correction of one patient's closed bite, in which the front teeth overlap the bottom abnormally. Each pair of pictures shows the teeth from a particular angle before and after correction. The pictures at the right were taken about 28 months after those on the left.

perimental reconstructions without touching an actual tooth of a patient. For example, the dentist can remove one or more teeth from the plaster model and reorganize neighboring teeth in the jaw bones to get an accurate representation of the effects of extracting teeth or forcing teeth into different developmental situations.

Orthodontic Appliances

Once a plan of orthodontic treatment has been determined by the dentist, he may choose from a dozen or more types of bands, braces, or other orthodontic appliances, some removable and some nonremovable, for shaping the teeth and jaws of

the patient. A typical orthodontic appliance may include small curved strips or loops of metal cemented to the surfaces of the teeth as anchors for arch wires which pass around the dental arch. Springs and specially designed rubber bands, called elastics, are sometimes used to bring about alignment of the two jaws, or to align teeth within a dental arch.

In addition to the appliances that are attached to and between the upper and lower dental arches, the dentist may prescribe the use of an elastic tape device with a strap that fits around the back of the patient's neck and is attached also to the arch wire inside the mouth, thus providing a force from outside the mouth to bring teeth into alignment.

Orthodontic appliances are custom-designed and built for the individual patient. This requires several rather long sessions or one all-day session in the dental chair while the appliance is being organized and properly anchored. Thereafter, the patient must return at regular intervals spaced a few weeks to a month apart so the dentist can make adjustments in the appliance, determine if any of the bands have pulled away from tooth surfaces, and prevent plaque from building up in places that the braces may make impervious to brushing.

The patient, meanwhile, must follow a diet that prohibits sticky foods or items that may damage the appliance or any of its parts. A conscientious program of oral hygiene including regular cleaning by the dentist or hygienist, also is necessary because, as indicated above, it is more difficult to do a thorough job of cleaning the teeth when orthodontic appliances are in the mouth.

Orthodontics for Adults

Although orthodontic treatment originally was applied only to children, the technique has been requested with increasing frequency for the correction of a variety of facial and dental disorders. Receding chins, buck teeth, sunken cheeks, sunken mouths, and other abnormalities have been treated successfully in adults beyond the age of 40. Orthodontists have observed that adult patients usually are more patient and cooperative during the

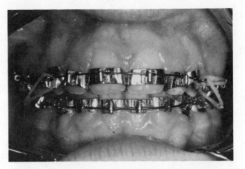

In this orthodontic appliance, arch wires are held in place by metal bands cemented to the surface of the teeth.

long periods of treatment than youngsters.

The upper age limit for orthodontic work has not really been established, but doctors at the National Institute of Dental Research believe it is possible to treat adult patients with protrusion of the upper jaw and related disfigurements until the age of 70. This is possible because the upper jaw does not completely unite with the frontal bone of the skull, according to the experts, until after the age of 70 in most people.

Orthodontic treatments can be relatively expensive and involve many visits to a dentist's office over a long period of time. Any parent of a prospective patient or a responsible older patient seeking orthodontic work for himself should have a frank discussion with the dentist regarding the time and money to be invested in the corrective procedures before making an agreement to begin the work. In nearly every case some arrangement can be made for covering the costs of dental work that is vital to the health and welfare of a patient.

CHAPTER 17

Aches, Pains, Nuisances, Worries

And Other Things You Can Live With But Could Get Along Very Well Without

None of the variety of discomforts discussed in this chapter is a laughing matter. The best thing about most of them is that they will pass, given your common-sense attention, or will disappear if you follow your doctor's advice. This includes taking the medications prescribed by your doctor exactly as directed. In a few cases, such as allergies or gout, long-term drug therapy may be necessary on a self-supervised basis, once treatment has been established by a doctor. Of course, when symptoms of any kind persist or get worse, you should waste no time in seeking a professional diagnosis.

There may be somebody, somewhere, who has never felt rotten a day in his life. But most of us are not so fortunate. Among the most common nuisance ailments are:

- Upper respiratory infections
- Allergies
- Occasional headaches
- Backaches
- Weight problems
- Weather discomforts
- Disturbances of normal sleep patterns
- Aching feet
- Indigestion.

The unpleasant feeling associated with any of these common disorders can almost always be banished with a modicum of care and thought. For example, allergic reactions to particular foods can be avoided by identifying the offending food and avoiding it. Self-diagnosis and self-discipline can often cope with weight problems. A backache may be cured by attention to posture, or adjusting your office chair. A sensible approach to clothing and exposure can often do away with weather discomforts.

But when symptoms do not respond to self-help—as when sporadic difficulty in sleeping burgeons

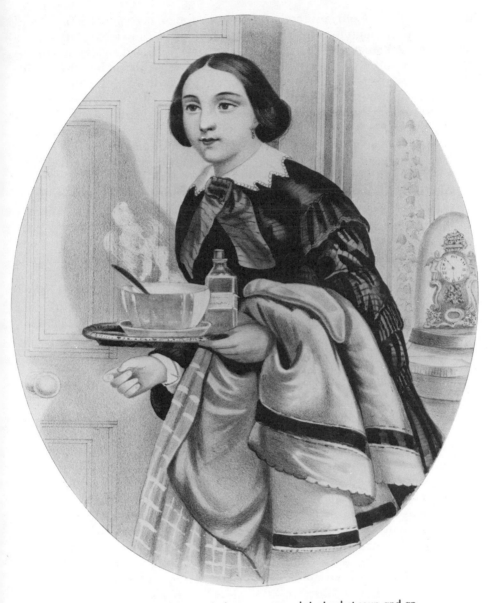

A Currier and Ives lithograph shows a woman bringing hot soup and an extra blanket for the patient with a cold—a treatment still in use.

into a string of near-sleepless nights, or when abdominal pain you interpret as indigestion is intense or frequent in spite of avoiding rich or heavy foods, it's time to see a doctor.

The Common Cold and Upper Respiratory Infections

Common cold is the label attached to a group of symptoms that can be caused by one or more of some 20 different viruses. Colds are considered highly contagious, but some doctors think that people don't entirely catch others' colds—in a sense they catch their own. While the viruses that carry the infection are airborne and practically omnipresent, somebody in good health is usually less susceptible to a cold than someone who is run down. Both environmental factors (such as air pollution) and emotional ones (such as anxiety or depression) seem to increase susceptibility.

SYMPTOMS: Symptoms differ from person to person and from cold to cold with the same person. Generally, a cold starts with sneezes, a running nose, teary eyes, and a stuffed head. Sometimes the nasal membranes become so swollen that a person can breathe only through the mouth; sometimes the senses of smell and taste simply disappear. The throat may be sore; a postnasal drip may cause a constant cough when the person is lying down at night.

When these symptoms are acute and are accompanied by fever and aching joints, the illness is usually referred to as influenza or "the flu." There are many different viruses that cause influenza, and new ones are always turning up. Unfortunately, there is as yet no medicine that can cure either a cold or a flu attack, although many people do get relief from symptoms by taking various cold remedies. Antibiotics are sometimes prescribed by doctors to prevent more serious bacterial diseases, such as pneumonia, from developing, but antibiotics are not effective against the cold viruses.

TREATMENT: Some people can get away with treating a cold with contempt and an occasional aspirin, and go about their business. Others are laid low for a few days. If you are the type who is really hit hard by a cold, it isn't coddling yourself to stay home for a couple of days. In any event, a simple cold usually runs its course, lasting anywhere from a few days to two weeks.

Discomfort can be minimized and recovery speeded by a few simple steps: extra rest and sleep, drinking more liquids than usual, and taking one or two aspirin tablets every four hours. Antihistamine preparations or nose drops should be avoided unless specifically prescribed by a physician.

A painful sore throat accompanied by fever, earache, a dry hacking cough, or pains in the chest are symptoms that should be brought to the attention of a physician.

PREVENTION: Although taking massive doses of vitamin C at the first sign of a cold is said by some authorities to prevent the infection from developing, there is not yet general agreement on the effectiveness of this treatment.

Actually, there are several common-sense ways of reducing the risk of infection, particularly for those people who are especially susceptible to catching a cold. For most people, getting a proper amount of sleep, eating sensibly, avoiding exposure to sudden chill, trying to stay out of crowds, and trying to keep emotional tensions under control can increase resistance to colds and other minor respiratory infections.

Inoculation against particular types of viruses is recommended by many physicians in special cases: for pregnant women, for the elderly, and for those people who have certain chronic heart and lung diseases. Flu shots are effective against a particular virus or viruses for a limited period.

Allergies

Discomforts of various kinds are considered allergies when they are brought on by substances or conditions that ordinarily are harmless. Not too long ago, perturbed allergy sufferers would say things like:

"I can't use that soap because it gives me hives."

"Smelling roses makes me sneeze."

"Eating almonds gives me diarrhea."

Nowadays, such complaints are commonly recognized as allergies.

SYMPTOMS: Allergic symptoms can range from itching eyes, running nose, coughing, difficulty in breathing, welts on the skin, nausea, cramps, and even going into a state of shock, depending upon the severity of the allergic individual's response. Almost any part or system of the body may be affected, and almost anything can pose an allergic threat to somebody.

ALLERGENS: Substances that trigger an allergic reaction are called *allergens*. The system of an allergic individual reacts to such substances as if they were germs, producing *antibodies* whose job it is to neutralize the allergens. But the body's defense mechanism overreacts: in the process of fighting off the effects of the allergens, various chemicals, particularly *histamines*, are dumped indiscriminately into the blood-

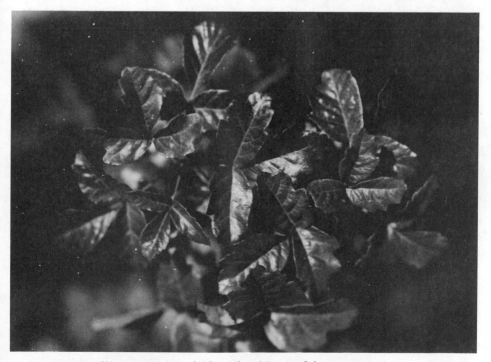

Western poison oak (shown here) is one of the common poisonous plants that cause allergic reactions in many people.

stream. It is the overabundance of these "good" chemicals that causes the discomforts associated with allergies.

Allergens are usually placed in the following categories:

• Those that affect the respiratory tract, or *inhalants*, such as pollens, dust, smoke, perfumes, and various airborne, malodorous chemicals. These bring on sneezing, coughing, and breathing impairment.

• Food substances that affect the digestive system, typically eggs, seafood, nuts, berries, chocolate, and pork. These may not only cause nausea and diarrhea, but hives and other skin rashes.

• Medicines and drugs, such as penicillin, or a particular serum used in inoculations.

• Agents that act on the skin and mucous membranes, such as insecticides, poison oak, and poison ivy, particular chemical dyes, cosmetics, soaps, metals, leathers, and furs.

• Environmental agents such as sunlight or excessive cold.

• Microbes, such as particular bacteria, viruses, and parasites.

TREATMENT: Some allergic reactions are outgrown; some don't develop until adulthood. In many cases, the irritating substance is easy to identify and then avoid; in others, it may take a long series of tests before the allergen is finally tracked down.

As soon as the source of the allergen is identified, the best thing for the allergic person to do is avoid it—if possible. But a person may find it more convenient to be relieved of the allergy by desensitization treatments administered by a doctor. Sometimes allergies that re-

sist these treatments are kept under control by medicines such as adrenaline, ephedrine, cortisone, or the antihistamines.

Any person subject to severe, disabling allergy attacks by a known allergen should carry a card describing both the allergic reactions and the allergen. Detailed information on the latest developments in the treatment of allergies is available from the Allergy Foundation of America, 801 Second Avenue, New York, New York 10017. See also *Allergies and Hypersensitivities*, p. 861.

Headaches

The common headache is probably as ancient as primitive man. The headache, a pain or ache across the forehead or within the head, may be severe or mild in character, and can last anywhere from under half an hour to three or four days. It may be accompanied by dizziness, nausea, nasal stuffiness, or difficulty in seeing or hearing. It is not a disease or illness, but a symptom.

Causes

Headaches in today's modern world can arise from any of a number of underlying causes. These include excessive drinking or smoking, lack of sleep, hunger, drug abuse, and eyestrain. Eyestrain commonly results from overuse of the eyes, particularly under glaring light, or from failure to correct defective vision.

Headaches can also be caused by exposure to toxic gases such as carbon monoxide and sulfur dioxide, which are common components in polluted air. Some headaches are symptoms of illness or disease, in-

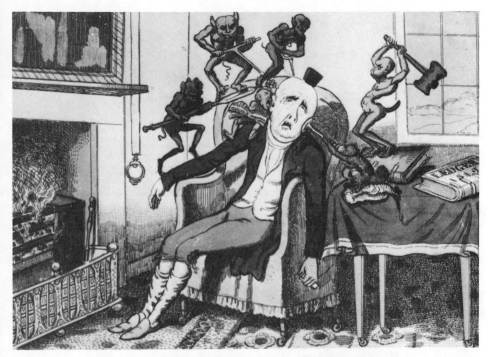

This 19th-century etching by George Cruikshank (1792–1878) vividly illustrates the diabolical misery of a headache.

cluding pneumonia, constipation, allergy, high blood pressure, and brain tumor. Finally, emotional strain or tension can cause headache by unconsciously constricting the head and neck muscles. Many of these causes give rise to the common physiological cause of headache—dilation of the blood vessels in the head.

Headaches may be suffered on an occasional basis, or they may be chronic. Chronic headaches are usually *tension headaches* or *migraine*.

Migraine

Migraine, also called *sick headache,* is a particularly severe intense kind of headache. An attack may last several days and necessitate bed rest. Dizziness, sensitivity to light, and chills may accompany a migraine headache.

The exact cause of migraine is unknown, but researchers suspect a hereditary link, since the majority of migraine patients have one or more close relatives with migraine.

Migraine headaches can be precipitated by changes in body hormone balance (as from oral contraceptives), sudden changes in temperature, exposure to bright light or noise, shifts in barometric pressure, or by the intake of alcoholic beverages or the abuse of drugs. An attack can also be triggered by allergic responses to certain foods or beverages, such as chocolate or milk, and by emotional stress. Women, who outnumber men by a 2 to 1 ratio in the incidence of migraine, may have an attack brought on by premenstrual tension. Many migraine sufferers

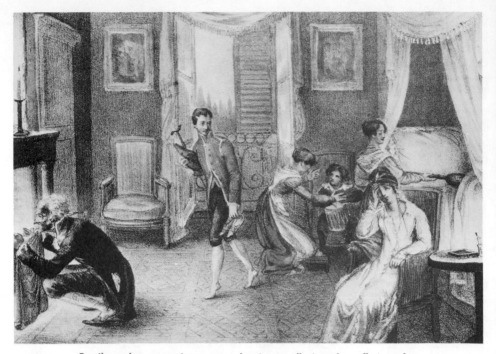

Family and servants tiptoe around trying to alleviate the suffering of a migraine patient (foreground) in a lithograph from the 1800s.

have been found to conform to a personality type characterized as compulsive; their standards of achievement are exacting, their manner of work meticulous, and they tend to avoid expression of their anxieties.

Anyone suffering from very severe or chronic headaches should see a doctor and get a complete physical checkup.

Tension Headaches

Tension headaches can be avoided by getting adequate amounts of sleep and exercise and by learning to cope with frustrations and anxieties. Find time to relax each day, and resist the temptation to be a perfectionist or overachiever in all things. Tension headaches can be helped by neck massage, use of a heating pad, or a long, hot bath.

Headache Relief

Aspirin is often effective against headaches, but should be taken according to directions. A double dose is dangerous, and is not doubly effective. A cup of coffee or other caffeine beverage may prove helpful, since caffeine helps constrict blood vessels. In some cases headaches can be helped by nothing more than a few deep breaths of fresh air. Excess use of alcohol and tobacco should be avoided. If you must skip a meal, have a candy bar, piece of fruit, or some soup to prevent or relieve a hunger headache.

Take care of your eyes. Do not read in dim or glaring light. Have your eyes checked regularly, and if you have glasses, wear them when you need them.

Backaches

"Oh, my aching back" is probably the most common complaint among people past the age of 40. Most of the time, the discomfort—wherever it occurs, up or down the backbone—can be traced to some simple cause. However, there are continuous backaches which have their origin in some internal disorder that needs the attention of a physician. Among the more serious causes are kidney or pancreas disease, spinal arthritis, and peptic ulcer.

SOME COMMON CAUSES: Generally a backache is the result of strain on the muscles, nerves, or ligaments of the spine. It can occur because of poor posture, carelessness in lifting or carrying heavy packages, sitting in one position for a long time in the wrong kind of chair, or sleeping on a mattress that is too soft. Backache often accompanies menstruation, and is common in the later stages of

The cause of a backache is often hard to pin down. A specialist examines a patient who has been complaining of chronic back pain.

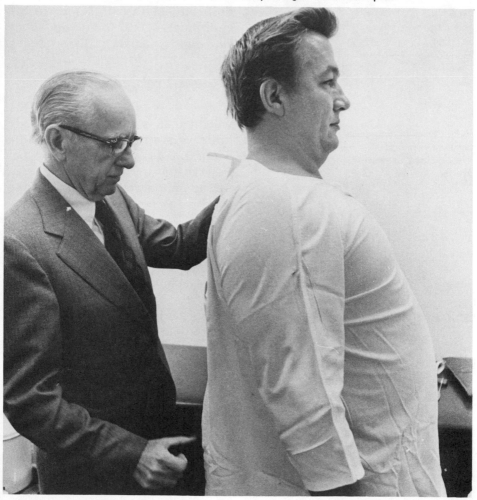

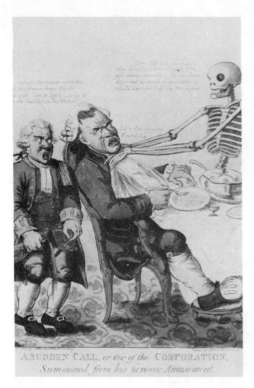

A SUDDEN CALL, or One of the CORPORATION, Summoned from his favorite Amusement

Death claims a man guilty of gluttony in a caricature published in 1799. Death says, "You have devoured as much in your time as would have fed half the . . . poor."

pregnancy. Emotional tension can also bring on back pain.

PREVENTION: In general, maintaining good posture during the waking hours and sleeping on a hard mattress at night—if necessary, inserting a bedboard between the mattress and bedsprings—are the first line of defense against backaches. Anyone habitually carrying heavy loads of books or groceries, or even an overloaded attaché case, should make a habit of shifting the weight from arm to arm so that the spine doesn't always get pulled in one direction. Workers who are sedentary for most of the day at a desk or fac-

tory table should be sure that the chair they sit in provides firm support for back muscles and is the right height for the working surface.

TREATMENT: Most cases of simple backache respond to rest, aspirin, and the application of heat, applied by a hot water bottle or heating pad. In cases where the pain persists or becomes more acute, a doctor should be consulted. He may find that the trouble is caused by the malfunctioning of an internal organ, or by pressure on the sciatic nerve (sciatica). With X rays he may also locate a slipped disk or other abnormality in the alignment of the vertebrae of the spine. See Back Pain and Its Causes, p. 1068.

Weight Problems

A few people can maintain the weight that is right for their body build without ever having to think about it. However, most experts believe that just about half the people in the United States may be risking shorter lives because they are too heavy. By one estimate, approximately one out of five American men and one out of four American women are ten percent or more overweight, a group that may be called the borderline obese.

There is no longer any reasonable doubt that, if you are overweight, you have statistically a greater chance of high blood pressure, diabetes, and atherosclerosis (lumpy deposits in the arteries). And since atherosclerotic heart disease alone accounts for 20 percent of deaths among adults in the United States, it is understandable why doctors consider weight truly a national problem.

CAUSES: In practically all cases, weighing too much is the result of eating too much and exercising too little. In many cases, the food eaten is of the wrong kind and leisure time is used for riding around in a car rather than walking, or for watching television rather than playing tennis.

Many people like to think that they weigh too much only because they happen to like good food; but the real explanations may be considerably more complicated. In some cases, overeating has been found to have emotional sources: feelings of inadequacy; the need to compensate for a lack of affection or approval, or an unconscious desire to ward off the attention of the opposite sex. Psychological weight problems of this kind can be helped by consulting a psychiatrist or psychologist.

TREATMENT: There are many overweight people who merely need the support and encouragement that comes from participating in a group effort, and for them, joining one of the various weight-control organizations can be extremely beneficial in taking off extra pounds and keeping them off.

Permanent results are rarely achieved by crash diets, faddish food combinations, or reducing pills. Not only are such solutions usually temporary, they may actually be harmful. See *Weight*, p. 718, for further information about weight problems.

Weather Discomforts

Using good sense about clothing, exercise, and proper diet is probably our best protection against the discomforts caused by extremes of temperature. Sometimes circumstances make this exercise of good sense impossible, with unpleasant but rarely serious results, if treatment is promptly administered. Following are some of the more common disorders resulting from prolonged exposure to excessive heat or cold, and what you can do to alleviate them.

Heat Cramps

In a very hot environment, a person may drink great quantities of water while "sweating buckets" of salty perspiration. Thus, the body's water is replaced, but its salt is not. This salt-water imbalance results in a feeling of faintness and dizziness accompanied by acute stomach cramps and muscle pains in the legs. When the symptoms are comparatively mild, they can be relieved by taking coated salt tablets in five-to-ten-grain doses with a full glass of tepid or cool—not iced—water. Salt tablets along with plenty of fluids should be taken regularly as a preventive measure by people who sweat a great deal during hot weather.

Sunburn

If you have not yet been exposed to much sun, as at the beginning of summer, limit your exposure at first to a period of 15 or 20 minutes, and avoid the sun at the hours around mid-day even if the sky is overcast. Remember, too, that the reflection of the sun's rays from water and beach sand intensifies their effect. Some suntan lotions give effective protection against burning, and some creams even prevent tanning; but remember to cover all areas of exposed skin and to reapply the lotion when it's been washed away after a swim.

TREATMENT: A sunburn is treated like any other burn, depending upon its severity. See *Burns*, p. 170. If there is blistering, take care to avoid infection. Extensive blistering requires a physician's attention.

Heat Exhaustion

This condition is different from heatstroke or sunstroke, discussed below. Heat exhaustion sets in when large quantities of blood accumulate in the skin as the body's way of increasing its cooling mechanism during exposure to high temperatures. This in turn lowers the amount of blood circulating through the heart and decreases the blood supply to the brain. If severe enough, fainting may result. Other symptoms of heat exhaustion include unusual pallor and profuse cold perspiration. The pulse may be weak and breathing shallow.

TREATMENT: A person suspected of having heat exhaustion should be placed in a reclining position, his clothing loosened or removed, and his body cooled with moist cloths applied to his forehead and wrists. If he doesn't recover promptly from a fainting spell, smelling salts can be held under his nose to revive

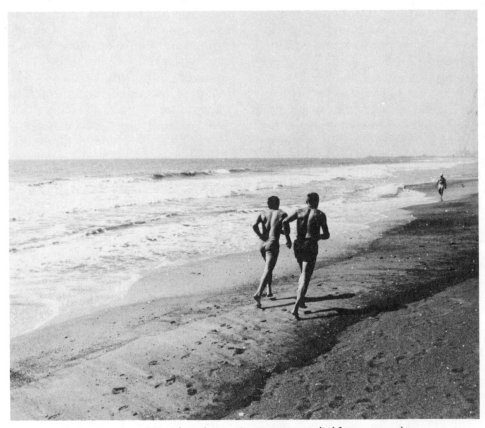

Vigorous exercise under a hot sun is not recommended for anyone who is not in good physical condition. Heat exhaustion is a real possibility.

him. As soon as he is conscious, he can be given salt tablets and a cool sugary drink—either tea or coffee— to act as a stimulant. Don't give the patient any alcoholic beverages.

Sunstroke or Heatstroke

Sunstroke is much more of an emergency than heat exhaustion and requires immediate attention. The characteristic symptom is extremely high body temperature brought on by cessation of perspiration. If hot, dry, flushed skin turns ashen gray, a doctor must be called immediately. Too much physical activity during periods of high temperature and high humidity is a direct contributing cause.

TREATMENT: See *Heatstroke*, p. 185, for a description of the emergency treatment recommended for this condition.

Chapped Skin

One of the most widespread discomforts of cold weather is chapped skin. In low temperatures, the skin's sebaceous glands produce less of the oils that lubricate and protect the skin, causing it to become dry. Continued exposure results in reddening and cracking. In this condition, the skin is especially sensitive to strong soaps.

TREATMENT: During cold, dry weather, less soap should be used when washing, a bath oil should be used when bathing, and a mild lotion or cream should be applied to protect the skin from the damaging effects of wind and cold. A night cream or lotion containing lanolin is also helpful, and the use of cleansing cream or oil instead of soap can reduce additional discomfort when cleansing chapped areas. The use of

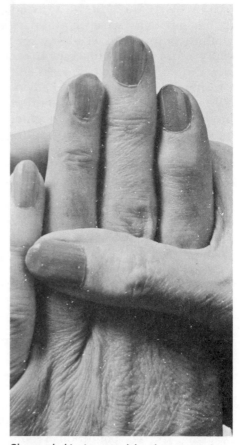

Chapped skin is caused by dryness resulting from the effect of cold weather on the sebaceous glands. The secretions of the glands are reduced at low temperatures.

a colorless lip pomade is especially recommended for children when they play out of doors in cold dry weather for any length of time.

Chilblain

A *chilblain* is a local inflammation of the skin brought on by exposure to cold. The condition commonly affects people overly sensitive to cold because of poor circulation. When the hands, feet, face, and ears are affected, the skin in these areas itches and burns, and may swell and turn reddish blue.

TREATMENT: The best way to avoid chilblains is to wear appropriate clothing during cold weather, especially warm socks, gloves, and ear coverings. The use of bed socks and a heating pad at night is also advisable. Cold wet feet should be dried promptly, gently, and thoroughly, once indoors. Rubbing or massaging should be avoided, since these can cause further irritation. People who suffer from repeated attacks of chilblains should consult a doctor for diagnosis of circulatory problems.

Frostbite

Frostbite is a considerably more serious condition than chilblains, since it means that a part or parts of the body have actually been frozen. The fingers or toes, the nose, and the ears are most vulnerable. If frostbitten, these areas turn numb and pale, and feel cold when touched. The dangerous thing about frostbite is that pain may not be a warning. If the condition is not treated promptly, the temperature inside the tissues keeps going down and eventually cuts off blood circulation to the overexposed parts of the body. In such extreme cases, there is a possible danger of gangrene.

TREATMENT: In mild cases, prompt treatment can slowly restore blood circulation. The frozen parts should be rewarmed *slowly* by covering them with warm clothing or by soaking them in lukewarm water. Nothing hot should be applied—neither hot water nor a heating pad. Nor should the patient be placed too close to a fireplace or radiator. Since the affected tissues can be easily bruised, they should not be mas-

saged or rubbed. If you are in doubt about restoring circulation, a doctor should be called promptly or the patient taken to a hospital for emergency treatment.

Sleep and the Lack of It

Until rather recently, it was assumed that sleep was the time when the body rested and recovered from the activities of wakefulness. Although there is still a great deal to learn about why we sleep and what happens when we are sleeping, medical researchers have now identified several different phases of sleep, all of them necessary over the long run, but some more crucial than others.

How much sleep a person needs varies a great deal from individual to individual; and the same individual may need more or less at different times. Children need long periods of unbroken sleep; the elderly seem to get along on very little. No matter what a person's age, too little sleep over too long a time leads to irritability, exhaustion, and giddiness.

Insomnia

Almost everybody has gone through periods when it is difficult or impossible to fall asleep. Excitement before bedtime, temporary worries about a pressing problem, spending a night in an unfamiliar place, changing to a different bed, illness, physical discomfort because of extremes of temperature—any of these circumstances can interfere with normal sleep patterns.

But this is quite different from *chronic insomnia*, when a person consistently has trouble falling asleep for no apparent reason. If despite all your common-sense approaches insomnia persists, a doctor should be consulted about the advisability of taking a tranquilizer or a sleeping pill. Barbiturates should not be taken unless prescribed by a physician.

The Vulnerable Extremities

Aches and pains in the legs and feet occur for a wide variety of reasons, some trivial and easily corrected, others serious enough to require medical attention. Those that originate in such conditions as arthritis and rheumatism can often be alleviated by aspirin or some of the newer prescription medications.

Gout

Gout, which is actually a metabolic disorder, is a condition that especially affects the joint of the big toe, and sometimes the ankle joint, causing the area to become swollen, hot, and acutely painful. Although the specific cause of gout is not yet clearly understood, the symptoms can be alleviated by special medication prescribed by a physician. An attack of gout can be triggered by a wide variety of causes: wearing the wrong shoes, eating a diet too rich in fats, getting a bad chill, surgery in some other part of the body, or chronic emotional anxiety, as well as the use of certain medicines such as diuretics ("water-pills"). See also p. 1060.

Fallen Arches

Fallen arches can cause considerable discomfort because the body's weight is carried on the ligaments of

Do your feet hurt? Then you can readily sympathize with the gout patient shown in this 1799 lithograph. Gout was once very common.

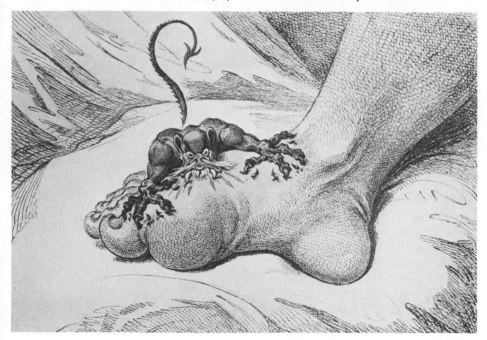

the inside of the foot rather than on the sole. When the abnormality is corrected by orthopedic shoes with built-in arches for proper support, the pressure on the ligaments is relieved. A doctor rather than a shoe salesman should be consulted for a reliable diagnosis. In some cases, the doctor may also recommend special exercises to strengthen the arch.

Flat Feet

Flat feet can usually be revealed by a simple test—making a footprint on level earth or hard-packed sand. If the print is solid rather than indented by a curve along the big-toe side of the foot, the foot is flat. Aching ligaments in the area of the instep are often a result, but can be relieved by proper arch supports inside the shoes. Corrective arch supports are particularly important for young children, for anyone who is overweight, and for anyone who has to stand a great deal of the time.

Blisters

Although blisters are sometimes a sign of allergy, fungus infection, or sunburn, they most commonly appear on the feet because of the friction of a shoe or of hosiery that does not fit properly. A *water blister* is a collection of lymph that forms inside the upper level of the skin; a *blood blister* goes down deeper and contains some blood released from broken capillaries. A normal amount of walking in shoes and hosiery that fit comfortably—neither too loose nor too tight—rarely results in blisters. When blisters do appear, it is best to protect them from further friction by the use of a sterile bandage strip.

TREATMENT: A blister that causes acute pain when walking can be treated as follows: after cleaning the area with soap and water, pat it dry and swab it with rubbing alcohol. Sterilize the tip of a needle in a flame, let it cool a little, and then puncture the edge of the blister, absorbing the liquid with a sterile gauze. The loose skin can be removed with manicure scissors that have been sterilized by boiling for ten minutes. The surface of raw skin should then be covered with an adhesive bandage. This procedure is best done before bedtime so that healing can begin before shoes are worn again.

If redness appears around the area of any blister and inflammation appears to be spreading, a doctor should be consulted promptly.

Bunions

A *bunion* is a deformation in the part of the foot that is joined by the big toe. The swelling and pain at the joint is caused by inflammation of the *bursa* (a fluid-filled sac) that lubricates the joint. Although bunions often develop because of wearing shoes that don't fit correctly, they most frequently accompany flat feet. Pain that is not too severe can be relieved by the application of heat; the condition may eventually be cured by doing foot exercises recommended by a physician, who will also help in the choice of correct footwear. A bunion that causes acute pain and difficulty in walking can be treated by a simple surgical procedure.

Calluses

A *callus* is an area of the skin that has become hard and thick as a re-

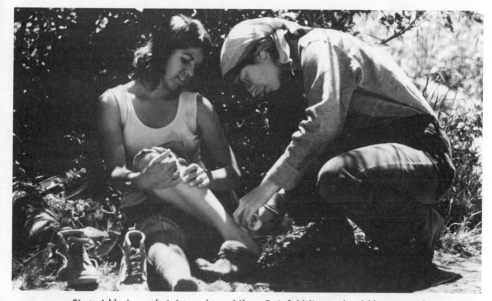

First aid being administered to a hiker. Painful blisters should be opened under sterile conditions and protected with a sterile bandage strip.

sult of constant friction or pressure against it. Pain results when the callus is pressed against a nerve by poorly-fitting shoes. A painful callus can be partially removed by rubbing it—very cautiously—with a sandpaper file or a pumice stone sold for that purpose. The offending shoes should then be discarded for correctly fitted ones. Foot care by a podiatrist is recommended for anyone with recurring calluses and corns (see below), and especially for those people who have diabetes or any disorder of the arteries.

Corns

A *corn* is a form of callus that occurs on or between the toes. When the thickening occurs on the outside of the toe, it is called a *hard corn*; when it is located between the toes, it is called a *soft corn*. The pain in the affected area is caused by pressure of the hard inside core of the corn against the tissue beneath it. The most effective treatment for corns is to wear shoes that are the right size and fit. Corns can be removed by a podiatrist or chiropodist, but unless footwear fits properly, they are likely to return.

TREATMENT: To remove a corn at home, the toes should be soaked in warm water for about ten minutes and dried. The corn can be rubbed away with an emery file, or it can be treated with a few drops of ten percent salicylic acid in collodion, available from any druggist. Care should be exercised in applying the solution so that it doesn't reach surrounding tissue, since it is highly irritating to normal skin. The area can then be covered with a corn pad to relieve pressure. This treatment may have to be repeated several times before the corn becomes soft enough to lift out. Diabetics or those suffering from any

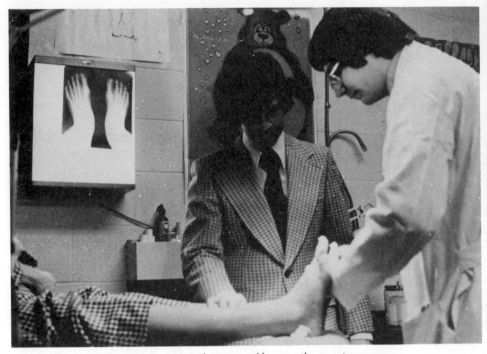

Corns can sometimes be removed by over-the-counter preparations, but diabetics should never treat their own corns.

circulatory disorder should never treat their own corns.

Housemaid's Knee

Housemaid's knee is actually a form of *bursitis*, in which the fluid-filled bursa in front of the kneecap becomes inflamed by injury or excessive pressure, as because of constant kneeling. When the inflammation is mild, it can usually be corrected by rest. In the acute stage, the knee becomes swollen and painful, particularly when bent. It is especially prone to infection if scratched, bruised, or cut. Acute housemaid's knee is usually treated by anti-inflammatory type drugs, injections of cortisone, or by surgery under local anesthesia in the doctor's office. Anyone whose daily activities involve a great deal of kneeling should make a habit of using a thick rubber mat.

Tennis Elbow

This disorder can affect not only tennis players but also people who have injured their elbow joint or subjected it to various stresses and strains. It may be a form of bursitis similar in nature to housemaid's knee, but it is more correctly called *tendinitis*, that is, an inflammation of the tendons which can affect any joint in the arms and legs. Rest and the application of heat usually relieve the painful symptoms. If the pain becomes acute, a doctor should be consulted.

Tenosynovitis

Tenosynovitis is an inflammation of a tendon sheath. One of the commoner sites of trouble is that of the wrist muscles. It can be caused by injury, infection, or constant use of the wrist muscles in piano-playing, typing, or some form of labor involving the wrist. The condition is usually treated by splinting the wrist and resting it for a while. Pain can be relieved with aspirin.

Writer's Cramp

Writer's cramp is a muscular pain caused by constant use of a set of muscles for a particular activity. The same set of muscles will function with no difficulty when the activity is changed. The best way to treat the discomfort is to give the muscles a rest from the habitual activity and to relieve the pain with heat and aspirin.

Other Muscle Cramps

A sharp cramp or pain in the leg muscles, and sometimes in the arm, can occur because blood circulation has been impaired, either by hardening of the arteries, or because of undue pressure, such as habitually sitting with one leg tucked under the upper thigh. The cramp is usually relieved by either changing the activity involved or by shifting the position of the affected limb. Constant or acute muscle cramps should be brought to the attention of a doctor.

The Exposed Integument

Common skin and scalp annoyances such as rashes, itches, dandruff, excessive perspiration, and infections of various kinds (such as athlete's foot and ringworm), as well as acne, wrinkles, and baldness, are discussed under *Skin and Hair,* p. 776.

Splinters

If lodged superficially in the hand,

a splinter will usually work its own way out, but a splinter of no matter what size in the sole of the foot must be removed promptly to avoid its becoming further embedded by pressure and causing infection. The simplest method of removal is to pass a needle through a flame; let the needle cool; then after the skin surface has been washed with soap and water or swabbed with alcohol, press the point of the needle against the skin, scraping slightly until the tail of the splinter is visible and loosened. It can then be pulled out with tweezers that have been sterilized in boiling water or alcohol.

Hangnails

Hangnails are pieces of partly living skin torn from the base or side of the fingernail, thus opening a portion of the underskin to infection. A hangnail can cause considerable discomfort. It should not be pulled or bitten off; but the major part of it can be cut away with manicuring scissors. The painful and exposed area should then be washed with soap and water and covered with a sterile adhesive bandage. Hangnails are likely to occur when the skin is dry. They can therefore be prevented by the regular use of a hand cream or lotion containing lanolin.

"Normal" Disorders of the Blood and Circulation

Almost everybody is bothered occasionally by minor disturbances of the circulatory system. Most of the time these disturbances are temporary, and in many cases where they are chronic they may be so mild as not to interfere with good health. Among the more common disturbances of this type are the following.

Anemia

Anemia is a condition in which there is a decrease in the number of red blood cells or in the hemoglobin content of the red blood cells. *Hemoglobin* is the compound that carries oxygen to the body tissues from the lungs. Anemia in itself is not a disease but rather a symptom of some other disorder, such as a deficiency of iron in the diet; excessive loss of blood due to injury or heavy menstrual flow; infection by industrial poisons; or kidney or bone marrow disease. A person may also develop anemia as a result of hypersensitivity (allergy) to various medicines.

In the simple form of anemia, caused by a deficiency of iron in the diet, the symptoms are rarely severe. There may be feelings of fatigue, a loss of energy, and a general lack of vitality. Deficiency anemia is especially common among children and pregnant women, and can be corrected by adding foods high in iron to the diet, such as liver, lean meat, leafy green vegetables, whole wheat bread, and dried peas and beans.

If the symptoms persist, a doctor should be consulted for diagnosis and treatment. For more information on anemia; see under *Diseases of the Blood,* p. 1111.

Varicose Veins

Varicose veins are veins that have become ropy and swollen, and are therefore visible in the leg, sometimes bulging on the surface of the skin. They are the result of a sluggish blood flow (poor circulation), often combined with weakened walls of the veins themselves. The condition is common in pregnancy and occurs frequently among people who find it necessary to sit or stand in the same position for extended periods of time. A tendency to develop varicose veins may be inherited.

Even before the veins begin to be visible, there may be such warning symptoms as leg cramps, feelings of fatigue, or a general achiness. Unless the symptoms are treated promptly, the condition may worsen, and if the blood flow becomes increasingly impeded, ulcers may develop on the lower area of the leg.

TREATMENT: Mild cases of varicose veins can be kept under control, or even corrected, by giving some help to circulation, as follows:

• Several times during the day, lie flat on your back for a few minutes, with the legs slightly raised.

• Soak the legs in warm water.

• Exercise.

• Wear lightly reinforced stockings or elastic stockings to support veins in the legs.

If varicose veins have become severe, a physician should be consulted. He may advise you to have injection treatment or surgery. See also p. 1124.

Chronic Hypertension

Hypertension, commonly known as *high blood pressure,* is a condition that may be a warning of some other disease. In many cases, it is not in itself a serious problem and has no one underlying specific cause: this is called *functional, essential,* or *chronic hypertension.* The symptoms of breathing difficulty, headache, weakness, or dizziness that accompany high blood pressure can often be controlled by medicines that bring the pressure down, by sedatives or tranquilizers, and in cases where overweight is a contributing factor, by a change in diet, or by a combination of these.

More serious types of high blood pressure can be the result of kidney disease, glandular disturbances, or diseases of the circulatory system. Acute symptoms include chronic dizziness or blurred vision. Any symptoms of high blood pressure call for professional advice and treatment. See *Hypertensive Heart Disease*, p. 1143.

Tachycardia

Tachycardia is the medical name for a condition that most of us have felt at one time or another—abnormally rapid heartbeat, or a feeling that the heart is fluttering, or pounding too quickly. The condition can be brought on by strong feelings of fear, excitement, or anxiety, or by overtaxing the heart with sudden exertion or too much exercise. It may also be a sign of heart disease, but in such cases, it is usually accompanied by other symptoms.

The most typical form of occasional rapid heartbeat is called *paroxysmal tachycardia*, during which the beat suddenly becomes twice or three times as fast as it is normally, and then just as suddenly returns to its usual tempo. When the paroxysms are frequent enough to be disturbing and can be traced to no specific source, they can be prevented by medicines prescribed by your physician.

Nosebleed

Nosebleeds are usually the result of a ruptured blood vessel. They are especially common among children, and among adults with high blood pressure. If the nosebleed doesn't taper off by itself, the following measures should be taken: the patient should be seated—he should not lie down—his clothing loosened, and a cold compress placed on the back of his neck and his nose. The soft portion of the nostril may be pressed gently against the bony cartilage of the nose for at least six minutes, or rolled wads of absorbent cotton may be placed inside each nostril, with part of the cotton sticking out to make its removal easier. The inserted cotton should be left in place for several hours and then gently withdrawn.

Fainting

Fainting is a sudden loss of consciousness, usually caused by an insufficient supply of blood and oxygen to the brain. Among the most common causes of fainting are fear, acute hunger, the sight of blood, and prolonged standing in a room with too little fresh air. Fainting should not be confused with a loss of consciousness resulting from excessive alcohol intake or insulin shock. A person about to faint usually feels dizzy, turns pale, and feels weak in the knees.

TREATMENT: If possible, the person should be made to lie down, or to sit with his head between his knees for several minutes. Should he lose consciousness, place him so that his legs are slightly higher than his head, loosen his clothing, and see that he gets plenty of fresh air. If smelling salts or aromatic spirits of ammonia are available, they can be held under his nose. With these procedures, he should revive in a few minutes. If he doesn't, a doctor should be called.

Troubles Along the Digestive Tract

From childhood on, most people are occasionally bothered by minor and temporary disturbances connected with digestion. Most of the disturbances listed below can be treated successfully with common sense and, if need be, a change in habits.

The Mouth

The digestive processes begin in the mouth, where the saliva begins chemically to break down some foods into simpler components, and the teeth and the tongue start the mechanical breakdown. Disorders of the teeth such as a malocclusion or poorly fitted dentures that interfere with proper chewing should be

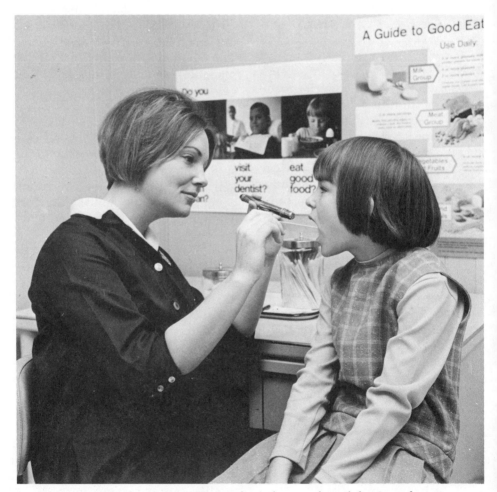

A school nurse examines a student's throat and mouth for signs of inflammation or other symptoms of illness. Contrary to popular impression, a coated tongue is not necessarily an indication of illness.

brought to the prompt attention of a dentist.

INFLAMMATION OF THE GUMS: Also known as *gingivitis*, inflammation of the gums is caused by the bacteria that breed in food trapped in the spaces between the gums and the teeth. The gums become increasingly swollen, may bleed easily, and be sore enough to interfere with proper chewing. The condition can be prevented by cleaning the teeth thoroughly and frequently, which includes the use of dental floss or the rubber tip on the toothbrush to remove any food particles lodged in the teeth after eating. Since gingivitis can develop into the more serious condition of *pyorrhea,* persistent gum bleeding or soreness should receive prompt professional treatment. See *The Teeth and Gums,* p. 805.

CANKER SORES: Canker sores are small ulcers inside the lips, mouth, and cheeks. Their specific cause is unknown, but they seem to accompany or follow a virus infection, vitamin deficiency, or emotional stress. They may be additionally irritated by citrus fruit, chocolate, or nuts. A canker sore usually clears up in about a week without special treatment. A bland mouth rinse will relieve pain and, in some cases, speed the healing process.

COATED TONGUE: Although a coated tongue is commonly supposed to be a sure sign of illness, this is not the case. The condition may occur because of a temporary lack of saliva.

GLOSSITIS: Glossitis, an inflammation of the tongue causing the tongue's surface to become bright red or, in some cases, glazed in appearance, may be a symptom of an infection elsewhere in the body. It may also be a symptom of anemia or a nutritional deficiency, or it may be an adverse reaction to certain forms of medication. If the inflammation persists and is accompanied by acute soreness, it should be called to a doctor's attention.

HALITOSIS OR BAD BREATH: Contrary to the millions of commercial messages on television and in print, bad breath cannot be cured by any mouthwash, lozenge, spray, or antiseptic gargle now on the market. These products can do no more than mask the odor until the basic cause is diagnosed and cured. Among the many conditions that may result in bad breath (leaving out such fleeting causes as garlic and onions) are the following: an infection of the throat, nose, or mouth; a stomach or kidney disorder; pyorrhea; respiratory infection; tooth decay; improper mouth hygiene; and excessive drinking and smoking. Anyone who has been made self-conscious about the problem of bad breath should ask his doctor or dentist whether his breath is truly offensive and if it is, what to do about it.

Gastritis

Gastritis, one of the most common disorders of the digestive system, is an inflammation of the lining of the stomach which may occur in acute, chronic, or toxic form. Among the causes of *acute gastritis* are various bacterial or viral infections; overeating, especially heavy or rich foods; excessive drinking of alcoholic beverages; or food poisoning. An attack of acute gastritis may be severely painful, but the discomfort usually subsides with proper treatment. The first symptom is typically sharp stomach cramps, followed by

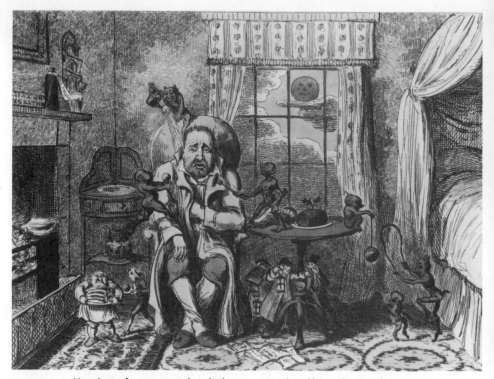

Morning-after remorse does little to counter the effects of overindulgence, as this 1825 etching by George Cruikshank so graphically illustrates.

a bloated feeling, loss of appetite, headache, and nausea. When vomiting occurs, it rids the stomach of the substance causing the attack but usually leaves the patient temporarily weak. If painful cramps persist and are accompanied by fever, a doctor should be consulted about the possibility of medication for bacterial infection. For a few days after an attack of acute gastritis, the patient should stay on a bland diet of easily digested foods, taken in small quantities.

TOXIC GASTRITIS: Toxic gastritis is usually the result of swallowing a poisonous substance, causing vomiting and possible collapse. It is an emergency condition requiring prompt first aid treatment and the attention of a doctor. See *Poisoning*, p. 150.

CHRONIC GASTRITIS: Chronic gastritis is a recurrent or persisting inflammation of the stomach lining over a lengthy period. The condition has the symptoms associated with indigestion, especially pain after eating. It can be caused by excessive drinking of alcoholic beverages, constant tension or anxiety, or deficiencies in the diet. The most effective treatment for chronic gastritis is a bland diet from which caffeine and alcohol have been eliminated. Heavy meals should be avoided in favor of eating small amounts at frequent intervals. A tranquilizer or a mild sedative prescribed by a doctor may reduce the tensions that contribute to the condition. If the discomfort continues, a physician should be consulted about the possibility of ulcers. See under *Diseases of the Digestive System*, p. 1155.

Gastroenteritis

Gastroenteritis is an inflammation of the lining of both the stomach and the intestines. Like gastritis, it can occur in acute or toxic forms as a result of food poisoning, excessive alcohol intake, viral or bacterial infections, or food allergies. Vomiting, diarrhea, and fever may be more pronounced and of longer duration. As long as nausea and vomiting persist, no food or fluid should be taken; when these symptoms cease, a bland, mainly fluid diet consisting of strained broth, thin cereals, boiled eggs, and tea is best. If fever continues and diarrhea doesn't taper off, a doctor should be called.

Diarrhea

Diarrhea is a condition in which bowel movements are abnormally frequent and liquid. It may be accompanied by cramps, vomiting, thirst, and a feeling of tenderness in the abdominal region. Diarrhea is always a symptom of some irritant in the intestinal tract; among possible causes are allergy, infection by virus or bacteria, accidentally swallowed poisonous substances, or excessive alcohol. Brief attacks are sometimes caused by emotions, such as overexcitement or anxiety.

Diarrhea that lasts for more than two days should be diagnosed by a physician to rule out a more serious infection, a glandular disturbance, or a tumor. Mild attacks can be

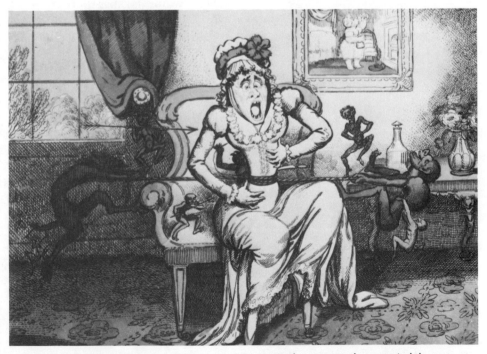

It must have been something she ate! Digestive demons attack an overindulgent lady of fashion in this 19th-century caricature by George Cruikshank.

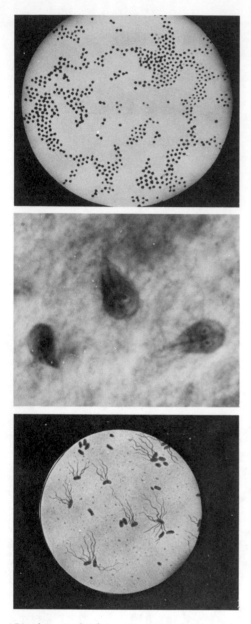

Diarrhea results from a variety of causes. In severe cases, a physician may do extensive testing and find one of these culprits responsible: *Staphylococcus aureus* bacteria *(top)*, *Giardia lamblia* protozoans *(center)*, or *Salmonella* bacteria *(bottom)*.

treated at home by giving the patient a light bland diet, plenty of fluids, and the prescribed dosage of a kaolin-pectin compound available at any drugstore.

Constipation

Many people have the mistaken notion that if they don't have a bowel movement every day, they must be constipated. This is not necessarily so. From a doctor's viewpoint, constipation is not determined by an arbitrary schedule of when the bowel should be evacuated, but by the individual's discomfort and other unpleasant symptoms. In too many instances, overconcern and anxiety about bowel movements may be the chief cause of constipation.

The watery waste that results from the digestion of food in the stomach and small intestine passes into the large intestine, or colon, where water is absorbed from the waste. If the waste stays in the large intestine for too long a time, so much water is removed that it becomes too solid and compressed to evacuate easily. The efficient removal of waste material from the large intestine depends on wavelike muscular contractions. When these waves are too weak to do their job properly, as often happens in the elderly or the excessively sedentary, a doctor may recommend a mild laxative or mineral oil.

TREATMENT: Constipation is rarely the result of an organic disorder. In most cases, it is caused by poor health habits; when these are corrected, the disorder corrects itself. Often, faulty diet is a major factor. Make sure that meals contain plenty of roughage in the form of whole-grain cereals, fruit, and leafy green vegetables. Figs, prunes, and dates should be included from time to time. Plenty of liquid intake is important, whether in the form of juices, soups, or large quantities of water. Scheduling a certain amount of exercise each day strengthens the abdominal muscles and stimulates muscle activity in the large intestine. Confronting the sources of worries and anxieties, if necessary with a trained therapist, may also be helpful.

An enema or a laxative should be considered only once in a while rather than as regular treatment. The colon should be given a chance to function properly without relying on artificial stimulation. If constipation resists these common-sense approaches, the problem should be talked over with a physician.

Hemorrhoids

Hemorrhoids, commonly called *piles,* are swollen veins in the mucous membrane inside or just outside the rectum. When the enlargement is slight, the only discomfort may be an itching sensation in the area. Acute cases are accompanied by pain and bleeding. Hemorrhoids are a very common complaint and occur in people of all ages. They are usually the result of straining to eliminate hard, dry stools. The extra pressure causes a fold of the membranous rectal lining to slip down, thus pinching the veins and irritating them.

Since hemorrhoids may be a symptom of a disorder other than constipation, they should be treated by a physician. If neglected, they may bleed frequently and profusely enough to cause anemia. Should a blood clot develop in an irritated vein, surgery may be necessary.

TREATMENT: Advertised cures should be avoided since they are not only ineffective but can cause additional irritation. Laxatives and cathartics, which may temporarily solve the problem of constipation, are likely to aggravate hemorrhoids.

If pain or bleeding becomes acute, a doctor should be consulted promptly. Treatment can be begun at home. Sitting for several minutes in a hot bath in the morning and again in the evening (more frequently if necessary) will provide temporary relief. Preventing constipation is of the utmost importance.

Anal Fissure

This is a condition in which a crack or split or ulcerated place develops in the area of the two anal sphincters, or muscle rings, that control the release of feces. Such breaks in the skin are generally caused by something sharp in the stool, or by the passage of an unusually hard and large stool. Although discomfort often accompanies a bowel movement when there is a fissure, the acute pain typically comes afterward. Healing is difficult because the injured tissue is constantly open to irritation. If the condition persists, it usually has to be treated by a minor surgical procedure. Intense itching in this area is called *anal pruritis.*

Minor Ailments in the Air Pipes

In addition to all the respiratory discomforts that go along with the common cold (see above, p. 829), there are various other ailments that affect breathing and normal voice production.

Bronchitis

Usually referred to as a chest cold, *bronchitis* is an inflammation of the bronchial tubes that connect the windpipe and the lungs. If bronchitis progresses down into the lungs, it can develop into pneumonia. Old people and children are especially susceptible to acute bronchitis. The symptoms include pain in the chest, a feeling of fatigue, and a nagging cough. If the infection is bacterial, it will respond to antibiotics. If it is viral, there are no specific medicines. The attack usually lasts for about ten days, although recovery may be speeded up with bed rest and large fluid intake.

CHRONIC BRONCHITIS: Chronic bronchitis is a condition that may recur each winter, or may be present throughout the year in the form of a constant cough. The condition is aggravated by smoking and by irritants, such as airborne dust and smog. The swollen tissues and abnormally heavy discharge of mucus interfere with the flow of air from the lungs and cause shortness of breath. Medicines are available which lessen the bronchial phlegm and make breathing easier. People with chronic bronchitis often sleep better if they use more than one pillow and have a vaporizer going at night.

Coughing

Coughing is usually a reflex reaction to an obstruction or irritation in the trachea (windpipe), pharynx (back of mouth and throat), or the bronchial tubes. It can also be the symptom of a disease or a nervous habit. For a simple, cough brought on by smoking too much or breath-ing bad air, medicines can be taken that act as sedatives to inhibit the reflex reaction. Inhaling steam can loosen the congestion (a combination of swollen membranes and thickened mucus) that causes some types of coughs, and hot drinks such as tea or lemonade help to soothe and relax the irritated area. Constant coughing, especially when accompanied by chest pains, should be brought to a doctor's attention. For a discussion of whooping cough and croup, see the respective articles under the *Alphabetical Guide to Child Care* beginning on p. 446.

Laryngitis

Laryngitis is an inflammation of the mucous membrane of the larynx (voice box) that interferes with breathing and causes the voice to become hoarse or disappear altogether. This condition may accompany a sore throat, measles, or whooping cough, or it may result from an allergy. Prolonged overuse of the voice, a common occupational hazard of singers and teachers, is also a cause. The best treatment for laryngitis is to go to bed, keep the room cool, and put moisture into the air from a vaporizer, humidifier, or boiling kettle. Don't attempt to talk, even in a whisper. Keep a writing pad within arm's reach and use it to spare your voice. Drinking warm liquids may help to relieve some of the discomfort. If you must go out, keep the throat warmly protected.

Chronic laryngitis may result from too many acute laryngitis attacks, which can cause the mucous membrane to become so thick and tough that the voice remains permanently hoarse. The sudden onset of hoarseness that lasts for more than two weeks calls for a doctor's diagnosis.

Hiccups

Hiccups (also spelled *hiccoughs*) are contractions of the diaphragm, the great muscle responsible for forcing air in and out of our lungs. They may be brought on by an irritation of the diaphragm itself, of the respiratory or digestive system, or by eating or drinking too rapidly. Common remedies for hiccups include sipping water slowly, holding the breath, and putting something cold on the back of the neck. Breathing into a paper bag is usually effective because after a few breaths, the high carbon dioxide content in the bag will serve to make the diaphragm contractions more regular, rather than spasmodic. If none of these measures helps, it may be necessary to have a doctor prescribe a sedative or tranquilizer.

The Sensitive Eyes and Ears

Air pollution affects not only the lungs but the eyes as well. In addition to all the other hazards to which the eyes are exposed, airborne smoke, chemicals, and dust cause the eyes to burn, itch, and shed tears. Other common eye troubles are discussed below.

Sty

This pimplelike inflammation of the eyelid is caused by infection, which may be linked to the blocking of an eyelash root or an oil gland, or to general poor health. A sty can be treated at home by applying clean compresses of hot water to the area for about 15 minutes at a time every two hours. This procedure should

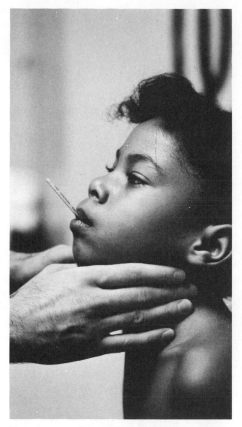

The presence of a respiratory infection calls for a check of the lymph nodes in the neck. Swollen glands are characteristic of a number of diseases, including scarlet fever.

cause the sty to open, drain, and heal. If sties are recurrent, a health checkup may be indicated.

Pinkeye

Pinkeye, an acute form of *conjunctivitis*, is an inflammation of the membrane that lines the eyelid and covers the eyeball, causing the eyes to become red and the lids to swell and stick together while sleeping. The condition may result from bacterial or viral infection—in which case it is extremely contagious—or from allergy or chemical irritation. A doctor should be consulted.

Conjunctivitis can be treated by washing the eyes with warm water, drying them with a disposable tissue to prevent the spread of infection, and applying a medicated yellow oxide of mercury ophthalmic ointment (as recommended by your physician) on the inner edges of the lids. This should be done upon rising in the morning and upon retiring at night. The eyes should then be closed until the ointment has spread. Apply compresses of hot water three or four times a day for five-minute periods.

Eyestrain

Eyestrain—with symptoms of fatigue, tearing, redness, and a scratchy feeling in the eyelids—can be caused by a need for corrective glasses, by a disorder of the eye, or by overuse of the eyes that brings about fatigue. One of the most common causes of eyestrain, however, is improper lighting. Anyone engaged in close work, such as sewing or minature model building, and at all times when reading, should have light come from behind and from the side so that no shadow falls on the book or object being scrutinized. The light should be strong enough for comfort—not dazzling. Efforts should be made to avoid a shiny or highly polished work surface that produces a glare. To avoid eyestrain when watching television, the picture must be in sharp focus; the viewer should sit at least six feet from the screen; and the room should not be in total darkness.

Ear Infections

Ear infections related to colds, sore throats, or tonsillitis can now be kept from spreading and entering the mastoid bone by the use of sulfa drugs and antibiotics. Any acute earache should therefore be called to a doctor's attention promptly. Aspirin can be taken for temporary relief from pain; holding a heating pad or a hot water bottle to the affected side of the face may also be helpful until proper medication can be prescribed.

Earwax

An excessive accumulation of earwax can sometimes cause pain as well as interfere with hearing. When the ear canal is blocked in this way, gently rotating a small wad of cotton may clean it. The ears should never be cleaned with sharp objects such as hairpins or matchsticks. If earwax has hardened too much to be removed with cotton, it can be softened by a few drops of hydrogen peroxide. When the wax is so deeply and firmly imbedded that it can't be removed at home, a physician may have to flush it out with a syringe.

Ear Blockage

A stopped-up feeling in the ear can be caused by a cold, and also by the change in air pressure experienced when a plane makes a rapid descent. The obstruction of the Eustachian tube can usually be opened by swallowing hard or yawning.

Ringing in the Ear

The general word for a large variety of noises in the ear is *tinnitus*. People who experience such noises describe the sounds in many ways: hissing, ringing, buzzing, roaring, whistling. When they are heard only occasionally for brief periods, without any other symptoms, they can be ignored. However, when they are constant, they should be considered a symptom of some disorder such as an infection, high blood pressure, allergy, or an improper bite (malocclusion). Sounds in the ears may also be caused by excessive smoking or drinking, or by large doses of aspirin or other medicines. In cases where the source of the ear disturbance can't be diagnosed and the noises become an unsettling nuisance, the doctor may recommend a sedative or tranquilizer.

The Path From the Kidneys

Cystitis

Cystitis is the general term for inflammation of the bladder caused by various types of infection. It is more common in women than in men. Infecting microbes may come from outside the body by way of the urethra, or from some other infected organ such as the kidney. When the bladder becomes inflamed, frequent and painful urination results.

Cystitis may also occur as a consequence of other disorders, such as enlargement of the prostate gland, a structural defect of the male urethra, or stones or a tumor in the bladder. Although there is no completely reliable way to prevent cystitis, some types of infection can be prevented by cleansing the genital region regularly so that the entrance of the urethra is protected against bacterial invasion. Cystitis is usually cured by medicines prescribed by a physician. For a detailed discussion of cystitis and related conditions affecting women, see *Disorders of the Urinary System*, p. 1008.

Prostatitis

Prostatitis is an inflammation of the prostate gland (present in males only), caused by an infection of the urinary tract or some other part of the body. It may occur as a result of venereal infection. The symptoms of painful and excessive urination generally respond favorably to antibiotics. *Acute prostatitis* is less common: the patient is likely to have a high fever as well as a discharge of pus from the penis. These symptoms should be brought to a doctor's attention without delay.

Excessive Urination

A need to empty the bladder with excessive frequency can be merely a nuisance caused by overexcitement or tension, or it can be the sign of a disorder of the urinogenital system. A doctor should be consulted if the problem persists.

The All-Important Feet

The *podiatrist* is the specialist who treats foot problems. Causes of foot ailments range from lack of cleanliness to ill-fitting shoes and over-indulgence in athletic activities (see "Care of the Feet," p. 627, "The Vulnerable Extremities," p. 841, and other sections on foot problems and foot care).

An ache, pain, or other disorder of the foot can be particularly annoying because it usually hampers mobility. A severe problem can keep a person bedridden, sometimes in the hospital, for substantial periods of time. As humans, we move about on our feet. They deserve the best of care from us, as their owners, and from the podiatrist in case a

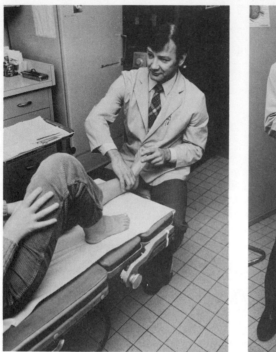 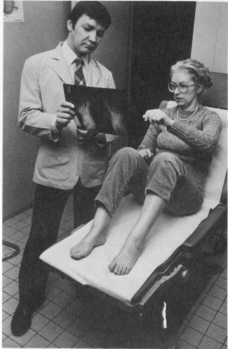

A podiatrist examines a patient with chronic foot problems and then uses X rays to explain the course of treatment he thinks is needed.

serious problem arises.

PODIATRICS, the science of foot care, has become more and more important as Americans have taken to athletics and exercises of various kinds. Most of these activities require the use of the feet. Increasing numbers of persons in the adult years are also taking up walking, jogging, or running as diversions or exercises.

Podiatrists believe that some persons "walk old"—they give the appearance, by the way they walk, of greater age than their chronological years. Others "walk young," or walk normally. Those who walk old may be inviting foot problems, and a fact of podiatric science is that every foot problem has its reflection in another part, or other parts, of the body.

By contrast, good foot and body posture often suggests that the owner of the feet enjoys good health in other parts of the body. Foot care may in effect help other body parts to function better. Because many problems with parts of the body remote from the feet make good foot posture and normal walking difficult or impossible, individuals with diverse problems, such as back pains, sometimes go to a podiatrist for treatment. The back pain may disappear when the feet have been brought into good working order.

Diabetes and the Feet

"Care" for the feet of diabetics means prevention. The diabetic tries to keep his feet so healthy that he avoids major problems. He knows that diabetes affects blood circulation, and that the leg and foot are extremely vulnerable to circulatory problems. Where blood cannot reach a limb or member, gangrene becomes a possibility.

FOOT CARE: What kind of care serves the diabetic best? Effective care means that the diabetic takes steps quickly to treat such problems as abrasions or ulcers that refuse to heal. Other conditions that warn of possible future problems are dry skin, numbness, and dried or brittle nails. Ulcers that appear in the skin of the foot and that appear to have roots in deeper layers of tissue serve as danger signals. Such ulcers may appear on the site of an injury, cut, or scratch. A physician will usually prescribe medication, dietary adjustments, or other measures.

Ulcers may result from neglect of a corn or callus. But such neglect itself indicates the risks that diabetics incur: they may neglect to have a foot problem such as a corn treated because their disease has, over time, reduced the sensitivity of their feet. They may lose much of their ability to feel pain, heat or cold, or stress in the foot. Because of such problems, diabetics generally follow certain rules of foot care, including the following:

• Give the feet a daily examination for cuts, bruises, or other abnormalities
• Use only prescribed medications in caring for the feet—and avoid over-the-counter preparations
• Visit a podiatrist regularly, as often as once a month, and avoid medical "treatment" of one's own feet or even cutting one's own toenails
• Wash the feet daily in warm, not hot, water, and dry them carefully, including the area between the toes
• Use a gentle lubricant on the feet after washing and drying—and never go barefoot
• Avoid the use of items of clothing that may interfere with circulation, including wrap-around garters and support hosiery
• Avoid "holey" socks, darned socks, or anything else that may irritate the soles of the feet
• Avoid constrictive boots or shoes

JOGGING AND RUNNING: The podiatrist usually tries to learn about a patient's work, his hobbies and sports, and other facts before undertaking treatment. In particular, the foot-doctor asks whether the patient runs or jogs or takes part in other strenuous exercises. With such background information, the podiatrist can suggest appropriate treatment.

A podiatrist will advise runners or joggers on the kind of footwear that would be best—especially if problems have been encountered or may be expected. Shoe inserts may be custom-designed if needed. The podiatrist may also advise runners and joggers to run on softer surfaces rather than cement. Jogging or running "in place," without forward movement, is to be avoided if possible; even when jogging inside the home or apartment, the jogger should move from room to room.

Podiatrists point out that even the more serious knee and ankle problems incurred in running and jogging can be treated. "Jogger's ankle," pain resulting from too much jogging and the attendant strain, can be controlled if the jogger will use moderation. Beginning joggers in particular should start slowly and gradually increase their level of participation. Runners' knee problems may be cured in many cases by treatment that enables the feet to carry the weight of the body properly. In part, the treatment requires practice in throwing the body weight onto the balls of the feet, not on the inner sides of the feet. The remainder of the body, including the knees, can be kept in proper alignment with the feet if the weight falls where it should.

Podiatrists also advise runners, joggers, and others taking part in sports to make certain *all* their clothing and equipment are appropriate. That applies especially in skiing, ice skating, and other sports requiring extensive foot use. Proper equipment helps runners and joggers avoid colds and similar respiratory problems.

With proper equipment, including good shoes, and a moderate approach, runners and joggers can avoid many other potentially troublesome physical difficulties that could require podiatric care. These others include fallen arches; corns, calluses, and bunions; and "aging feet" that grow weaker from lack of proper foot attention.

CHAPTER 18

Allergies and Hypersensitivities

Allergy is a broad term used to describe an unusual reaction of the body's tissues to a substance which has no noticeable effect on other persons. About 17 out of every 100 persons in America are allergic, or hypersensitive, to one or more substances that are known to precipitate an unusual reaction. Such substances, known as *allergens*, include a variety of irritants, among them mold spores, pollens, animal dander, insect venoms, and house dust. Some individuals are allergic to substances in soap, which produce a skin irritation. Others react to the smell of a rose by sneezing. Still others react with an outbreak of hives, diarrhea, or other symptoms to allergens in foods.

How Allergens Affect the Body

Allergic symptoms can range from itching eyes, running nose, coughing, difficulty in breathing, and welts on the skin to nausea, cramps, and even going into a state of shock, depending upon the severity of the particular individual's sensitivity and response. Almost any part or system of the body can be affected, and almost anything can pose an allergic threat to somebody.

The Role of Antibodies

The system of an allergic individual reacts to such substances in the way it would react to an invading disease organism: by producing *antibodies* whose job it is to neutralize the allergen. In the process of fighting off the effects of the allergen, the body's defense mechanism may overreact by dumping a chemical mediator, *histamine*, indiscriminately into the individual's bloodstream. It is the overabundance of this protective chemical that causes the discomforts associated with allergies.

At the same time, the antibodies can sensitize the individual to the

861

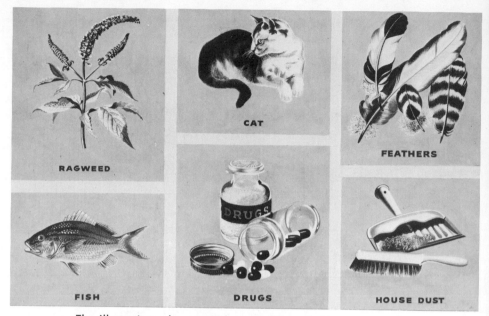

RAGWEED

CAT

FEATHERS

FISH

DRUGS

HOUSE DUST

The illustrations above provide a sampling of the enormous number of creatures and substances that can cause allergic reactions.

allergen. Then, with each new exposure to the allergen, more antibodies are produced. Eventually the symptoms of allergy are produced whenever the allergen is encountered. Most allergic reactions, including hay fever, asthma, gastrointestinal upsets, and skin rashes, are of the type just described; their effect is more or less immediate. A second type, known as the delayed type, seems to function without the production of antibodies; contact dermatitis is an example of the delayed type.

Eosinophils

Some individuals seem to be sensitive to only one known allergen, but others are sensitive to a variety of substances. Persons who suffer acute allergic reactions have abnormally high levels of a type of white blood cell called *eosinophil*. The eosinophil contains an enzyme

that may have some control over the allergic reaction, and varying degrees of the enzyme's efficiency appear to account for individual differences in the severity of allergic reactions.

Allergic Symptoms in Children

Many of the common allergies appear during the early years of life. It has been estimated that nearly 80 percent of the major allergic problems begin to appear between the ages of 4 and 9 years of age. Allergic youngsters may have nasal speech habits, breathe through the mouth, have coughing and wheezing spells, or rub their eyes, nose, and ears because of itching. A not uncommon sign of allergic reaction in a child may be dark circles under the eyes caused by swelling of the mucous membranes to such an extent that blood does not drain properly from the veins under the lower eyelids.

Nose twitching and mouth wrinkling also are signs that a youngster has allergic symptoms.

Common Allergens

The allergens responsible for so many unpleasant and uncomfortable symptoms take a variety of forms too numerous and sometimes too obscure for any book to enumerate. Discussed below are some of the more common types of allergens.

Foods

Foods are among the most common causes of allergic reactions. While nearly any food substance is a potential allergen to certain sensitive individuals, those most frequently implicated are cow's milk, orange juice, and eggs, all considered essential in a child's diet. However, substitute foods are almost always available. Many natural foods contain vitamin C, or ascorbic acid, found in orange juice. Ascorbic acid also is available in vitamin tablets. All of the essential amino acids and other nutrients in cow's milk and eggs also can be obtained from other food sources, although perhaps not as conveniently packaged for immediate use. Other common food offenders are chocolate, pork, seafoods, nuts, and berries. An individual may be allergic to the gluten in wheat, rye, and oats, and products made from those grains.

Inhaled Allergens

Allergens also may affect the respiratory tract, bringing on sneezing, coughing, and breathing impairment. The substances involved can be pollens, dust, smoke, perfumes, and various airborne chemicals.

MOLD SPORES: A person also can become allergic to a certain mold by inhaling the spores, or reproductive particles, of fungus. In the nose, the

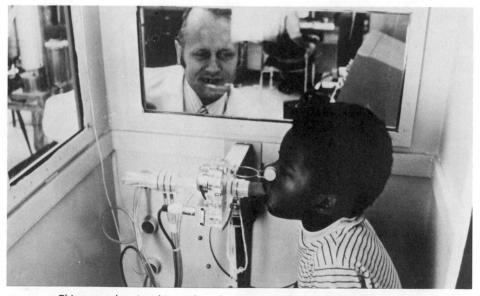

This young boy is taking a lung function test. Such tests provide accurate measurements which are of great value in asthma and allergy evaluations.

mold spores trigger a reaction in cells of the tissues beneath the mucous membranes which line the nasal passages. This in turn leads to the symptoms of allergy. Because they are small, mold spores can evade the natural protective mechanisms of the nose and upper respiratory tract to reach the lungs and bring on an allergic reaction in that site. Usually, this leads to the buildup of mucus, wheezing, and difficulty in breathing associated with asthma.

Less frequently, inhaling mold spores can result in skin lesions similar to those of eczema or chronic hives. In all but the very warmest

A very common allergy in many parts of the United States is hay fever, which is caused by ragweed pollen (shown greatly magnified).

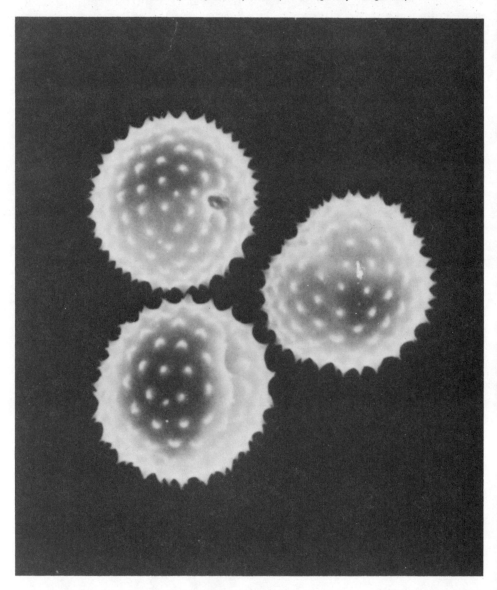

areas of the United States, molds are seasonal allergens, occurring from spring into late fall. But unlike pollens, molds do not disappear with the killing frosts of autumn. Actually, frost may help increase the activity of molds, which thrive on dying vegetation produced by cold temperatures.

DUST AND ANIMAL HAIR: House dust and animal hair (especially cat and dog hair) are also responsible for respiratory allergies in many people. Asthma attacks are often triggered by contact with these substances. Symptoms of dust allergy are usually most severe in the spring and fall, and tend to subside in the summer.

MAN-MADE ALLERGENS: An example of respiratory allergy caused by man-made allergens is the complaint known as "meatwrappers' asthma," which results from fumes of the price-label adhesive on the polyvinyl chloride film used to package foods. The fumes are produced when the price label is cut on a hot wire. When the fumes are inhaled, the result is burning eyes, sore throat, wheezing and shortness of breath, upset stomach, and other complaints. Studies show that exposure to the fumes from the heat-activated label adhesive for as little as five minutes could produce airway obstruction in food packagers.

Another source of respiratory allergy is the photochemical smog produced by motor vehicle exhaust in large city areas. The smog is composed of hydrocarbons, oxides of nitrogen, and other chemicals activated by the energy of sunlight. When inhaled in the amounts present along the nation's expressways, the smog has been found to impair

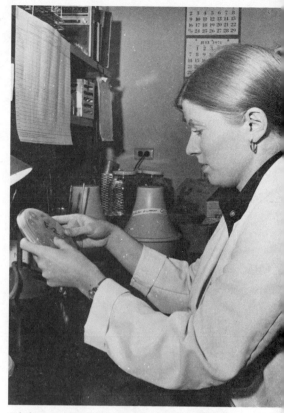

A laboratory technician conducting an experiment designed to test the allergic reaction of patients to various antibiotics.

the normal function of membranes in the lungs.

Drugs

Medicines and drugs, such as penicillin, or serums used in inoculations, can cause allergic reactions. Estimates of the incidence of allergy among those receiving penicillin range from one to ten percent. The National Institutes of Health has calculated that just three common drugs —penicillin, sulfonamides, and aspirin—account for as much as 90 percent of all allergic drug reactions. The allergic reactions include asthmatic symptoms, skin rash, shock, and other symptoms similar to tissue reactions to other allergens. Medical scientists theorize that chemicals in certain drugs probably combine with protein molecules in the patient's body to form a new substance which is the true allergen. However, it also has been noted that some persons show allergic reactions to placebo drugs, which may contain sugar or inert substances rather than real drugs.

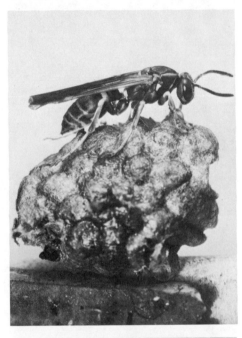

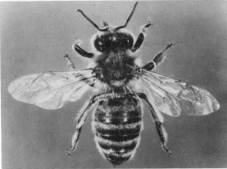

Stings of the wasp *(top)* and bee *(bottom)* can cause serious allergic reactions in susceptible individuals, who should take extra precautions to avoid them.

Insect Venom

Insect stings cause serious allergic reactions in about four of every 1,000 persons stung by bees, fire ants, yellow jackets, wasps, or hornets. A single sting to a sensitive person may lead to a serious drop in blood pressure, shock, and possibly death. There are more than 50 reported fatalities a year, and experts suspect that other deaths occur as a result of insect stings but are listed as heart attacks, stroke, or convulsions.

Sensitivity tests of persons who might be acutely allergic to insect stings have been difficult to develop because allergic individuals reacted in the same way as nonallergic persons to skin tests performed with extracts from insect bodies. More recently, doctors have found that using pure insect venom produces a reaction that determines whether a person is allergic to the sting. Medical scientists also have isolated the major allergen in an insect venom for use in diagnosing and treating patients' who are particularly sensitive to stings.

Skin Allergies

Allergies affecting the skin take many forms, the most common being eczema, urticaria (hives), angioedema (swelling of the subcutaneous tissues), and contact dermatitis. Among the most common causes are foods, cosmetics, fabrics, metals, plants and flowers, plastics, insecticides, furs and leather, jewelry, and many industrial chemicals. Studies of patients who seem to be especially sensitive to skin allergies show that they have

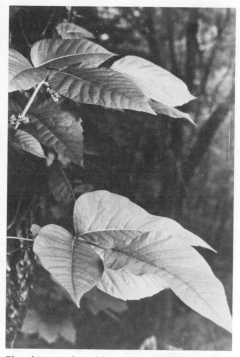

The shiny-surfaced leaves of the common poison ivy plant grow in clusters of three.

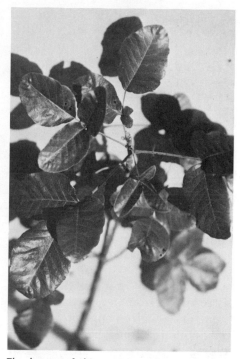

The leaves of this western poison oak plant have a thick, leathery appearance.

higher than average amounts of a body protein called *immunoglobulin E* in their systems.

In certain instances, a person who is sensitive to an allergen in a plant food also may be allergic to the pollen of the plant. The fava bean, for example, produces severe reactions when eaten by individuals who are allergic to the food; inhaling the pollen of the growing plant can cause similar reactions.

Poisonous Plants

Poison ivy, poison oak, and poison sumac contain an extremely irritating oily resin which sensitizes the body; repeated contact seems to increase the severity of the allergic reactions. About 50 percent of the population that comes in contact with the resin will experience a se-

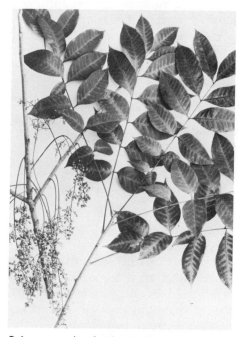

Poison sumac has featherlike leaves and hanging clusters of small, grayish fruit.

vere form of dermatitis and up to ten percent will be temporarily disabled by the effects. Exposure to the resin may come from direct contact with the plant, by contact with other objects or animals that have touched the plant, or by inhaling smoke from the burning plant.

Cosmetics and Jewelry

A wide variety of cosmetics and jewelry can cause allergic reactions through skin contact. Even jewelry that is presumably pure gold can contain a certain amount of nickel which will produce a mild reaction that causes a skin discoloration, sometimes aided by chemical activity resulting from perspiration in the area of jewelry contact. Among cosmetics that may be involved in allergic reactions are certain permanent-wave lotions, eyelash dyes, face powders, permanent hair dyes, hair spray lacquers, and skin tanning agents. Of course, not all persons are equally sensitive to the ingredients known to be allergens, and in most cases a similar product with different ingredients can be substituted for the cosmetic causing allergic reactions. For more information on skin allergies, see *Disorders of the Skin,* p. 792.

Environmental Allergies

Environmental agents such as sunlight, excessive cold, light, and pressure are known to produce allergic reactions in certain individuals. Cold allergy, for example, can result in hives and may even lead to a drop in blood pressure, fainting, severe shock, and sometimes death. Research into the causes of cold allergy has shown that cold urticaria, or hives, results from a histamine released from body tissues as they begin to warm up after a cold stimulus. Extremely high histamine levels coincide with episodes of very low blood pressure, the cause of fainting.

Although reaction of the body tissues to the invasion of microbes, such as bacteria, viruses, and other microorganisms, generally is not thought of as an allergic situation, the manner in which the body musters its defenses against the foreign materials is essentially the same as the way the antibodies are mobilized to neutralize other allergens. Thus, there is a similarity between infectious diseases and allergies.

Temporary Allergies

Occasionally, a change in the body's hormonal balance may trigger a hypersensitivity to a substance that previously had no effect on the individual. Pregnant women are especially susceptible to these temporary allergies, which almost always disappear after childbirth. Some women, on the other hand, experience complete relief during pregnancy from allergies that have plagued them since childhood.

People who suffer from seasonal allergies, such as hay fever, often have heightened allergic reactions to dust, animal dander, and even certain foods, such as chocolate and pineapple, during the season when ragweed pollen or other airborne allergens are plentiful.

Diagnosis of Allergies

Some allergic reactions are outgrown; some don't develop until adulthood; some become increasingly severe over the years because each repeated exposure makes the body more sensitive to the allergen. In many instances, the irritating substance is easily identified, after which it can be avoided. In other cases, it may take a long series of tests before the offending allergen is tracked down.

Medical History

If a person suspects he may have an allergy, the first thing he should do is consult a doctor to see if the help of an allergy specialist should be sought. The doctor or allergist will first take a complete medical history and check the patient's general health. Not infrequently the source of an allergy can be found by general questioning about the patient's life style. For example, the reaction may occur only on or immediately after the patient eats seafood. Or a patient may have an apparently chronic allergy, but is not aware that it may be related to daily meals that include milk and eggs. A patient who keeps several cats or sleeps every night with a dog in the bedroom may not realize that an asthmatic condition actually is an allergic reaction to dander from the fur of a pet animal.

The history taken by the doctor will include questions about other known allergies, allergies suffered by other members of the family, variations in symptoms according to the weather, time of day, and season of the year. The symptoms may be related to a change in working conditions or the fact that the symptoms, if perhaps due to house dust, diminish during periods of outdoor exercise. A person sensitive to cold may unwittingly exacerbate the symptoms with cold drinks while another person who is sensitive to heat may not realize that symptoms can be triggered by hot drinks but relieved by cold drinks, and so on.

Skin Testing

If the patient is referred to an allergy specialist, the allergist will continue the detective story by conducting skin tests.

SCRATCH TEST: Based on information in the medical history of the patient and the allergist's knowledge of molds, pollens, and other airborne allergens in the geographical area, he will conduct what is called a *scratch test*.

A diluted amount of a suspected allergen is applied to a small scratch

An allergy specialist applies seven substances to a patient's arm for skin testing. He will then perform a scratch test for each substance.

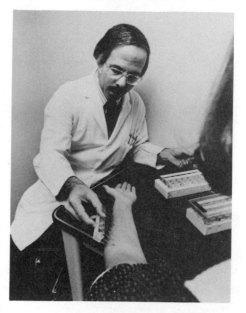

on the patient's arm or back. If the results of the scratch test are inconclusive, a more sensitive test may be tried.

INTRACUTANEOUS TEST: In the *intracutaneous* test, a solution of the suspected allergen is injected into the underlayer of skin called the dermis. The intracutaneous test also may be used to verify the results of a positive scratch test. With either test, a positive reaction usually consists of a raised reddish welt, or *wheal*. The welt should develop within 15 or 20 minutes if that particular allergen is the cause of the symptoms.

CULTURE PLATES: If the allergen has been identified, or if the allergist still suspects a substance in the environment of the patient despite negative or inconclusive tests, the patient may be given a set of culture plates to place around his home and office or work area. If the allergen has been identified, the culture plates can help the doctor and patient learn where his exposure to the substance takes place. If the allergen is not known, the cultures may pick up samples of less common allergens which the specialist can test.

MUCOSAL TEST: Another kind of approach sometimes is used by allergists when skin tests fail to show positive results despite good evidence that a particular allergen is the cause of symptoms. It is called the mucosal test. The allergist using the mucosal test applies a diluted solution of the suspected allergen directly to the mucous membranes of the patient, usually on the inner surface of a nostril or by aerosol spray into the bronchial passages. In

A physician puts drops of pollen extract in a patient's eye to find the pollen strength he reacts to—which in turn determines treatment.

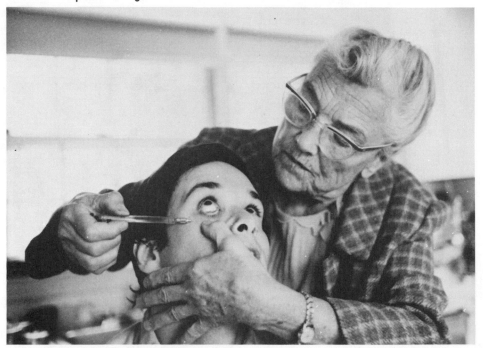

some cases, the allergic reaction occurs immediately and medication is administered quickly to counter the effects. Because of the possibility of a severe reaction in a hypersensitive patient, the mucosal test is not employed if other techniques seem to be effective.

Relief From Allergies

AVOIDANCE: For a patient sensitive to a particular type of allergen, such as molds, complete avoidance of the substance can be difficult, but some steps can be taken to avoid undue exposure. For example, the mold allergy sufferer should avoid areas of his home, business, or recreational areas that are likely spots for mold spores to be produced. These would include areas of deep shade or heavy vegetation, basements, refrigerator drip trays, garbage pails, air conditioners, bathrooms, humidifiers, dead leaves or wood logs, barns or silos, breweries, dairies, any place where food is stored, and old foam rubber pillows and mattresses.

MEDICATION: To supplement avoidance measures, the allergist may prescribe medications that will significantly reduce or relieve the irritating symptoms of the allergic reaction. Antihistamines, corticosteroids, and a drug called cromolyn sodium are among medications that may be prescribed, depending upon the nature and severity of the patient's reactions to the allergen.

IMMUNOTHERAPY: If avoidance measures and medications do not control the symptoms effectively, the allergist may suggest *immunotherapy*. Immunotherapy consists of injections of a diluted amount of the allergen, a technique similar to that used in the skin tests. A small amount of a very weak extract is injected once or twice a week at first. The strength of the extract is gradually increased, and the injections are given less frequently as relief from the symptoms is realized. The injections are continued until the patient has experienced complete relief of the symptoms for a period of two or three years. However, some people may have to continue the injections for longer time spans. Even though the treatments may relieve the symptoms, they may not cure the allergy.

IDENTIFICATION CARDS: Any person subject to severe disabling allergy attacks by a known allergen should carry a card describing both the allergic reaction and the allergen. Detailed information can be obtained from the Allergy Foundation of America, 801 Second Avenue, New York, New York 10017. See also *Allergic Respiratory Diseases*, p. 1192, and *Asthma Attack*, p. 165.

CHAPTER 19

Physicians and Surgeons and Their Diagnostic Procedures

Perhaps a few words are called for in explanation of the title of this chapter. *Medicine* is the umbrella term for the entire profession dealing with the maintenance of health and treatment of disease. In a narrower sense, however, it is often used in distinction to *surgery,* which deals with the correction of disorders or other physical change by operation or by manual manipulation. Thus the term *medical* is often used in distinction to *surgical,* and a *physician,* who treats his patients by medical means, may likewise be distinguished from a *surgeon.* The term *physician,* however, is also used broadly to apply to any authorized practitioner of medicine, including surgeons.

The two kinds of physicians most likely to be encountered when we have an undefined symptom or ailment that requires professional diagnosis and treatment are general or family practitioners and internists. These are the generalists of the medical profession, physicians who treat a wide variety of disorders and illnesses. Unlike other specialists, they usually do not require a referral from another doctor and are the first to interview a person about his condition and any complaints he may have.

The General Practitioner

The *general practitioner* or GP is about the closest thing we have to the old country doctor who hung out his shingle in front of his small-town house and made midnight carriage rides to deliver babies. The GP not only delivers babies, but also listens to our problems, treats skin rashes,

872

sets broken bones, sees children through difficult diseases, dispenses antibiotics and pain-killers, and does all the other things we expect a doctor to do. He may also perform appendectomies.

Internal Medicine

The *internist* is really a specialist in the branch of medicine called internal medicine. He usually refers surgery, and may also refer special problems affecting specific body systems, to physicians specializing in such areas. The internist's training is longer and more intensified than that of the GP. In addition, most internists spend one or two years of study in a subspecialty, such as cardiology (heart), hematology (blood), etc. An internist is usually associated with at least one major hospital, its specialists, and its operating and laboratory facilities.

The field of an internist has been defined as "medical diagnosis and treatment"—obviously a very broad definition, to which must be added the observation that one of the responsibilities of the internist is to know when his knowledge is insufficient and when he should refer a patient to another specialist.

An internist should not be confused with an *intern* (or *interne*), who is a medical school graduate serving a year in residence at a hospital. The intern is, in a sense, an apprentice doctor, putting the finishing practical touches on the knowledge he has accumulated in medical school by first-hand diagnosis and treatment of patients under the supervision of an experienced doctor.

The medical profession officially recognizes and licenses physicians and surgeons to become specialists in 19 fields (listed below). Before becoming a certified specialist in any of these fields, a doctor must qualify in training and pass examinations supervised by a board made up of physicians already practicing that specialty. This training is known as *residency* training.

Subspecialties of Internal Medicine

There are also a number of subspecialties in which an internist may develop a special interest, such as *cardiology*, the study of the diseases of the heart, or *gastroenterology*, dealing with disorders of the digestive tract. Both cardiology and gastroenterology are unusual subspecialties in that passing of examinations is required for certification as a *cardiologist* or a *gastroenterologist*.

There are a number of other subspecialties of internal medicine, some having a quite familiar ring. *Allergology*, the treatment and diagnosis of allergies, is the interest of the *allergist*. The circulatory system (heart and blood vessels) is the special concern of the *cardiovascular specialist*. *Endocrinology* is the study of the endocrine system and its glands; the specialist is an *endocrinologist*. The study of blood chemistries and treatment of blood diseases, such as anemia and leukemia, are called *hematology*, the province of the *hematologist*. The study of the connecting and supporting tissues of the body is called *rheumatology*, and the specialist is a *rheumatologist*.

Apart from these subspecialties, a number of internists have satisfied the requirements of boards for both internal medicine and one of the other special branches of medicine.

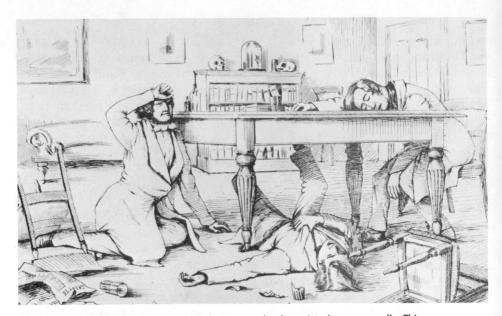

Doctors at one time tested new remedies by trying them personally. This nineteenth century drawing shows scientists taking chloroform.

Specialties Approved by the American Medical Association

The following major specialties are recognized by the American Medical Association:

ANESTHESIOLOGY: The *anesthesiologist*, especially during major surgery, administers a patient's state of anesthesia (loss of the sensation of pain) either in parts of or all of the body.

COLON AND RECTAL SURGERY: *Proctology* is the field dealing with diseases of the rectum and colon.

DERMATOLOGY: The *dermatologist* is a specialist in the diagnosis and treatment of skin diseases.

INTERNAL MEDICINE: The role of the *internist*, a kind of general specialist, is discussed above.

NEUROLOGICAL SURGERY: The neurological surgeon deals with the diagnosis, treatment, and surgical management of disorders and diseases of the brain, spinal cord, and nervous systems.

OBSTETRICS AND GYNECOLOGY: A physician can be an *obstetrician*, a *gynecologist*, or both. The obstetrician's specialty is pregnancy and childbirth; the gynecologist specializes in the care and treatment of women and their diseases, especially of the reproductive system. In practice, he usually treats women who are not pregnant.

OPHTHALMOLOGY: The *ophthalmologist* is a specialist in medical and surgical treatment of the eye.

ORTHOPEDIC SURGERY: The *orthopedist* or *"orthopod"* specializes in diagnosing, treating, and surgically correcting, where possible, disorders and injuries associated with the bones, joints, muscles, cartilage, and ligaments.

OTOLARYNGOLOGY: The *otolaryngologist* is a specialist, with surgical competence, in practically all the cavities of the head except those holding the eyes and the brain. He is the doctor of the ear, nose, and throat, often abbreviated to ENT.

PATHOLOGY: The pathologist investigates the course and causes of diseases with a mastery of the laboratory devices and techniques at his disposal.

PEDIATRICS: The pediatrician specializes in all medical aspects of child care.

PHYSICAL MEDICINE AND REHABILITATION: This specialist deals with the full or partial restoration of use and function to body parts that have been affected by disease or injury, or have been defective at birth.

PLASTIC SURGERY: The plastic surgeon specializes in operations designed to give a more normal appearance to parts of the body that are disfigured or that the owner feels are unsightly.

PREVENTIVE MEDICINE: This specialist is concerned with predicting and preventing disease, usually in one specific institution or sector, such as an industry or an urban community.

PSYCHIATRY AND NEUROLOGY: Broadly speaking, the psychiatrist deals with the subjective feelings of his patients; the neurologist deals with the objective facts of the nervous system.

RADIOLOGY: The radiologist is an expert in using electromagnetic radiations (e.g., X rays) for the diagnosis and treatment of diseases.

SURGERY: The general surgeon has been trained to perform surgery anywhere on the body, but he usually specializes in a particular area.

THORACIC SURGERY: A thoracic surgeon specializes in operations involving the organs of the chest, or thoracic cavity.

UROLOGY: The urologist specializes in the diagnosis, treatment, and surgical management of diseases affecting the male urinogenital tract and the female urinary tract.

A pediatrician examines a patient with a sore throat. Pediatrics as a specialty deals with all types of disease experienced by children.

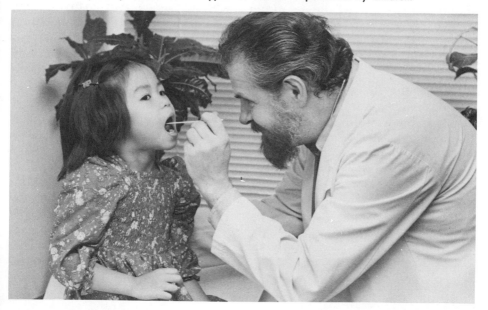

THE PHYSICAL EXAMINATION

The use of physical examinations to determine the health of people is not new. Medical literature reveals that periodic health examinations were required of the Spartans of ancient Greece. American doctors have encouraged periodic examinations of children and adults as a preventive health measure since the beginning of the Civil War. But only in the last few decades has the general public accepted the idea that many physical disorders can be detected in the earliest stages by an examining physician and corrective measures prescribed to insure the maximum number of productive years for the patient. Heart disease, cancer, diabetes, hypertension, and glaucoma are just a few examples of diseases that a doctor can detect during a routine physical examination long before disabling symptoms begin to be noticeable to the patient. The Pap test for women is a specific example of an examination technique that can predict the development of cervical cancer several years before the woman might notice signs and symptoms of the insidious disease.

On the other hand, physical examinations may determine that bothersome symptoms do not herald a dangerous disease. A man who suffers from abdominal pains and fears he has stomach cancer would be relieved to learn after an examination that the problem is only nervous tension, which can be corrected by other means. Heart palpitations and breathlessness similarly might be found through a doctor's examination to be due to anxiety rather than heart disease.

The Importance of Periodic Physicals

Health examinations for most Americans unfortunately tend to be sporadic. During infancy and upon entering school, there may be detailed physical examinations, followed by possibly additional checkups during later childhood when required by the local educational system, and finally, a thorough examination for persons entering the military service or applying for a job or insurance policy. But there may follow a period of 30 to 40 "lost years" for many persons before they feel the need for a checkup because of the symptoms of one of the degenerative diseases that may appear when they have reached their 50s or 60s. Unfortunately, statistics show that nearly 30 percent of chronic and disabling diseases begin before the age of 35 and about 40 percent appear between the ages of 35 and 55, with evidence that many chronic disabilities actually developed more or less unnoticed by the patients during the "lost years" when periodic physical examinations were considered unnecessary.

Periodic physical examinations are now encouraged for persons of all age groups with four objectives:
• to detect abnormalities so that early diagnosis and treatment can prevent disability and premature death, especially from chronic diseases
• to improve the individual's understanding of health and disease
• to establish good relations between patient and doctor as a basis for continuing health maintenance

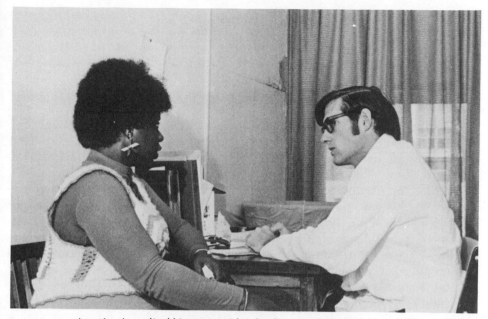

A patient's medical history provides the doctor with valuable information that can help him in diagnosing illness and prescribing treatment.

• to provide specific preventive health measures such as immunizations and advice about such life style matters as cigarette smoking and weight control.

General Diagnostic Procedures

A typical physical examination will include a careful health appraisal by an examining physician, including a detailed health history of the patient and study of the patient's body appearance and functions, an X ray of the chest area, and electrocardiogram of the heart in some cases, and laboratory analysis of blood and urine samples. Other appropriate procedures, such as a Pap test smear, may be added to the routine. Since no two persons are exactly alike and the differences between patients are likely to increase with advancing years, the examining doctor's interest in a set of signs and

symptoms may vary with different patients as he pieces evidence together to come up with a complete evaluation of a particular patient.

Medical History

The examination almost invariably begins with the *medical history* and includes details which may seem trivial or unimportant to the patient. But the information sometimes can provide important clues to a physician compiling data about a patient. This information usually includes the age, sex, race, marital status, occupation, and birthplace of the patient. The examiner also may want to know about any previous contacts with the doctor's medical group, clinic, hospital, or other medical facility, in the event that previous medical records of the individual are on file.

SYMPTOMS: The doctor may ask a simple, obvious question, like

"What is bothering you?" or "Why did you want to see a doctor?" The answer given may become for examining purposes the chief complaint and usually will involve any current or recent illness. If there is a current or recent illness to discuss, the doctor will want to know more about it: when did it begin, how did it begin, and how has it affected you? If the doctor asks about *symptoms*, he usually is probing for information about what the patient feels, and where. A symptom may be a pain, ache, bloated feeling, and so on. A *sign* is, in medical terminology, what somebody else, such as the doctor, observes; signs and symptoms usually go together in solving a medical problem.

The doctor's view of the importance of some symptoms may not be the same as the patient's. The doctor may try to pursue complaints that may not seem important to the patient but actually can be more significant than the chief complaint. The doctor's training and experience give him some advantages in concluding, for example, that a 45-year-old woman who has had a chronic cough for several years probably does not have lung cancer, even though that may be her chief concern.

PAST ILLNESSES: Other questions included in the medical history would be a list of childhood diseases, adult diseases such as pneumonia or tuberculosis, broken bones suffered, burns or gunshot wounds, unconsciousness as a result of an injury, a description of past operations, information about immunizations, medicines taken and side effects experienced from medications, and, for women, information about preg-nancies, if any. Family history questions would cover information about the parents and blood relatives, including a variety of diseases they may have suffered.

LIFE STYLE AND ATTITUDE: Next, the doctor may review the body systems, asking questions about any difficulties experienced with the head, eyes, ears, mouth, nose, lungs, heart, etc. Changes in body weight, hair texture, appetite, and other factors will be recorded, along with information about occupation, military service, and travel in foreign countries. Life style questions could cover sleeping habits, sex life, use of coffee, tea, alcoholic beverages, vitamin tablets, sleeping pills, tobacco, exercise, and social activities. In addition to the answers given, the doctor may record how the answers to questions are presented by a patient, since the patient's attitude can offer additional insight into the person's mental and physical health. For example, a patient who tries to dominate the examination interview or who answers the doctor's questions with a response like "What do you mean by that?" may reveal more by the quality than the content of the answers.

Observation

After the medical history has been recorded or updated, the doctor may begin a general inspection of the patient's body, beginning with the head and neck and working down to the feet. The doctor looks for possible deformities, scars or wounds including insect bites, or pulsations or throbbing areas. Bruises, areas of skin peeling or flaking, areas of heavy skin pigmentation or loss of pigmentation, hair distribution, per-

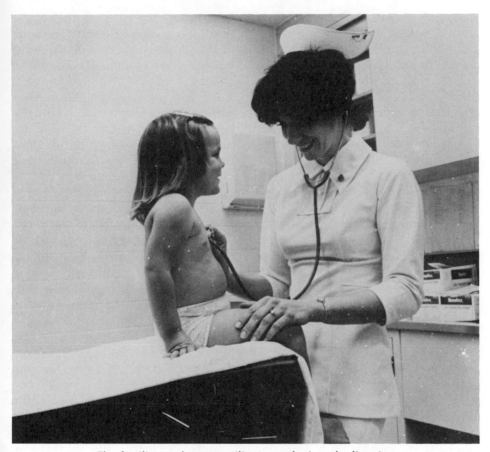

The familiar stethoscope utilizes auscultation, the listening
to sounds within the body, to check the condition of the lungs.

spiration or goose bumps, firmness or slackness of the skin, warts, calluses, and other features are noted.

Palpation

The doctor usually checks the exterior of the body by a method known as *palpation,* which means feeling with the fingers and hands. Because some parts of the hand are more sensitive to warmth and others are more sensitive to vibrations, the doctor may shift from finger tips to palms at various times in his search for health clues. Rough vibrations from a disorder in the respiratory system, the trembling sensation of

blood encountering an obstruction, or the grating feeling of a bone deformity can be detected during palpation. The doctor also can tell from palpation where areas are tender or abnormally warm to the touch. If he finds a raised area of the skin, he can tell by palpation whether there is a growth within or beneath the skin.

Percussion and Auscultation

In addition to palpation, the examining physician may apply *percussion,* or tapping, of certain body areas. Tapping the chest, for example, gives the doctor some information from the sounds produced about the condition of the lungs. He also uses a related technique of *auscultation,* or listening to sounds within the body, either with his ear against the body or through a stethoscope, the familiar Y-shaped instrument used to amplify internal sounds.

In percussion, the doctor usually places one hand on the surface of the patient's body with the fingers slightly spread apart and taps on one of the fingers with the middle finger of the other hand. By moving the lower hand around on various areas of the chest surface while tapping one finger on the other, the doctor can get a fairly accurate "sound picture" of the condition of organs within the chest. He can outline the heart and the distance moved by the diaphragm in filling and emptying the lungs by listening for changes in percussion sounds that range from resonance over hollow spaces to dullness over solid or muscular areas. Lack of resonance over a normally resonant area of the lung might indicate fluid, pneumonia, or perhaps an abnormal mass. Percussion may also give the first sign of enlargement of organs such as the liver, heart, or spleen.

During auscultation, the doctor listens for normal or abnormal breathing sounds. He can usually detect specific aberrations in lung function by noises made as the air rushes in and out of the lungs through the bronchi. A sound of frictional rubbing can suggest a rough surface on the lining of the pleura, a membrane surrounding the lung tissue; a splashing or slapping sound would indicate the presence of fluid in the lungs. In auscultation of the heart, the doctor listens for extra heartbeats, rubbing sounds, the rumbling noises of a heart murmur, or the sounds of normally functioning heart valves opening and closing.

An experienced physician may use his stethoscope for listening to sounds beyond the chest area. He may listen to the sounds of blood flowing through vessels of the neck, bowel sounds through the wall of the abdomen, and the subtle noises made by joints, muscles, and tendons as various limbs are moved.

During examination of the chest, the doctor usually asks the patient to perform certain breathing functions: take a deep breath, hold your breath, inhale, exhale, etc. On one or more of the exhalation commands, the doctor may make a quick check of the air exhaled from the lungs to determine if there is any odor suggesting a disease that might be unnoticed by the patient. Just as the doctor learns to recognize the meaning of percussion and auscultation sounds, he learns the meaning of certain odors of bacterial activity or other disorders.

Body Structure and Gait

Weight and height are checked as part of any routine examination. These factors are important in a health examination for children to determine the rate of growth, even though youngsters of the same age can vary considerably in height and weight and still be within the so-called normal range. Sudden changes in the rate of growth or abnormal growth may be signs that special attention should be given to possible problems. Adults also can vary greatly in weight and height, but special concern may be indi-

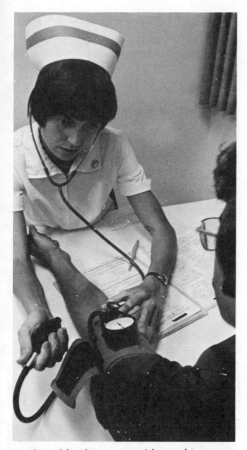

In taking blood pressure with a sphygmomanometer, a stethoscope is used to listen for the heartbeat as pressure is released.

cated by the doctor if the individual is exceptionally tall, short, fat, or skinny. In addition to a possible disease associated with unusual stature, the facts and figures obtained about body build can be important because certain disorders tend to develop in individuals of a particular body structure. Posture also provides clues to the true condition of a patient; a person who has a slouch or who holds one shoulder higher than the other may have an abnormal spinal curvature. The doctor may watch the patient's manner of walking because a person's gait can

suggest muscle, bone, or nervous-system disorders; a person who seems to lean forward and take short steps, for example, may have muscles that do not relax normally during movement of the legs.

Blood Pressure

Blood pressure is measured with the help of a device called a *sphygmomanometer* and the stethoscope. The sphygmomanometer has either a dial with a face that shows the blood pressure reading in millimeters of mercury, or a column of mercury in a glass tube with numbers alongside it. Either kind of device also has attached to it an inflatable cuff, which is wrapped around the upper arm; a rubber bulb is used to inflate the cuff and increase pressure in it so that it can control the blood flow in the arm. The doctor places the bell-shaped end of the stethoscope on a point on the inside of the elbow where the pulse can be felt. The bulb is squeezed to increase the cuff pressure until the heartbeat, in the form of the pulse, can no longer be heard through the stethoscope. The reading on the sphygmomanometer at that stage may be well over 200. Then the doctor slowly deflates the cuff and lets the reading on the gauge fall gradually until he hears the first beat of the heart. The reading on the gauge at that point is recorded as the *systolic pressure*. The doctor continues to relax the pressure in the cuff and watches for the reading at the point where the thumping of the heart disappears. That number is recorded as the *diastolic pressure*.

If the systolic pressure is, for example, 130 and the diastolic pressure is 72, the doctor may make a notation of "BP 130/72," which is the patient's blood pressure at the time of the examination. The records also may indicate whether the patient was sitting or lying down at the time and whether the pressure was taken on the right arm or the left arm. Sometimes the pressure is checked on both arms. If the patient appears tense or anxious, which could produce a higher than normal blood pressure reading, the doctor may encourage the patient to relax for a few minutes and try again for a more meaningful reading.

Pulse Rate

The pulse itself usually is studied for rate and quality, or character, which means the force of the pulse beat and the tension between beats. The pulse beat for small children may be well over 100 per minute and still be considered normal. But in an adult who is relaxed and resting any pulse rate over 100 suggests that something is wrong. An adult pulse rate of less than 60 also might indicate an abnormal condition.

Eyes

Inspection of the eyes, is usually done with the aid of an *ophthalmoscope*, by means of which the doctor can visualize the retina on the back inner surface of each eye, and its associated arteries, veins, and nerve fibers. Distended retinal veins may be a sign of a variety of disorders, including diabetes or heart disease;

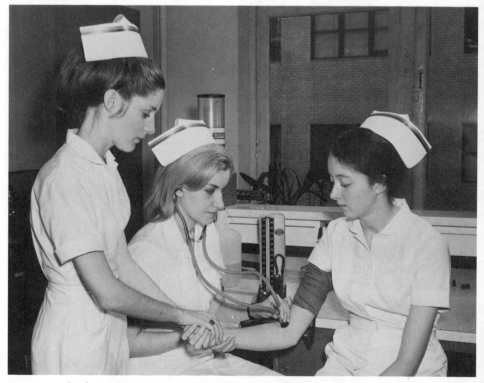

Student nurses practice taking pulse and blood pressure readings. The sphygmomanometer here utilizes a column of mercury rather than a dial.

signs of hardening of the arteries also may be observed in the eyes before other indications are found elsewhere in the body. The condition of retinal blood vessels may, in addition, signal the development of hypertension.

Mouth, Nose, and Ears

The mouth, nose, and ears are inspected for signs of abnormalities. A device called an *otoscope* is inserted in the outer ear to examine the external auditory canal and eardrum. If the patient wears dentures, the doctor may ask that they be removed during examination of the mouth so that the health of the gums can be checked. The condition of the tongue, teeth, and gums can reveal much about the health habits of the individual. An inadequate set of teeth, for example, can indicate that certain important food items that require chewing are being avoided. Tobacco stains obviously are a sign of tobacco use.

X Rays

A chest X ray is usually a routine part of the examination; the X ray usually covers the chest area, showing the condition of the heart and lungs. The finished X-ray picture looks something like a large photographic negative but the film is designed so that areas filled with gas, such as the lungs or fatty tissues, appear almost transparent, and bone or solid metal objects appear sharply opaque. Muscle, blood, and other objects, including gall bladder stones, can be identified through a hazy kind of contrast between opaque and translucent. A number of special kinds of X rays may be ordered if the doctor wants to make a

more detailed check of some possible disorder involving a specific body cavity, such as a peptic ulcer in the stomach wall.

Electrocardiogram

An increasing number of health examinations today include an electrocardiographic study of the heart. An *electrocardiogram*, or *EKG*, is made as a kind of "picture" traced by a pen on a moving sheet of paper, with the movements of the pen controlled by electrical impulses produced by the heart. All muscle activity produces tiny electrical discharges, and the rhythmic contractions of heart muscle result in a distinctive pattern of electrical pulsations which form the electrocardiogram picture. The tracing appears to the patient as simply a long wavy line, but the doctor can identify each of the wave crests and dips in terms of different parts of the heart muscle contracting or relaxing in proper sequence, or—if the heart is not functioning normally—not in proper sequence.

The electrocardiogram is recorded by attaching electrodes, or leads, to the chest, arms, and legs, in a series of differing arrangements depending upon the kind of heart picture the doctor wants to record. The wires from the electrodes are connected to the machine that translates the heartbeat rhythms into the electrocardiogram. There is no danger of electrical shock because the only electricity flowing through the wires is the current produced continuously by the human body as part of its natural functions.

It is always an advantage for the patient to have an electrocardiogram taken early in adult life and

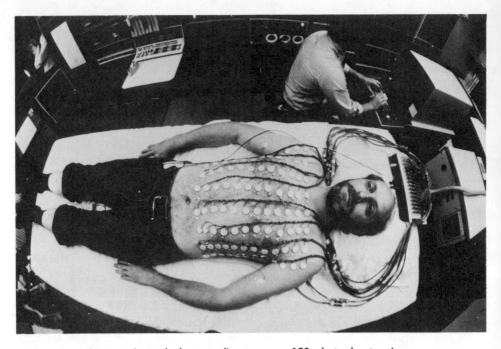

An experimental electrocardiogram uses 190 electrodes to give a clearer picture of the heart's movements than the traditional EKG.

when in a good state of health, because that record can serve as a benchmark for comparing electrocardiograms made later in life when the condition of the heart may have changed. This rule applies to all other health examination records as well.

Urinalysis

No patient health evaluation is complete without the findings of laboratory tests of blood and urine. The doctor or his assistant may give special instructions about food and water intake well in advance of the time for delivering a urine specimen because those factors can influence the chemical makeup of the sample. The time of day of the collection also can affect the composition of the urine sample; urine voided early in the morning is likely to be more acid in content, while urine collected after a meal may be more alkaline. Thus, for a routine physical, the doctor may advise that a urine sample be taken at his office at 9 a.m. but that nothing be eaten since the previous evening meal. The doctor also may want not the first, but the second specimen of the day. In some cases, depending upon the patient's complaint, the doctor may request a collection of all the urine voided during a period of 12 or 24 hours.

CHEMICAL CONTENT OF THE URINE: A typical urine sample is, of course, mostly water. But it also may contain about two dozen identifiable minerals and other chemicals, including sodium, potassium, calcium, sulfur, ammonia, urea, and several different acids. A urine sample can range in color from pale straw to dark amber, depending upon the concentration.

It also can be other colors, including orange or blue, or even colorless, depending upon foods eaten, medications taken, diseases, or exposure to toxic substances.

APPEARANCE AND ACIDITY: The urine sample's general appearance, including color, is noted by the laboratory technician. The sample also is tested for acidity or alkalinity, normal urine being just slightly on the acid side of neutral. Urine that is definitely acidic can be a sign of a variety of disorders, including certain metabolic problems. Urine that is markedly on the alkaline side of neutral also can suggest a number of possible disorders, including an infection of the urinary tract. Alkalinity could also be caused by certain medications, or even by the patient's use of large doses of bicarbonate of soda. Foods rich in protein can make the urine more acidic, while citrus fruits and some vegeta-bles may tend to make a patient's urine more alkaline.

WHAT THE URINE SHOWS: A thorough analysis of a person's urine can turn up some clues to the condition of almost every part of the body and verify or rule out the presence of myriad physical disorders. The specific gravity of the urine, for example, can indicate the general health of the urinary tract; protein (albumin) tests may tell something about the condition of the kidneys and prostate and, in a pregnant women, indicate toxemia; glucose (sugar) in the urine could suggest diabetes; the presence of ketone bodies could be a sign of metabolic disorders; bilirubin (bile) in the urine could be a sign of liver disease, and so on. Various urine tests check for the presence of red blood cells or white blood cells, tissue cells from the lining of organs, various hormones, traces of drugs taken, fat bodies,

Examining a patient's urine is a time-honored method of diagnosing disease, as is evident in this sixteenth century woodcut from Italy.

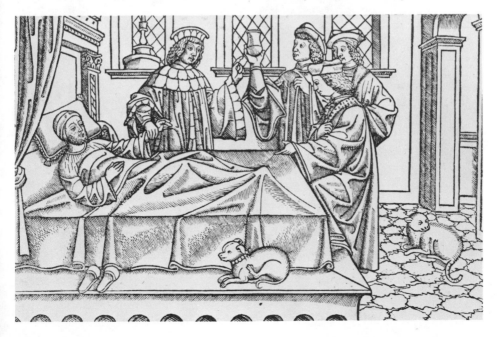

parasites, indications of renal calculi (kidney stones), and a variety of bits of tissue, often microscopic, called *casts*. One kind of cast might be a sign of heart failure or shock, another might be a warning of heavy-metal poisoning, a third might indicate a kidney infection.

Blood Tests

Laboratory blood studies also can reveal bits of information about organ systems throughout the body. For a simple blood test, a few drops may be drawn from a capillary through a finger prick; more detailed blood tests can require the equivalent of a couple of teaspoonfuls of blood drawn from a vein in the arm. The amount of blood taken for a laboratory test is not harmful; a normal body manufactures a couple of ounces of new blood every day, several times the amount used for a laboratory test.

RED CELLS: For a count of red blood cells (RBC), or *erythrocytes*, a small part of the original blood sample may be diluted and a bit of the solution placed on a special microscope slide that enables the technician to estimate the average number of red blood cells per cubic millimeter of blood. The normal RBC range for a man is in the neighborhood of 4.8 to 5.8 million red blood cells per cubic millimeter of blood; for a woman, the RBC count is about 4.4 to 5.4 million. For a child, the normal figure is slightly less than that of a woman.

The blood sample also may be checked for the level of hemoglobin, an iron-protein substance that gives the blood its red color and makes it possible for blood to carry

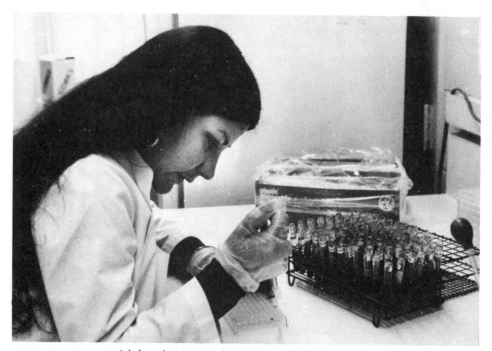

A lab technician conducting a test of blood samples.

oxygen to all parts of the body. A below-normal level of hemoglobin could be a sign of anemia due to a number of possible causes, including actual loss of blood from hemorrhage, vitamin deficiencies, lack of iron in the diet, or a disease.

WHITE CELLS: White blood cell (WBC), or *leukocyte,* counts are made the same way as RBC counts. The total normal WBC count for both men and women ranges from 5,000 to 10,000 per cubic millimeter. A higher count would indicate the presence of an infection or other disease problem.

OTHER FACTORS: Other blood studies may be performed for information about the coagulation characteristics of a patient's blood sample, levels of calcium, sodium, potassium, and other chemicals present, presence of certain enzymes, acidity of the blood, levels of sugar, bilirubin, urea nitrogen, cholesterol and other fatty substances, alcohol and other drugs, and proteins, including albumin.

Not all of these tests are performed during a routine physical examination, but they could be used if needed to track down the cause of an otherwise elusive set of symptoms. By comparing the results of two blood enzyme tests, for example, it would be possible to sort out symptoms of six different kinds of liver disease as well as a heart attack and infectious mononucleosis. The results might not be the final answer to a medical problem, but the laboratory test data could be important pieces of the jigsaw puzzle that the doctor needs to complete the health picture that begins to take form when the patient enters the doctor's office for a physical examination.

Specialties and Their Diagnostic Procedures

If a definite diagnosis cannot be made on the basis of the medical history and preliminary physical examination, more specialized tests are employed. These are usually made under the direction of a specialist. These specialists and some of the most important of their diagnostic procedures—there are literally hundreds of them—are described below, arranged according to the major body systems.

The Skeleton and the Muscles

The *orthopedic surgeon,* or *orthopedist,* is the major specialist in the diagnosis, treatment, and surgical correction of diseases and injuries of the bones, joints, and musculature. Because the healthy functioning of muscles is closely involved with the nervous system, the *neurologist* is frequently consulted. The branch of internal medicine called *rheumatology* is specially concerned with the joints.

The teeth and their supporting structures are, of course, the concern of *dentistry* and the *dentist.* The *orthodontist* is a dentist specializing in the alignment of teeth and their proper positioning in the mouth. A *pediatric dentist* specializes in teeth problems of young people up to the time that the second set of teeth erupt. An *oral surgeon* (dental surgeon) performs surgery within the oral cavity, including tooth extraction. He and the orthodontist have had additional training after receiving the dental degree, and the oral surgeon may have a medical degree (M.D.) as well. The *periodontist* treats gum disorders.

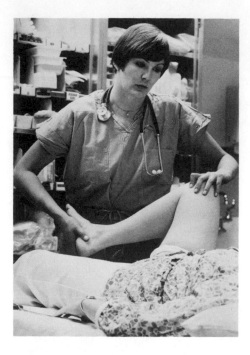

Orthopedic surgery, which deals with bone defects and diseases, was long considered a specialty for men only; recently women have entered the field.

DIAGNOSTIC PROCEDURES: *X rays* are probably relied upon more than any other technique for special investigations of the bones, joints, and teeth. They can reveal a tiny tooth cavity, a hairline fracture of a major bone, a bony deposit, or an eroded surface around a joint. *Serum analysis*—laboratory investigation of the clear portion separated from a person's blood sample—can also reveal underlying chemical irregularities that accompany or precede bone and joint diseases.

Synovial aspiration (also called *synovial fluid exam*) involves the withdrawal of a tiny amount of fluid (synovial fluid) with a needle inserted into a joint. The laboratory analysis of the fluid can diagnose gout and some forms of arthritis.

Electromyography can give an electrical tracing of muscle nerve function and reveal the presence of disorders.

Muscle biopsy is the surgical excision of a small piece of muscle tissue for laboratory examination and tests.

Skin, Hair, and Nails

The *dermatologist* is the principal specialist. *Skin biopsy,* the removal of a piece of skin tissue for laboratory testing and microscopic study, is used for difficult diagnoses.

The Nervous System and the Brain

The *neurosurgeon,* sometimes popularly referred to as a brain surgeon, is qualified for diagnosis, treatment, and surgery of the brain and nervous system. The term *neurologist* is generally restricted to a physician who does not perform surgery. The neurologist may be an internist having neurology as a subspeciality.

DIAGNOSTIC PROCEDURES: A *spinal fluid exam* or spinal tap involves the withdrawal by special needle under sterile conditions, and subsequent laboratory examination, of a small amount of cerebrospinal fluid for the diagnosis of polio, meningitis, brain tumors, and other conditions. The *electroencephalogram* (EEG) gives a picture of, and shows irregularities in, a person's "brain waves." The *echoencephalogram* uses ultrasonic waves, rather than the electric currents of the EEG, to investigate the functioning of the brain. A *brain scan* calls for the injection of a radioactive element into the brain tissue or fluid and records its movements on a photographic plate.

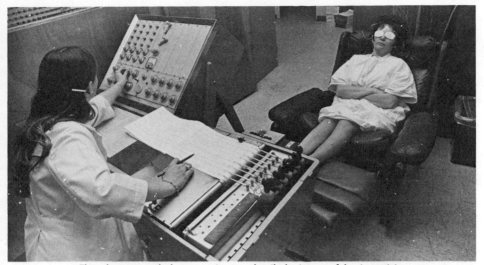

The electroencephalogram gives a detailed picture of brain activity.
Electrodes placed on the patient's head record brain waves in detail.

Recently, an X-ray technique utilizing a computer and known as *CAT scanning* (for *computerized axial tomography*) has proved to be most effective for visualizing "slices" of the brain that would otherwise be inaccessible, and no injection is necessary. Sometimes called a *brain scanner,* the device takes a series of pictures as it is rotated around the patient. From data fed into a computer, the computer generates composite pictures of the brain.

The *cerebral arteriogram* is a method of visualizing and assaying

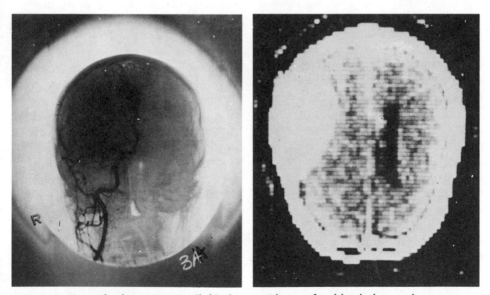

A cerebral arteriogram *(left)* shows evidence of a blood clot on the surface of a patient's brain. A CAT scan *(right)* of the same individual clearly shows the clot as a white area in the upper left section of the scan.

brain damage by injecting a dye into the blood vessels serving the brain and then X-raying them. It is especially useful in judging the severity and location of hemorrhages and strokes. A *pneumoencephalogram* is an X-ray picture of the brain taken after air or gas has been injected into the ventricles of the brain.

The Circulatory System, the Heart, and Blood

The *cardiologist* is an internist who has special knowledge in the diagnosis and medical treatment of heart disease. The *hematologist* is an internist who has special training in the techniques of diagnosing and treating diseases of the blood (including lymph) and bone marrow.

The *thoracic surgeon* is a surgeon who has satisfied the requirements of licensing boards for both general surgery and thoracic (chest cavity) surgery. He has special training in the surgical treatment of defects and diseases of the heart and large blood vessels. The *vascular surgeon* is a general surgeon specializing in the surgical treatment of diseases of blood vessels.

DIAGNOSTIC PROCEDURES: The *electrocardiogram* graphically records the electrical activity of the heart associated with contraction of the cardiac muscle. It can provide valuable information regarding disorders of or damage to the heart muscle (i.e. heart attack), disturbances in rhythm, or enlargement of any of the four chambers of the heart. A *vectorcardiogram* is similar to the electrocardiogram, but more specifically attuned to the magnitude and direction of the electrical currents of the heart. Abnormalities not apparent on the electrocardiogram may often be revealed by a vectorcardiogram.

The *phonocardiogram* is a recording on paper of the heart sounds, which enables the physician to evaluate murmurs and abnormal heart sounds with more accuracy than by listening with the stethoscope. The timing of the murmur with relation to the specific events of heart muscle contraction may also be precisely evaluated. The *echocardiogram* provides a paper tracing of sound waves which are directed towards, and subsequently bounced back from, various internal heart structures. The technique is useful in diagnosing abnormalities of the heart valves, as well as abnormal collections of fluid in the sac (pericardium) enveloping the heart.

The *fluoroscope* visualizes the heart in action by use of X rays. It is useful in the evaluation of heart and vessel pulsation as well as valve or vessel calcification. Plain *chest X rays* may reveal enlargement of the heart, abnormal calcification of vessels or heart valves, and signs of a congestive heart valve. These are only three examples of the great number of abnormalities that can be revealed by a routine chest X ray.

The *cardiac X-ray series* are a number of X rays of the chest taken in several positions as the patient swallows a liquid, for example, barium sulfate, which makes the esophagus stand out on the X ray. This is usually called a barium swallow. Indentation of the esophagus by abnormally enlarged heart chambers may be revealed by this technique. "Barium meals" are also important in the radiologic diagnosis of disorders of the esophagus, stomach, and small intestine.

Cardiac catheterization is the in-

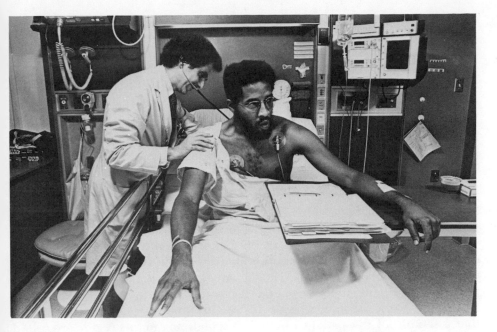

A physician examines a heart patient to see if he is ready to be transferred out of the hospital's cardiac intensive care unit.

sertion of a small tubular surgical instrument, via a vein in the arm or artery of the leg, through the blood vessels, directly into the right or left side of the heart. This procedure is employed to confirm suspected intracardiac (within the heart) anomalies, determine intracardiac pressures, and take blood samples. Catheterization enables the physician to confirm suspected defects in the walls dividing the heart chambers or to estimate the severity of a lesion and the need for corrective surgery.

Angiocardiography (or simply *angiography*), if warranted, is performed at the same time as cardiac catheterization. Its principle involves the injection of a contrast material (e.g., a substance visible on a fluoroscopy screen or X-ray film) by means of the catheter, with consequent visualization of the heart and major blood vessels. Angiog-

raphy is not limited to investigation of the heart chambers but can reveal abnormalities of large vessels such as the aorta, coronary arteries, and renal arteries.

CAT scanning, mentioned above on p. 889, is becoming an increasingly important diagnostic tool and may in many cases make angiocardiography unnecessary. Sometimes called a *body scanner,* the CAT scanner takes a series of computer-assisted X-ray pictures as it slowly rotates around the patient, thus providing cross-sectional pictures of the target organ. It is a painless and safe procedure, and is capable of providing pictures of areas of the body that would be very difficult to visualize by any other means.

HEMATOLOGICAL (BLOOD SAMPLING) DIAGNOSTIC TECHNIQUES: Routine laboratory tests performed in all hospital admissions are the *peripheral smear* and *complete blood count.* Approximately 5 milliliters (ml) of blood are *aspirated* (withdrawn by suction) from a vein, typically in the crease of the elbow. From this sample, a determination of the patient's hemoglobin and percentage of red corpuscles per milliliter of plasma may be calculated. Microscopic analysis of the number and character of the red cells, white cells, and platelets provides additional essential information. See also p. 886.

If an abnormality such as decreased hemoglobin or overpopulation of white cells is noted on complete blood count and peripheral smear, the physician might request that a sample of the patient's bone marrow be obtained for evaluation —a procedure called *bone marrow biopsy.* Following local anesthesia of the operative site, typically the hip bone, a biopsy needle is inserted into the marrow of the bone and a small sample of marrow is withdrawn. If performed by an experienced physician, the patient feels only some pressure and very slight pain as the marrow sample is aspirated.

In suspected cases of *neoplastic* diseases—diseases involving abnormal growths that may be or may become malignant—a *lymph node biopsy* (surgical excision and microscopic examination of lymph node tissue) is performed. A *lymphangiogram* is used when tumors of the lymphatic system are suspected. A dye or contrast material visible on an X ray is injected into a lymphatic vessel, usually one on the top of the foot. X rays of the abdomen taken over the next several days are studied for abnormalities in the size and structure of internal lymph nodes.

There are numerous other hematological tests, including radioactive (radio-isotope) tests, which are used in special situations when diagnosis by other means is inadequate.

The Digestive System and the Liver

The internist is generally able to treat most gastrointestinal disorders. The *gastroenterologist* is an internist who has special knowledge of disorders of the digestive tract. *Colon and rectal surgeons* operate on the large intestine, rectum, and anus; *proctology* deals with the diagnosis and treatment of disorders in this area. Surgeons and internists specializing in this region are called *proctologists.*

DIAGNOSTIC PROCEDURES: Examination can be made of the esophagus, stomach, and duodenum, and sometimes of the entire length of the small intestine, by using a sequence of many fluoroscope, motion-picture, and X-ray pictures. This is called the *gastrointestinal series,* or simply the *GI series.* So that the internal walls of the digestive organs will stand out clearly in the pictures, the patient eats nothing for eight hours before, and when the examination begins, he is asked to swallow a glassful of chalky, sticky barium sulfate. The GI series is one of the first tests administered when an ulcer or cancer is suspected in the stomach or duodenum.

Gastric analysis is the extraction and study of stomach juices for clues to intestinal disorders.

A *barium enema* is the injection via the anus of a barium solution; it usually precedes X-ray examination of the large intestine for signs of

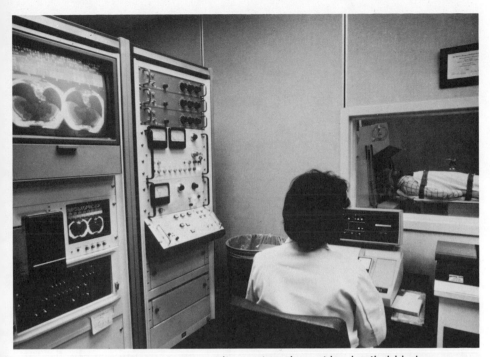

CAT scanning, an important diagnostic tool, provides detailed black-and-white or full-color TV images of a cross-section or "slice" of the body.

cancer or other diseases. *Stool exams,* laboratory studies of the feces, may also reveal cancer as well as the presence of parasitic worms and amebas.

There are a wide variety of slender, hollow, tubular instruments, equipped with a light and a lens to enable the physician to see into the GI tract: the *esophagoscope* for insertion by way of the mouth into the esophagus; the *gastroscope* for inspection of the stomach; the *gastroduodenal fiberscope* for inspection of the stomach and duodenum. "Scopes" inserted via the anus include the *proctosigmoidoscope* for visual examination of the rectum and lower colon, and the *colonoscope* for investigating farther up the large intestine. These are called *fiberoptic* instruments because they transmit light by means of a bundle

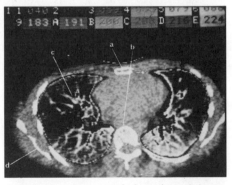

A CAT scan of a normal chest shows (a) sternum, (b) spine, (c) lung, (d) shoulder blade. Panel above indicates tissue densities.

of fibers of glass or plastic which permit observation of curved interior spaces of the body that would otherwise be inaccessible.

Special tests for the liver's health and function include the removal of a tiny piece of liver tissue, by means of a long needle inserted

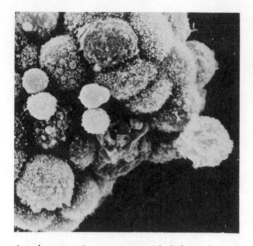

An electron microscope provided this enlarged photo of malignant cells obtained in a *biopsy*—surgical removal of tissue for purposes of diagnosing possible disease.

through the skin, and the tissues' subsequent laboratory examination; this procedure is called *needle biopsy of liver* and often is used to confirm diagnosis of cirrhosis. An injection of a chemical called *BSP*, followed later by analysis of a blood specimen, is used to investigate liver function. A *liver scan*, like a brain scan, employs a radioactive substance to visualize the function of the organ.

X-ray examination of the gall bladder, resulting in a *cholecystogram*—*cholecyst* is a medical name for gall bladder—is used to diagnose gall bladder disease and to locate gallstones. A dye is swallowed before the test.

The Respiratory System and the Lungs

The internist handles most non-surgical disorders, and the thoracic surgeon specializes in surgical procedures involving the respiratory organs.

DIAGNOSTIC PROCEDURES: In the *sputum exam* a number of bacteriological, chemical, and microscopic tests are performed on the sputum (saliva, often mixed with mucus or other substances); these tests can detect a hidden abscess in the respiratory tract, pneumonia, tuberculosis, and other lung diseases.

Practically everybody is aware of the value of *chest X rays* in the diagnosis of diseases and disorders of the lungs, heart, and ribs. Many diseases of the lungs and respiratory system are also revealed by tests administered on the skin. For example, the skin's reaction to a substance called PPD (*p*urified *p*rotein *d*erivative) is used in diagnosing tuberculosis. *Bronchoscopy* is inspection of the bronchial tubes with the tube and scope instrument called the *bronchoscope*.

Special tests that measure lung volume, capacity, and function have become more common as doctors have become conscious of the adverse effects of air pollution and the growing incidence of irreversible diseases such as emphysema.

The Endocrine Glands

There is no AMA-licensed specialty, but the internist-endocrinologist is the expert.

DIAGNOSTIC PROCEDURES: There are a great many tests, using both blood and urine samples, that suggest or confirm the excess or insufficiency of a specific hormone in the body. In turn, these tests point to the overactivity or underactivity of one of the hormone-secreting endocrine glands.

The Sense Organs—Eye, Ear, Nose

The two specialists in this area are both licensed to perform surgery in their special areas of competence. The *ophthalmologist* is the eye doctor. The *otolaryngologist* is the ear, nose, and throat specialist.

DIAGNOSTIC PROCEDURES: We are all familiar with the lettered test charts that determine whether we are nearsighted or farsighted or have some other defect in our eye's focusing apparatus, such as an astigmatism. Color charts to test for color blindness are also commonly used.

With the *ophthalmoscope* and the *slit-lamp microscope,* which magnifies a beam of concentrated light, the ophthalmologist can examine the structures within the eye in great detail. The *retinoscope* reveals the actual structural abnormalities that account for nearsightedness or farsightedness. The *gonioscope* enables the ophthalmologist to inspect the angle between the cornea and the iris, which is of importance in diagnosing glaucoma. The fluid pressure itself within the anterior chamber can be measured by an extremely delicate spring-balance gauge called a *tonometer.* Finally, *perimeter* can be used to map boundaries of the visual field; the narrowing of these boundaries ("tunnel vision" is the extreme example) is a symptom of glaucoma

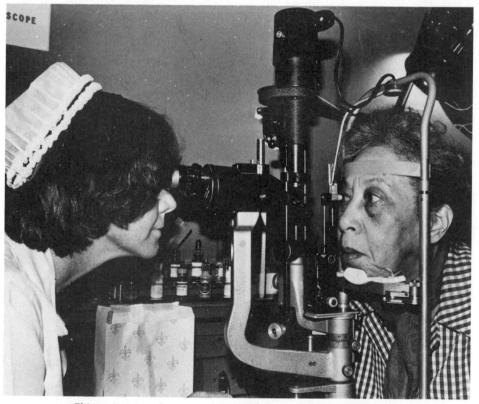

This patient is undergoing a test for glaucoma with a device known as a tonometer, which measures fluid pressure within the eye.

and other eye disorders.

Hearing and hearing loss are measured by a device called the *audiometer*, with which a physician can measure accurately the whole range of vibrations heard as sound by the human ear. The *otoscope* is an instrument for examining the external auditory canal and eardrum.

The Urinogenital System and the Kidneys

The *urologist* is the acknowledged specialist. He does not deal, however, with the female reproductive organs, which are the specialty of the obstetrician and gynecologist.

DIAGNOSTIC PROCEDURES: The collective name for a number of tests that analyze the contents or urine is *urinalysis*. These include tests of the urine's physical properties, as well as chemical and microscopic analysis. Telltale signs of diseases of the kidneys and bladder often show up in urine, and sugar in the urine may be an indication of diabetes. *Urine culture* is a test for microbial infections of the urinary tract. See also p. 568.

Pyelograms are X-ray examinations of the interior of the kidney (kidney pelvis) and of the tube (ureter) carrying urine away from the kidney to the bladder. Pyelograms may involve the injection of a substance into the patient's bloodstream to facilitate viewing of the kidney area.

The special hollow tube, lens, and light instrument called a *cystoscope* is used to view the inside of the bladder after being inserted up the urethra. *Voiding cystometrics* test the condition and capacity of the bladder by pumping water into it, measuring the resulting pressures, and timing the onset of the desire to void.

The technique of *needle biopsy*, discussed in respect to the liver under *The Digestive System and the Liver*, p. 892, is also used to examine kidney and prostate tissue.

For a discussion of diagnostic procedures for the female reproductive system, see *The Gynecological Examination*, p. 988. Diagnostic procedures are also discussed under *Surgery*, p. 900.

Patients' Rights

Diagnostic procedures have raised many questions centering on patients' rights. The questions concern both physicians and hospitals, and relate to the general right of a patient to know what is happening to him or her and why.

Efforts to develop lists of specific rights that the patient enjoys have gone far beyond the specific area of diagnosis and treatment. The lists touch on such matters as the patient's need to maintain privacy, his or her right to be informed of any surgical or other procedures to be performed, and the right to refuse treatment to the extent permitted by law. One such "Bill of Rights" was issued by the American Hospital Association in 1973. It noted in part:

Equitable and humane treatment at all times and under all circumstances is a right. This principle entails an obligation on the part of all those involved in the care of the patient to recognize and to respect his individuality and his dignity. This means creating and fostering relationships founded on mutual acceptance and trust.

Like other statements on patients' rights, the AHA list stressed *informed consent*. That meant the need on the part of the patient to be able to agree to medical and surgical treatment on the basis of complete, accurate information. Informed consent as a principle provided the foundation for many other specific or general rights. These include:

• The right to considerate and respectful care

• The right to take part in planning for one's own care

• The right to have records kept confidential

• The right to full explanation of the hospital bill

Questions to Ask the Doctor

The various rights suggest some of the questions the patient may want to ask the doctor—either at the time of the first visit or later. For example, most patients want to know the results of diagnostic tests and procedures. Patients may also ask about planned treatments, the risks and chances of success or failure with particular types of treatment, and the period of time for which the patient may be hospitalized.

Many other factors become important. Where one patient may want to know about alternative forms of care or treatment, another may ask about the surgeons who may perform an operation, the specialists who may be called in, and so on. Typically, most questions relate to the patient's situation: how far it has progressed, whether danger to life or health is involved, the doctor's estimate of the chances of recovery, and other points. Doctors themselves suggest that patients ask questions to find out . .

1. whether hospitalization, if it has been recommended, is really necessary;

2. whether consultation with another doctor or other doctors may be called for;

3. whether—if necessary—medical terms or wordings can be clarified; and

4. whether, in case the patient is in doubt, the doctor understood what the patient reported about symptoms, history, prescriptions already taken, and similar data.

Common sense usually indicates what other questions the patient should ask the doctor. The patient may have to make allowances for medical procedures. For instance, a thorough physical examination always requires that the patient undress—but no invasion of privacy is intended. Most important, the patient's right to free communication should be respected, and the patient should understand that it is.

Diagnostic Tests and Patients' Rights

Many diagnostic tests and procedures have been discussed. Many others could be listed.

One reason is that as medical costs have risen in recent years, some persons have questioned the necessity of various diagnostic tests. Consumer advocates have insisted that patients in some hospitals have been charged for tests that only increased their hospital bills. In some cases the tests were given in *batteries*, or sets. The question that has come up: Did the patients actually understand all those tests and what they involved?

Cost, as both outsiders and members of the medical profession admit, has definitely become a factor in medical care. An electro-cardiogram may cost only $20 or $30; but a computerized axial tomography (CAT) scan can cost $500 to $600.

Another reason why questions about patients' rights have been raised centers on the nature of test batteries and the time available to doctors. The batteries can be complex, and the physician may often be short of time. He may find it difficult or impossible to explain every test he has ordered—and to do so in enough detail so that the patient knows what each test requires and what it means in terms of discomfort, risk, and cost.

Hospital admission tests may be simple or complex. They may involve only "vital signs" tests of temperature, pulse rate, respiratory rate, and blood pressure. But they can include the *admission labs*—screening tests done by automated machines. These tests may include a urinalysis (UA), a complete blood count (CBC), and serum chemistries—Simultaneous Multiple Analyzer tests of 12 (SMA-12) or 24 (SMA-24) factors. The SMA-12 would typically call for chemical analyses for calcium, inorganic phosphorus, glucose, and nine other body elements.

Admission labs usually also include a test for syphilis, a chest X-ray, and an EKG. The latter is often considered essential for patients over 40. Together, the admission labs tell the physician a number of important facts about the state of the patient's health.

Literally dozens of other tests could be noted. All involve some degree of risk and discomfort for the patient. But for most admission tests, both risk and discomfort are minimal. When the patient agrees to undergo them in batteries, is his or her right of informed consent being violated?

The Doctor's Challenge

That question cannot be answered in a single word. The doctor faces a dilemma in nearly all cases. He or she has to ask how much information can and should be transmitted—and how much the patient can absorb without becoming confused. He or she has also to ask what degree of risk is involved in any test or series of tests. Then the doctor has to weigh the advantages of having test readings against the disadvantages involved in not having those test results. For a woman under 35, a test for cancer such as the mammogram may entail some risk if administered regularly (annually). For an older woman the risk is considered minimal.

With some tests, the risk for the patient is slight to virtually nonexistent. But all tests given in batteries involve some risk, however minor. Does that mean that administration of tests in batteries increases the risk element significantly? It may, say those who argue against administration of tests by sets or groups.

The protocols or understandings on patients' rights establish fairly loose standards. That applies particularly in the area of information to be given to the patient. Thus the physician has to make a judgment decision in many cases. He or she tries to find out what the patient wants to know and whether all the needed information is readily available. The doctor may even have to do some "homework" to answer the patient's questions.

Authorities agree that doctors should spend time with patients and their families to the extent necessary to clarify procedures, risks, and prognoses. Doctors are also advised to talk to patients in a direct and honest manner, and in layman's terms. By such means the patient's rights are protected. The doctor also finds out what he or she needs to know to make an accurate diagnosis.

CHAPTER 20

Surgery

WHAT YOU SHOULD KNOW BEFORE UNDERGOING SURGERY

Almost everyone can expect to be wheeled into an operating room at some point in his lifetime. Surveys of hospitals during the 1970s indicated that about 12,000,000 people in the United States were surgery patients in a typical year. The range of surgical procedures performed every year is vast—correction of broken bones, organ transplants, facial uplifts, hernia repairs, hysterectomies, Caesarian sections, vasectomies, appendectomies, and so on. It is obviously impossible for a work of this sort to describe more than a fraction of the thousands of surgical procedures and their variations that are widely performed. For a representative sampling of some specific surgical procedures, see *Common Surgical Procedures*, beginning on p. 926.

The seriousness of surgical procedures within the same category can vary widely. For example, one case of inguinal hernia may be repaired quickly and simply in a young man physically able to leave the hospital on the same day he arrived. Another inguinal hernia case could be a real emergency if a portion of the small intestine were to become trapped in the hernia sac protruding into the abdominal wall, resulting in the death of the bowel-tissue cells. Easy generalizations about the seriousness of a given procedure are simply not warranted.

Types of Surgery

Surgery is sometimes categorized according to whether it is vital to life, necessary for continued health, or desirable for medical or personal reasons. Although there are many ways in which surgical procedures are classified, the following breakdown is one that is widely accepted among surgeons.

Emergency Surgery

Most disorders requiring surgery do not improve by delaying the trip to the hospital. Some can be planned and scheduled so as to coincide with periods in which a few days in the hospital will be unlikely to interfere with job or family responsibilities. But unfortunately there are also unpredictable events that precipitate an immediate need for surgery. An automobile accident, a fire, a violent crime, or even a sudden change in a chronic medical problem like a perforated ulcer or a strangulated hernia, can create situations in which the life of the patient depends upon the time it takes to get the victim into the hands of a trained surgeon. Emergency surgery cases typically involve the treatment of gunshot and stab wounds, fractures of the skull and other major bones, severe eye injuries, or life-threatening situations such as obstruction of the windpipe caused by choking on a piece of food.

Emergency surgery may be one of the most common routes for patients entering the operating room. Accident patients, according to one estimate, require four times as many hospital beds as cancer patients and more hospital beds than all heart patients. They account for more than a half-million deaths and disabilities in America each year. They present tremendous challenges to surgeons

A physician is ready to examine a patient arriving in the emergency room with a severe wound that will undoubtedly need emergency surgery.

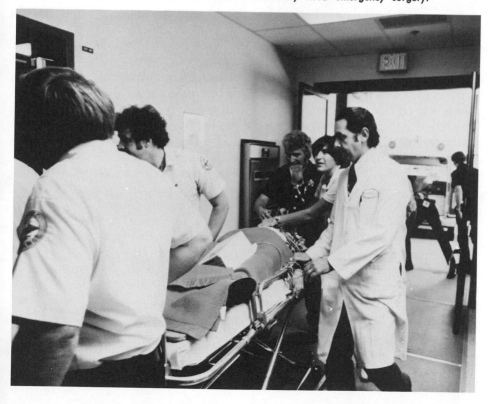

because emergency room patients frequently have multiple injuries involving several organ systems. Such victims are often unconscious or otherwise unable to communicate coherently about their injuries, and there may be little or no time to obtain medical histories or information about their blood types, allergies to medicines, etc.

When possible, vital information about the patient and the circumstances surrounding the injury or sudden need for surgery is obtained by medical personnel who question anybody who might provide one or more clues. Efforts to maintain life are begun even while blood samples are taken for laboratory analysis and X-ray photographs made of the chest, abdomen, and other body areas that may be involved. Many *heroic* measures—extreme measures taken when a life is in immediate peril—may be used in critical cases; for example, resuscitation, induction of anesthesia, and surgery might proceed simultaneously as soon as a diagnosis is made. When several teams are working on the patient at the same time, a general surgeon may be called upon to coordinate the multiple operating room procedures.

The Emergency Room

As the first part of the hospital to which patients with emergency problems are admitted, the emergency room (ER) plays a key role in making total medical care available. Not all patients admitted to the emergency room will require surgery; in fact, estimates place the number of *nonemergency cases* encountered in the typical emergency room at 50 to 75 percent. That means one-half to two-thirds of all ER patients cannot be classified as true emergency cases. But the ER staff has to be prepared to deal with cuts and bruises as well as with major emergencies that can, at worst, result in death.

The emergency room may or may not be part of the hospital's outpatient department. In either case, the ER remains what has been called a "stepchild" of the hospital system: it has its own record-keeping and admission procedures, and in general operates fairly independently of the rest of the hospital. But the ER physician makes the initial decisions regarding the seriousness of an emergency. He or she also provides initial treatment, and may ask for immediate tests of various kinds to make possible rapid diagnoses.

The patient reporting to the emergency room becomes an "emergency outpatient." He is thus distinguished from the "general outpatient" who receives various hospital services on an outpatient basis and is the responsibility of the hospital for further care and treatment. The emergency outpatient is different also from the "referred outpatient" who is referred by a doctor and who remains the doctor's responsibility while utilizing hospital services.

The inpatient, by contrast, is formally admitted to the hospital and assigned to a ward and bed. Special types of records are kept. Where the outpatient typically occupies a bed for a few hours, if at all, an inpatient may remain for weeks or even months. Once the emergency outpatient moves on to utilize the hospital's regular clinical or medical servic—including surgery—he or she ceases to be the responsibility of the outpatient department and becomes an inpatient.

Like all medical costs, the fees for emergency outpatient care have been rising steadily. In the early 1980s the basic per-visit fee reached $25 to $35. Other charges were regularly made for tests according to schedules that varied from hospital to hospital. For example, of the chemical analyses that could be ordered, a bilirubin test might cost $7.50 to $10. A complete blood count (CBC) might cost $12 to $15. Depending on the area of the body examined, an X-ray could cost from $50 to $90.

Urgent Surgery

Next in priority for the surgeon are cases in which an operation is vital but can be postponed for a few days. A person injured in an automobile accident, but conscious and suffering a minor bone fracture may be classed as an urgent rather than emergency surgery case, and the delay would give surgeons and other medical personnel time to study X rays carefully, evaluate blood tests and other diagnostic data, and otherwise plan corrective therapy while under less pressure. A penetrating ulcer of the stomach likely would be classed as urgent surgery, but the ulcer case would become emergency surgery if it were to rupture through the stomach wall. An acute, inflamed gall bladder, kidney stones, or cancer of a vital organ would be examples of urgent surgery cases.

Elective Surgery

Elective surgery is usually subdivided into three categories: required, selective, and optional.

REQUIRED SURGERY: Physical ailments that are serious enough to need corrective surgery, but which can be scheduled a matter of weeks or months in advance, generally are designated as required surgery cases. Conditions such as a chronically inflamed gall bladder, cataracts, bone deformities, or diseased tonsils and adenoids would be examples of conditions that require surgery. Also in this classification might be cases of uncomplicated inguinal hernia, hiatal hernia, and surgery of the reproductive organs that do not need immediate attention.

SELECTIVE SURGERY: Selective surgery covers a broad range of conditions which are of no real threat to the health of the patient but nevertheless should be corrected by surgery in order to improve his comfort and well-being. Certain congenital defects such as cleft lip (harelip) and cleft palate would be included in this classification, as well as removal of certain cysts and nonmalignant fatty or fibrous tumors. Selective surgery also might include operations to correct crossed eyes in children so that normal binocular vision can develop properly.

OPTIONAL SURGERY: Of the lowest priority are operations that are primarily of cosmetic benefit, such as removal of warts and other nonmalignant growths on the skin, blemishes of the skin, and certain cases of varicose veins. Optional surgery also includes various kinds of plastic surgery undertaken for cosmetic effect. Among popular types of plastic surgery are operations to change the shape of female breasts; this would include the correction of unusually large or pendulous breasts as well as the enlargement of unusually small breasts. Other common plastic surgery procedures are *rhinoplasty*, or nose shaping; *otoplasty*, the correction of protuding ears; *blepharoplasty*, the removal of bags under the eyes; and *rhytidoplasty*, known popularly as a facelift. Rhytidoplasty is relatively simple, virtually painless, and effective; because the benefits usually are temporary, it is an operation which many patients volunteer to undergo more than once. For fuller information on these procedures, see *Plastic and Cosmetic Surgery*, p. 976.

Since the end of World War II, there has been a proliferation of surgical specialties. The general surgeon of past eras who handled all kinds of operations is gradually being replaced by a battery of highly specialized experts who may work only on the nervous system, the eye, the ear, the bones and muscles, and so on. When warranted, a patient's case may be handled by several different surgical specialists. The result has been safer, more effective surgical treatment for the average patient.

Pre-operative Procedures

Preparation of a patient for surgery involves a variety of procedures determined by the urgency of the operation, the anatomical area involved, the nature of the disease or injury requiring surgery, the general condition of the patient, and other factors. Emergency surgery of an accident victim in critical condition obviously requires a greatly accelerated pace of preparing the patient for the operating room; medical personnel may cut away the clothing of the victim in order to save precious minutes. An operation on the intestine, on the other hand, may require a full week of preparation, including the five or so days needed to sterilize the bowel with drugs and evaluate laboratory tests. However, most pre-op procedures, as they are commonly called, generally follow a similar pattern designed to insure a safe and sound operation. Even in a case of emergency surgery, certain information must be compiled to help guide the surgeon and other hospital staff personnel in making the right decisions affecting proper care of the patient during and after the operation.

Medical History

This pattern begins with a medical history of the patient. The medical history should reveal the general health of the patient and any factors that might increase the risk of surgery. Perhaps one of his parents or another close relative suffered from heart disease or diabetes; such facts might suggest a predisposition of the patient to problems associated with those disorders. The data should also show whether the patient has a tendency to bleed easily, and whether he has been following a special diet such as a sodium-restricted diet.

It is important that the patient reveal quite frankly to his own doctor, the surgeon, and the anesthetist the names of any drugs or other medications used. It also is vital that the medical personnel have a complete record of any patient experiences, including allergic reactions to certain drugs, that might help predict drug sensitivities that could complicate the surgery. The simple fact that a patient suffers from asthma or hay fever might indicate that he may be more sensitive than other individuals to drugs that might be administered.

ALLERGIC REACTIONS: Some patients are allergic to penicillin or other antibiotics. Others may be sensitive to aspirin or serums. Still others could be allergic to iodine, Merthiolate, or even adhesive tape. All of these factors should be brought to the attention of the medical staff, if they are known and if they apply to the patient about to undergo surgery.

MEDICATIONS CURRENTLY BEING USED: Among medications routinely used by the patient that should be brought to the attention of the surgeon and anesthetist are insulin for diabetes, digitalis drugs for heart diseases, and cortisone for arthritis. Depending upon various factors relating to the individual case, the patient may be directed to continue using the medication as usual, change the size of the dose before or after surgery, or discontinue the drug entirely for a while.

A patient who has been taking certain sedatives or drinking alcoholic beverages regularly for a prolonged period before surgery may have developed a tolerance for the anesthetic used, which means that he would require a larger than usual dose to get the desired effect. A patient who has been using epinephrine-type eye drops for glaucoma may be asked to increase the dosage before surgery as an adjustment to

one of the drugs used in conjunction with a general anesthetic.

Diuretics, tranquilizers, and anticoagulant drugs are among other medications commonly used by patients that could affect the manner in which a surgical procedure is carried out. When possible, the patient should take a sample of the medication, a copy of the prescription, or the pharmacist's label from a container of the medication to the hospital so the medical staff can verify the type of drug used.

PSYCHOLOGICAL EVALUATION: Of increasing importance in recent years has been a psychological evaluation of the patient. Individuals with a past history of mental disease or patients whose complaints may be based on psychoneurotic factors may react differently to surgery than persons who could be described as psychologically well-balanced. The pre-operative interviews also may seek to obtain information about the patient's use of drugs of abuse or alcohol; a patient who has developed a physical dependence upon alcohol could develop withdrawal symptoms after suddenly being separated from alcoholic beverages during his hospital stay.

Physical Examination

In addition to the medical history evaluation, the surgeon will need vital information about the physical condition of the patient. This requires a complete physical examination, including a chest X ray, an electrocardiogram of the heart activity, a neurological examination, and a check of the condition of the blood vessels in various areas of the body. Other body areas may be checked as

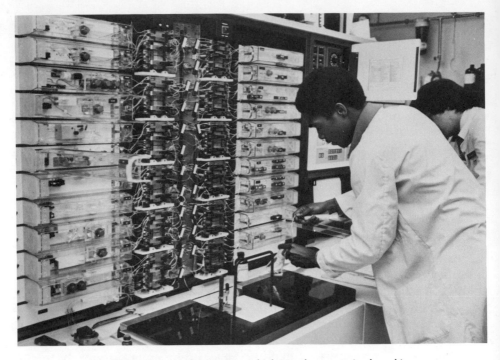

A wealth of tests precedes surgery. A high-speed computerized machine can analyze 150 blood samples an hour, making up to 20 tests on each.

warranted by complaints of the patient or by the type of surgery to be performed. An examination of the rectum and colon may be suggested, for example, if the medical history includes problems related to the digestive tract. Adult women patients usually receive a Pap test and possibly a pelvic examination. Samples of blood and urine are taken for laboratory analysis, including blood typing in the event a transfusion is needed. The laboratory tests for older patients frequently are more detailed and may include an examination of a stool sample.

Many hospitals and surgeons will accept information obtained from a pre-op examination conducted several days or more before admission to the hospital for surgery, especially for elective surgery. By completing the blood and urine tests, physical examination, X rays, electrocardiograms, and medical history interview in advance of the trip to the hospital, the patient can reduce the length of the hospital stay. In some instances, the patient may be able to report to the hospital the night before the surgery is scheduled or even a few hours ahead of actual surgery. However, additional blood and urine samples may be taken immediately after admission to recheck the body chemistry, and a brief physical examination may be made to make sure the patient does not have any open wounds or infections that might complicate the chances of recovery or introduce a dangerous strain of bacteria into the sterile environment of the operating room.

Preparation for Anesthesia

After the patient is settled in his assigned bed, he is visited by the anesthetist who will be working with the surgeon. The anesthetist usually has an advance copy of all the information obtained by the surgeon and other doctors who have examined the patient, along with laboratory reports of blood chemistry, etc. He may want to review the information with the patient and examine him briefly to learn more about his particular problem. If the patient uses a medication that might interfere with the intended effects of the anesthetic to be used, the anesthetist will make a decision regarding the best way to avoid a possible chemical conflict during surgery.

Other Preparations

In a typical case of elective surgery, the patient can expect to experience the actual pre-operative preparations on the afternoon or evening before surgery is scheduled. If blood transfusions may be required, there will be a final check by the hospital staff to make sure enough units of the correct cross-matched type are available.

If the surgery involves the lower digestive tract, or is an abdominal operation that may result in a disturbance of normal bowel function, the patient can expect to be given an enema. However, enemas are not administered routinely to surgery patients who are being prepared for other kinds of operations. An exception to the rule would be patients who complain of constipation.

Legal Authorization

Before the pre-operative prepara-

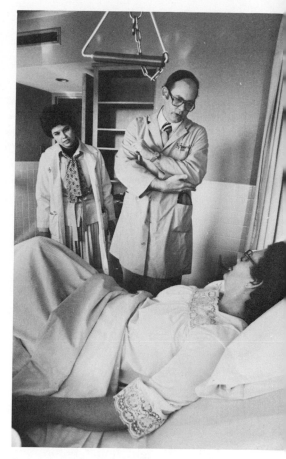

A surgeon explains what he will do and why to a patient the night before her surgery. The patient can also expect visits from the anesthesiologist and any specialists consulting her doctor.

tions are completed, chances are good that a member of the hospital staff will make sure that the patient has signed a permit authorizing the operation. The permit is a legal form describing the operation to be performed, or a special diagnostic or therapeutic procedure other than surgery if that is the purpose of the hospitalization. The statement may be signed by a close relative or legal guardian if for some reason the patient is unable to take responsibility for this action. For example, a parent will be asked to sign a permit authorizing an operation on his or her child.

Exceptions may be made in cases of emergency surgery where the patient is unable to sign a permit and a relative or guardian cannot be located in time. But there are in-house procedures of consultation among staff members who accept the responsibility. Laws regarding permission to perform surgery may vary locally; and in some communities, for example, a married patient cannot authorize surgery that may affect his or her reproductive organs without consent of the spouse. Abortion, likewise, may be illegal in some areas without the husband's consent.

Pre-op Meals

A light but adequate evening meal is served if the surgery is scheduled for the following morning, but no solid food is permitted for 12 hours before surgery. No fluids are allowed during the eight hours before surgery. Children and patients with certain diseases, such as diabetes, may be given special orders regarding nutrients. An infant, for example, may be allowed sweetened orange juice up to four hours before surgery in order to prevent the child from developing restless anxiety because of hunger.

Preparation of the Skin Area

The area of the skin around the surgery site is carefully prepared beginning the evening before the operation. A member of the hospital staff may assist or direct the cleaning of the area with soap and warm water. The cleansing may be done in a shower or tub, or simply with a pan of water and soap brought to the patient's bedside. The cleaned skin area is usually scrubbed again in the operating room as further protection against possible infection.

SHAVING: Whether or not the skin area is to be shaved depends upon the amount of hair present. If there is no hair, the tiny nicks or cuts made by a razor would constitute an unnecessary hazard of infection. Where hair is present, however, shaving is essential in order to make available a very clean skin surface. Also, it is important that no hair or hair fragments be close enough to the surgical incision to fall beneath the skin; the bit of hair beneath the skin could cause a serious infection after surgery. Thus, to clean an area for an inguinal hernia the patient's abdomen may be shaved and scrubbed from a point above the navel down to the mid-thigh level.

Sedation

After all these pre-op steps have been completed, the patient usually is given a bedtime sedative or other medication and additional sedatives plus special medications in the morning, about 30 minutes to an hour before surgery is scheduled to begin.

The Surgical Team

Most surgical operations are performed not by the surgeon alone, but by a surgical team. Depending upon the complexity of the surgical procedure involved, the surgeon may have one or more assistants working with him. The assistants may be interns or hospital residents who participate in the operation as a part of their advanced training in

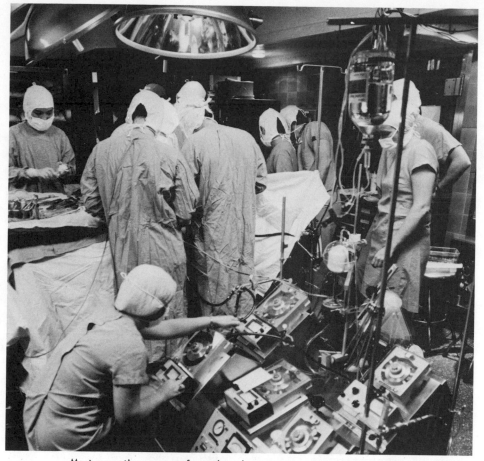

Most operations are performed not by a surgeon alone but by a surgical team, as seen here, with the anesthesiology unit in the foreground.

surgical techniques, or they may be other surgeons who are specialists in a particular field. An abdominal surgeon or orthopedic surgeon, for example, may be assisted by a neurosurgeon if the operation is likely to require a special knowledge of the nervous system as it affects another organ system.

The Anesthetist

The anesthetist, who is also likely to be a physician, specializes in maintaining the proper degree of anesthesia in the patient, while also helping to maintain the body's life systems. The job of the anesthetist is more complicated than one might suppose, because in addition to making the patient unaware of pain during the operation—sometimes by making him unconscious, sometimes without affecting consciousness— the muscles and nervous reflexes must be kept in proper state for the type of surgery to be performed. Each of the various functions—muscle relaxation, reflex paralysis, etc.— requires a different anesthetic drug. Their performance must be perfectly coordinated to prevent complications during the operation. In some

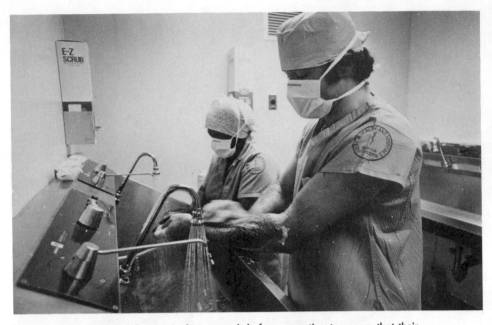

Members of a surgical team scrub before operating to ensure that their hands are sterile—free of germs that could infect the patient.

cases, it may be necessary for the patient to remain awake during the procedure so that he can follow instructions of the surgeon in moving certain muscle groups. At the same time, the patient must have an anesthetic that eliminates pain. Obviously, the anesthetist must prepare a different combination of drugs for a child, an elderly person, a pregnant woman in labor, or a man with a heart disease.

Other Members of the Surgical Team

As noted earlier, there are occasions when several surgeons are working more or less simultaneously on an accident victim with injuries to multiple organ systems. In such cases of emergency surgery, a general surgeon may supervise and coordinate the work of the other surgeons. The nursing staff in the operating room also may be headed by a Chief

Operating Room Nurse, whose responsibility is to supervise and coordinate the activities of the scrub nurses who assist the surgeon in the actual operation and the supply and circulating nurses who aid the rest of the surgical team by making available as needed the various towels, drapes, sponges, sutures, instruments, and other equipment.

One or more of the nurses wear gowns and gloves that have been sterilized so they can work directly with the surgeon and hand him equipment or supplies that he requests. Such a nurse is called a *scrub nurse* because she scrubs her hands and arms for ten minutes before the operation—just as the surgeon does. Other nurses in the operating room, who do not wear sterilized gowns and gloves, are not permitted to handle equipment directly but may be permitted to pick up sterilized materials with an instrument that has been sterilized. One or more orderlies, who are responsible for lifting the patient and keeping the operating room in tidy condition, complete a typical surgical team.

Operating Room Equipment

When the operating room is in use by the surgical team, an impressive array of equipment is mobilized. The center of activity, of course, is the operating table, a massive metal device equipped with numerous levers and gears to permit the surface of the table to be raised, lowered, tilted to various angles, or to raise or lower the head, feet, or other parts of the patient's body. The table is equipped with straps to hold the patient firmly in place during the surgical procedure.

Above the operating table is a very large and powerful lamp with lenses designed to focus a bright, shadowless light on the area in which the surgical team is working. Additional lights also are available to provide illumination at various sides or angles not adequately lighted by the overhead lamp.

Near the head of the operating table is a cart containing tanks of gases used as general anesthetics, plus oxygen tanks and equipment for administering anesthetics and monitoring the life processes of the patient.

Also in the operating room are a variety of other wheeled carts, small tables, and stands containing myriad instruments, suction machines to clear mucus from the patient's throat and blood and other fluids from the incision area. Several stands in the area hold basins which, during an operation, can be filled with sterile solutions for rinsing hands, cleaning

instruments, or moistening towels and sponges used by the surgeon and his assistants. One tall metal stand near the operating table is designed to hold bottles of intravenous fluids or containers of blood for transfusions. Another special stand is used to collect sponges used in the operation. One cart contains jars or bottles of alcohol and other solutions, soap, and gauze pads, all of which are available for careful cleansing and sterilizing of the skin around the area of the incision just

A table holding surgical instruments is placed conveniently near the operating table in the operating room. Of course, the instruments have all been sterilized, along with the other equipment in the room.

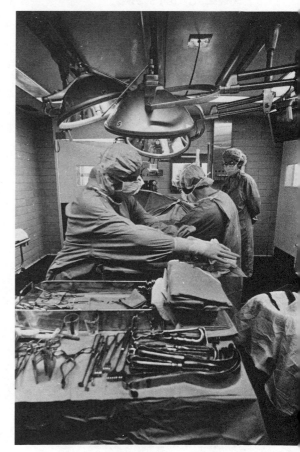

before the surgeon begins the actual operation.

A large clock on the wall of the operating room is intended for timing various functions and procedures involved in an operation, such as the number of minutes that have elapsed since sterilization of certain instruments was started. For many patients the clock is the last thing they see in the operating room before they begin the deep sleep of anesthesia; patients who remain conscious under a local anesthetic like to keep one eye on the clock face so they can tell how much time the operation requires.

Anesthetics and How They Are Used

Anesthesia is a word derived from ancient Greek, meaning "without perception," or a loss of sensation. During a major or minor operation, as in having a tooth extracted by a dentist, it is helpful to both the patient and the doctor if there is a lack of sensation during the procedure. But eliminating pain isn't the only consideration in the choice of anesthetic and other drugs used in conjunction with it. The age of the patient, chronic ailments, the site of the operation, and the emotional status of the patient are among factors considered. If a patient has undergone surgery previously and had an adverse effect from a particular kind of anesthesia, this information would have an important influence on the choice of an alternative type of anesthetic.

For many types of surgery, the kind of anesthetic chosen may be the result of an agreement among the surgeon, the patient, and the anesthetist. Some patients, given a choice, would prefer to remain conscious during an appendectomy or hernia repair; others would rather not. The surgeon frequently recom-

A doctor administers ether to a patient before surgery in an old print depicting instruction for surgeons at a Boston hospital.

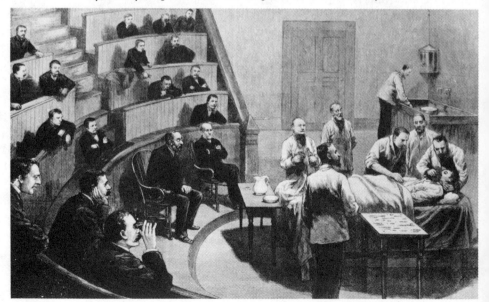

mends the use of a general anesthetic because the procedure may require more time than the patient can be comfortable with in an operating room situation. Therefore, patients should realize that when a surgeon recommends a general anesthetic for an operation in which a local or spinal anesthetic might be adequate, it is for their own welfare.

General Anesthetics

General anesthetics are those that produce "sleep," or unconsciousness, along with *analgesia*, or absence of pain. They also cause a kind of amnesia in that the patient remembers nothing that occurs during the period in which the anesthetic is effective. At the same time, general anesthetics produce a certain loss of muscle tone and reflex

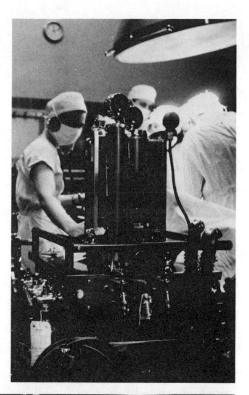

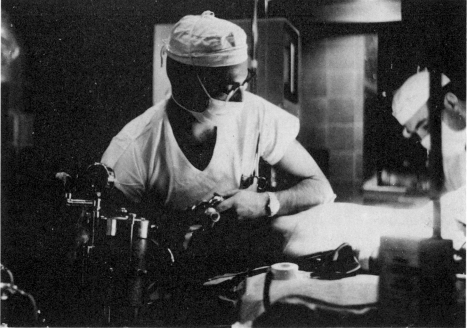

(Top) A gas-type anesthetic, such as nitrous oxide or cyclopropane, can be delivered under compression from tanks or cylinders. (Bottom) The liquid forms of gases may be dripped through a mask over the patient's face.

action. A general anesthetic, however, should not interfere significantly with such normal bodily functions as respiration and circulation, nor should it produce permanent damage to body tissues.

HOW THEY WORK: General anesthetics cause the patient to fall into a kind of sleep state by depressing the central nervous system, an effect that is reversible and lasts only until the drug has been eliminated by the body tissues. The general anesthetic reaches the central nervous system rather quickly because it is introduced directly or indirectly into the bloodstream. The use of a gas to produce anesthesia is an indirect method of producing unconsciousness.

A gas-type anesthetic, such as nitrous oxide or cyclopropane, can be delivered under compression from tanks or cylinders, or it may be stored in the operating room as a liquid that is converted to a vapor, like ether or halothane. The compressed gas anesthetics are administered with the help of an anesthetic machine. The liquid forms of gases may be dripped through a mask over the patient's face; or the liquid may be vaporized and directed to the patient by anesthetic equipment. Whether the source of the anesthetic is compressed gas or a volatile liquid, the purpose is the same: to get the anesthetic into the patient's lungs. There the gas enters the bloodstream through the walls of the blood vessels of the tiny sacs that make up the lungs.

KINDS OF GENERAL ANESTHETICS: Nearly a dozen different kinds of gases are available as general anesthetics. Each has certain advantages and disadvantages and interacts differently with other drugs used by the patient. The effects of each on chronic diseases of the patient must be weighed. Some gases induce anesthesia more rapidly than others; some are tolerated better by patients. These are among the many factors that can determine which gas or mixture of gases might be selected by the anesthetist for a particular surgical procedure.

INTRAVENOUS ANESTHETICS: Not all general anesthetics come in the form of compressed gases or volatile liquids. Several commonly used general anesthetics are administered intravenously, by injection into the bloodstream. The group includes barbiturates, such as thiopental, and narcotics, such as morphine. Ketamine is a general anesthetic drug that can be injected into the muscles as well as into the bloodstream. The intravenous anesthetics may be used instead of the gaseous general anesthetics or in combination with them. Thiopental is often administered to a patient first, to bring on sleep quickly, after which an inhaled general anesthetic is applied. Like the gaseous general anesthetics, each of the injected general anesthetics has its own peculiarities and may have different effects on different individuals. The rate of recovery from thiopental anesthesia varies according to the ability of a patient's body tissues to eliminate the drug; narcotics can affect the patient's respiration; ketamine may produce hallucinations in some patients.

Regional Anesthetics

Regional anesthetics include *local anesthetics* and *spinal anesthetics*. They are more likely to be used than general anesthetics when the patient is ambulatory and the surgery involves removal of moles or cysts, plastic surgery, certain eye, ear, nose, and throat procedures, and certain operations such as hernia repair that generally are uncomplicated. Regional anesthetics also may be recommended by the surgeon for operations to correct disorders in the arms or legs.

The surgical procedure may require that the patient remain conscious so he can follow instructions of the surgeon in manipulating muscles or bones to test the function of a body part being repaired. In such cases, a regional anesthetic would be preferred; a regional also would be advised for a patient with severe heart or lung disease that might be complicated by the effects of a general anesthetic. A restless child, on the other hand, might be given a general anesthetic for a relatively minor operation because the youngster would not be likely to remain motionless for the duration of the operation.

TOPICAL ANESTHETICS: Regional anesthetics generally are administered by infiltration of a drug into the tissues involved or into the nerve trunks leading into the area of incision. A simple kind of regional anesthesia is the topical application of a substance to a sensitive membrane of a body organ. For example, the eye drops applied by an opthalmologist may anesthetize a patient's eyes to make it easier for him to examine them. Topical anesthetics are not very effective when applied to the skin, which forms a tough barrier against most invasive substances, but they can effectively anesthetize the inner surfaces of the mouth, nose, throat, and other inner body surfaces. The anesthetic might be administered by sprays, gargles, or by direct application. Topical anesthetics commonly are used to prepare the throat and upper lung passages for examination with medical instruments.

LOCAL ANESTHETICS: Local anesthetics, which are similar to those used by the dentist, are usually injected by a hypodermic needle into the tissues surrounding the area to be operated on. The injection of an anesthetic into the tissue area sometimes is referred to as a *field block*. A variation of this technique is the *nerve* or *plexus block*, in which a hypodermic needle is used to inject the drug into the region of one or more key nerve trunks leading to the site of the incision. Local anesthetics are not recommended by most surgeons if there is an inflammation or infection of the tissues around the surgery site. The drugs used for local anesthetics can lower the patient's resistance to the infection while at the same time the inflammation may reduce the effectiveness of the drug as a pain-killer.

INTRAVENOUS ADMINISTRATION: Sometimes a regional anesthetic is administered intravenously by injecting it into a vein that runs through the site of the surgery. The drug is confined to the area, such as an arm or leg, by applying a tourniquet about the limb. Because of the possible dangers in suddenly releasing a potent anesthetic drug into the general bloodstream after the operation is ended, the tourniquet is intermittently tightened and released to slow the flow to a mere trickle. A sudden release also would quickly end the pain-killing effect in the area of the incision.

SPINAL ANESTHETICS: Spinal anesthesia is similar to a nerve trunk or plexus block method of eliminating pain sensation in a region of the body, except that the nerves receive the drug at the point where they leave the spinal cord. The drugs may be the same as those used as local anesthetics. They are injected either by hypodermic needle or catheter into tissues surrounding the spinal cord. Although there are several variations of spinal anesthesia—each involving the precise layer of tissue or space around the spinal cord that is the immediate target area of the injection—for all practical purposes the objective is the same. They are all intended to produce a lack of sensation in the spinal nerves along with a loss of motor function so there will be no movement of the body area to be operated on during surgery.

The spinal anesthetic may affect not only the targeted nerve system but neighboring spinal nerves as well, generally all the spinal nerves below the point of drug injection. For its purposes, spinal anesthesia can be a highly effective alternative to a general anesthetic. However, side effects are not uncommon. Severe headache is one of the most frequent complaints of patients. Temporary adverse effects can occur after use of other regional anesthetics as well and may be due in part to individual allergic reactions to the drug used.

Care After Surgery

The last thing you may remember as a patient, before receiving a general anesthetic, is being wheeled into the operating room and lifted by hospital orderlies onto the operating table. You may not see the surgeon, who could be scrubbing for the operation or reviewing the information compiled on your case. The anesthe-

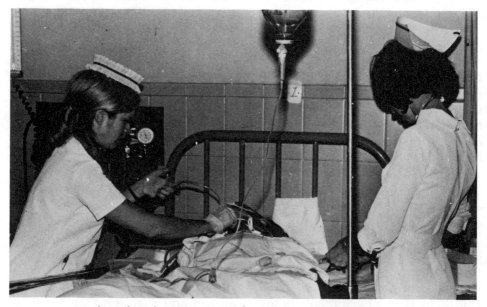

As patients in recovery rooms begin to regain consciousness, nurses apply oxygen masks to their faces to assist respiration.

tist and a few nurses may be in the operating room. You are feeling relaxed and drowsy because of the pre-anesthetic medications. A tube may be attached to your arm to drip an intravenous solution into a vein. The anesthetist may administer a dose of a drug such as sodium pentothal, a not unpleasant medication that brings on a deep sleep within a matter of seconds.

The Recovery Room

You will probably remember nothing after that point until you gradually become aware of the strange sounds and sights of a recovery room. The recovery room may contain a number of patients who have undergone surgery at about the same time, especially in a large hospital. Each is reclining in a bed equipped with high railings to prevent a groggy, confused patient just recovering from a general anesthetic from falling onto the floor.

Nurses move briskly about the room, checking the conditions of the various patients. As each patient gains some awareness of the situation, a nurse puts an oxygen mask over his face and explains the purpose: to help restore the tiny air sacs of the lungs to their normal condition. During administration of the anesthetic, the air sacs can become dry and partially collapsed. The humidified oxygen mixture helps restore moisture to the inner surfaces of the lungs; by breathing deeply of the oxygen the patient expands the air sacs to their normal capacity. Before the use of oxygen masks in the recovery room and deep breathing techniques for patients recovering from the effects of an anesthetic gas, there was a much

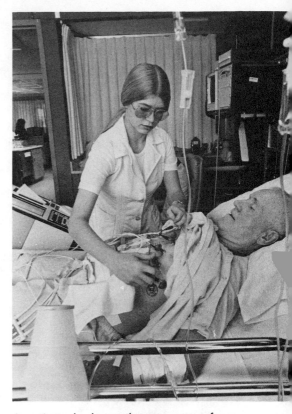

A patient who has undergone surgery for a coronary bypass needs careful and thorough monitoring afterwards, usually in a cardiac intensive care unit.

greater danger of pneumonia developing as a post-operative complication.

Nurses assigned to the recovery room are given a report on each patient arriving from the operating room and instructions about such matters as the position of the patient in the bed. One patient may have to lie flat on his back, another on his side, a third in a sitting position, and still another with the head lower than the feet. If the patient has received a general anesthetic, the nurses may be instructed to turn him from one side to the other at regular intervals until he is able to turn himself.

The patient's blood pressure, pulse, and respiration are checked at regular intervals by the recovery room nurses, who also watch for any signs of bleeding or drainage from the area of incision. The surgeon is notified immediately of any signs of complications. Since the recovery room usually is located next to the operating room, the surgeon can quickly verify any threatened complication and attend to the problem without delay. Most surgical patients will remain in the recovery room for a few hours at the most, and when they appear to be able to manage somewhat on their own they are returned to their beds in the regular nursing area of the hospital.

The Intensive Care Unit

Critically ill patients or those with heart, lung, kidney, or other serious disorders usually are assigned to an intensive care unit where each bed may be isolated from the others in a glass booth designed to provide privacy and quiet during the recovery period. Patients can still be clearly observed from the central nursing station.

Patients in an intensive care unit are given continuous care by nurses. Electronic equipment is used to monitor pulse, blood pressure, heartbeat, and, when needed, brain function and body temperature. Other devices are available for making bedside measurements of bodily function and to obtain laboratory data such as blood chemistry without moving the patient from his bed.

Pain

Most surgical patients will be concerned about how much pain they will feel after leaving the operating room. It is not unusual to expect greater pain than is actually experienced; the incision may cause no more discomfort than the problem that required surgical therapy. Obviously, a minor operation will result in less painful discomfort than a major operation. Generally, the pain or discomfort associated with a surgical incision may last for one or two days, then subside over a period of perhaps three or four days. After that an occasional twinge may be felt in the area of the incision when shifting the body puts extra stress on the muscles or other tissues involved in the operation. During the hospital stay medications will be available to help relieve any serious pain resulting from the operation.

Signs of Recovery or Complication

While the patient may be concerned about pain following surgery, the physicians and nurses are more likely to direct their attention toward other signs and symptoms that will help them to gauge the rate of recovery, such as the patient's body temperature, skin coloring, urine output, and his ability to cough. The health professionals are well aware that surgery, and drugs or anesthetics administered in conjunction with surgery, can be disruptive to normal bodily activities. The major operation is more likely to cause changes in the patient's physiology than a minor operation.

Vital Signs

Nurses can be expected to make regular checks of temperature, pulse, and respiration because these common measures of body functions (sometimes called *vital signs*) can provide early-warning signals of possible post-operative complications. A patient may have a temperature of 100°F. even after a major operation, but because of increased metabolic activity of the body following surgery a slightly elevated thermometer reading is considered normal. The pulse and respiration also may be slightly above the patient's rate before surgery, but the mild change again is due to a normal stress reaction of the body. However, a temperature rising above 100°F. and/or a significantly faster pulse or respiration rate suggests that a complication may have developed.

If a nurse seems interested in the patient's ability to cough, it is because the cough reflex helps the patient get rid of mucus accumulation in his lungs, especially after the use of a general anesthetic. If coughing is difficult, a plastic tube may be inserted into the patient's throat to help clear the breathing passages. Normal breathing can also be restored by steam inhalation, aerosol sprays of water or special medications, or positive pressure breathing equipment that forces air into the lungs. Failure to expand the air passages of the lungs leads to serious respiratory complications.

Urine output is also checked. This is just one more way of watching the rate of recovery of a patient and alerting the staff to any signs of complications. If for some reason the patient is unable to pass urine, a *catheter*, or plastic tube, is inserted into the bladder to drain it. The volume of urine drained is collected and measured.

The Incision Area

Some blood may accumulate under the skin in the area of the incision or in nearby tissues, causing a discoloration of the skin. But this effect is seldom a serious matter, and the discoloration gradually vanishes. In some cases of excess blood accumulation, the surgeon may simply remove one or two sutures and drain away the blood. Any continued bleeding about the incision would, of course, be a complication.

A more common complication is infection of the incision area by bacteria that enter the wound. An infection may develop any time from one day to one week after an operation. However, most post-operative infections of incision wounds are easily controlled by antibiotics, drainage, or natural defenses against disease. The surgeon or other physicians will make regular inspections of the incision during the first few days after surgery to make sure it is healing properly.

Post-operative Nourishment

A light meal may be offered the patient a few hours after surgery. The patient may or may not feel like eating, especially if he still feels a bit nauseated from the effects of a general anesthetic. At this stage fluid intake is probably more important, especially if the patient has not been allowed to have even a sip of water since the previous evening. If the surgery was not performed on the stomach or intestinal tract, a small amount of water or tea may be permitted within a few hours after the operation. It is unlikely in any case that the patient will feel a great desire for fluid because intravenous solutions may have been dripping slowly into a vein since he entered the operating room. Intravenous solutions can satisfy hunger as well as thirst, since they may contain proteins, carbohydrates, and essential vitamins and minerals dissolved in a finely formulated broth. Perhaps unnoticed by the patient, the amount of fluid intake will be routinely measured by members of the hospital staff.

Ambulation

Ambulation—getting the patient out of bed and moving about—is an important part of post-operative care. Experience has shown that recovery from surgery is more effective if the patient spends increasing amounts of time each day in simple physical activity. The degree of ambulation depends upon the magnitude of the surgery and the general physical health of the patient. But in a typical case of hernia surgery or an appendectomy, the patient may be asked, on the first or second day after the operation, to sit on the edge of his bed and dangle his legs for a while. On the second or third day, he may be allowed to walk about the room, and may in fact prefer to walk to the bathroom rather than use a bedpan or urinal. On the following day, he may walk up and down the halls with the help of a nurse or other hospital staff member.

Each patient is encouraged to handle the ambulation phase of recovery at his own pace, and there

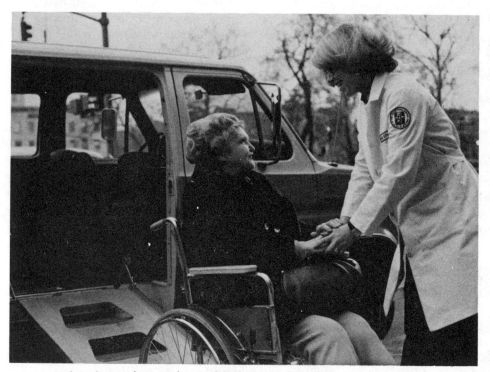

A patient on her way home after discharge from the hospital. Her surgeon will have outlined a detailed plan for recovery procedures at home.

are few hard and fast rules. Of two persons entering the operating room on the same day for the same kind of elective surgery, one may feel like walking to the bathroom a few hours after surgery while the second may prefer to remain in bed and use a bedpan a week after surgery. The surgeon and attending physicians may encourage and in some cases even insist upon early ambulation, however, because it reduces the rate of complications.

Back at Home

Dressings used to cover the incision are changed regularly, as the incision is inspected once each day, more frequently if warranted. If the patient is anxious to be discharged from the hospital as early as possible, the surgeon may give him instructions for changing his own dressings. The surgeon will also outline a plan for recovery procedures to be followed after he leaves the hospital. The plan will include a schedule of visits to the surgeon's office for removal of stitches that may remain and a final inspection of the incision. The surgeon will also offer his advice on how the patient should plan a return to normal activities, including a return to his job and resumption of sports or recreational programs.

Special Diets

Proper foods are as important as proper medicines in helping a patient recover from surgery. Despite the common complaints about hospital meals, the nutrients that are provided in certain special diets for surgical patients are as carefully prescribed and prepared as are some medications that are served in pill or capsule form.

Surgical nutrition has become increasingly important in recent years because of an awareness by physicians that an operation, minor or major, is not unlike an organic disease that creates physiological stresses and a nutritional imbalance in the patient's body. To help compensate for alterations in the patient's physiology as it recovers from the effects of surgery, special diets may be ordered.

Bland Soft Diet

A bland soft diet frequently is ordered for patients who are unable to handle a regular diet but whose condition is not serious enough to require a liquid diet. The foods are selected because they are low in cellulose and connective tissue; they are bland, smooth, and easily digested. The choice of food, nevertheless, represents as great a variety as one might be served in a restaurant or at home, except for an absence of spices and other substances that would be stimulating to the gastrointestinal tract. Included in the surgical soft diet might be lean meat, fish, poultry, eggs, milk, mild cheese, cooked tender or pureed fruits and vegetables, refined cereals and breads with butter or margarine, plus gelatin deserts, puddings, custards, and ice cream. See pp. 732–735.

Liquid Diet

Liquid diets for surgical patients may be prepared with or without milk. They are usually ordered for patients with impaired function of the gastrointestinal tract. A liquid diet without milk may include a cereal gruel made with water, clear bouillon or broth, gelatin, strained fruit juice, and coffee or tea. Liquid diets with milk are similar but may also include creamed soups, sherbets, ice cream, cereal gruel made with milk instead of water, cocoa and beverages of milk or cream. Beverage options permitted are tomato juice and some carbonated beverages such as ginger ale.

Diets Following Particular Kinds of Surgery

PEPTIC ULCERS: A special diet for peptic ulcer patients may include a half-and-half mixture of milk and cream, plus mashed potatoes, eggs, toast and butter, pureed vegetables, cottage cheese, rice, plain puddings and gelatin desserts. But meat soups, tea, coffee, raw vegetables, and fried foods are prohibited.

RECTAL SURGERY: Following rectal surgery, and other procedures in which it is necessary to prevent bowel movements for a period of several days, a low residue diet is ordered. A low residue diet (or *minimal residue diet*, as it is also called) might offer eggs, poached or boiled, rice, soda crackers, cereals made with water, butter, bouillon or clear broths, carbonated beverages, tea, coffee and certain meats including oysters, sweetbreads, and tender bits of beef or veal. See pp. 749–750. An alternative low residue diet is the bland soft diet with all milk-containing items eliminated.

GALL BLADDER SURGERY: Gall bladder surgical patients may expect a modified fat diet that eliminates as much as possible fats and gas-producing food items. It includes foods that provide protein and carbohydrate sources of energy to re-place fats and includes primarily fish, poultry, lean cuts of beef, cottage cheese, cereal products and bread, and certain fruits and vegetables. However, foods prohibited are mainly pork products and fatty cuts of other meats, cream, chocolate, melons, apples, fried foods of any kind, onions, cabbage, turnips, cucumbers, radishes, green peppers, and dried beans and peas. See pp. 741–743.

RESTRICTED SALT INTAKE: Chronic heart failure patients and those with liver ailments or edema are placed on a low-sodium diet before and after surgery. The low-sodium diet is fairly simple in that it is prepared mainly with foods from which sodium or salt either is naturally absent or has been removed. Many salt-free or low-sodium foods are available commercially from manufacturers that also supply special dietetic foods for persons suffering from diabetes. See pp. 737–740.

FRACTURES OR BURNS: Special consideration is given the diets of patients who are recovering from accidents that result in fractures or burns. Because of complex body responses to such injuries, there may be an abnormal loss of nitrogen from the tissues and a breakdown of muscle tissue, which is a rich source of nitrogen, an important component of protein. As a result, adequate amounts of protein need to be provided to surgical patients with burn injuries and broken bones.

Potassium Loss

Normal body stores of potassium also may be diminished during and immediately after surgery, but potassium can be replaced in the tissues by including in the meals adequate amounts of meats, fish, poultry, bananas, raisins, figs, dates, and prunes, as well as dried peaches and dried apricots. Prune, tomato, orange, and pineapple juices also are a rich source of potassium for post-operative patients.

Replacement of Water Losses

While water is not always thought of as a food, it is an important part of the gastronomic intake of the surgical patient; adequate amounts of water need to be provided the person recovering from an operation. The post-operative patient usually requires larger than normal amounts of water even though he may not feel inclined to help himself to as much fluid intake as he would at home or on the job. In addition to normal water losses through perspiration, urine, and breathing, there may be additional water losses through vomiting. Water replacement may be provided through sufficient amounts of fruit juices and other beverages offered during meals and between meals.

Apprehensions About Surgery

Most people feel anxious when faced with the need for surgery. This is to be expected. After all, a certain amount of anxiety normally accompanies any prolonged or incapacitating illness or infirmity. When surgery is the recommended therapy, it's natural for the patient to feel some anxiety about the surgery even if he's optimistic about a favorable result.

Factors That Reduce the Risk of Modern Surgery

Much of the risk of surgery these days is eliminated through the careful pre-operative screening examinations reviewed earlier. A patient with a chronic disease who might have been a surgical risk a generation ago may have one or more options not available in past years, such as regional anesthetics that allow surgeons alternatives to general anesthetics that would be less than satisfactory. Antibiotics and other backup medications are available to control possible complications after surgery. Recovery room techniques and intensive care units with electronic monitoring of vital life systems provide added insurance of safe recovery. And, of course, surgeons today have the added experience of many millions of successful operations involving a range of procedures such as kidney and heart transplants, open heart surgery, and replacement of important organ parts with plastic substitutes. These and other procedures, including the implanting of electronic heart pacemakers, were beyond the dreams of surgeons of past years.

Surgery for the Older Patient

With the rapid increase in the proportion of older people in the population, the surgical patient is more likely to be an older person with problems associated with aging. An older man who underwent surgery to remove his prostate gland before World War II had a life expectancy of a few years after the operation. Today, such procedures in older men are considered routine cases with little or no effect on longevity. It is not unusual nowadays to find men and women in their 70s and 80s who have undergone five or six major operations since

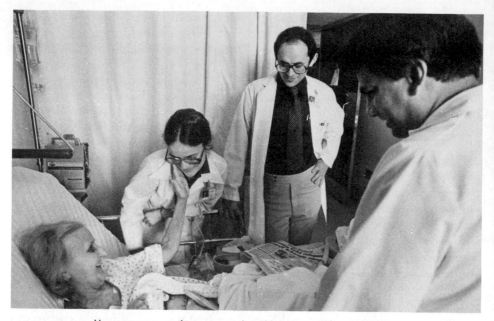

Many surgery patients are senior citizens; special preoperative and postoperative techniques for the aging have been developed.

reaching the traditional retirement age and without any significant restrictions on their physical activities.

Part of the reason for the greatly improved outlook for surgery on older patients may be that older persons today are simply in better health because of the improved medical care available. Thus they are better surgical risks than their parents would have been at the same age. Advanced pre-operative and post-operative care has also improved the outlook for the older patient. He may be admitted to the hospital a few days earlier than the younger patient for more intensive examinations, and he may remain a few days longer for post-operative care. Convalescence for the older patient may take longer, and in some instances the recovery may not be as complete as that of a younger person. But in general, modern surgical techniques are likely to offer a safe and effective therapy for people of advanced age with complaints that can be corrected by an operation.

In addition to the physical benefits, surgery may improve the mental capacity, personality, and sensitivity of older persons who had been depressed about a disorder before surgery. The patient who complained that he is "no longer the person he used to be" physically may have assumed that his medical problem was simply a result of growing old and overlooked the possibility that the complaint was due to a disease that might respond to treatment.

Surgery for the Child

A child, on the other hand, may have his own reasons to be apprehensive about the trip to a hospital for surgery. Most children seem to worry that the operation will hurt or that other procedures, such as taking a blood sample for testing, will be painful.

TELLING THE TRUTH: Many surgeons recommend that the child be told as realistically as possible, in terms he can understand, what can be expected. The youngster should not be given a sugar-coated story about the operation which might give the impression that he is embarking upon a happy adventure. At the same time, the child should not be frightened by suggestions that he may be given drugs to make him unconscious while he is strapped to a table so that strangely masked and gowned strangers can cut him open with sharp knives.

Children are more likely to appreciate surgery if they are told that a friendly person will help them go to sleep; that the operation will hurt a little but the pain will go away after a while; and that the operation will make them feel better or help correct a problem so they can be more active like other children. A small child should always understand that he may have to remain overnight at the hospital without his parents, but that he will have other adults to take care of him and there probably will be other children at the hospital to keep him company.

A volunteer at Children's Memorial Hospital in Chicago uses puppets to explain to a young patient what will happen to her in surgery.

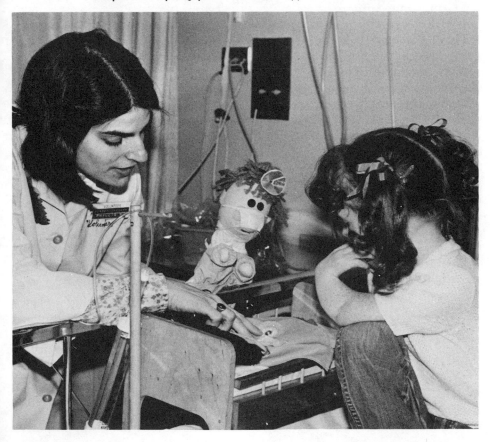

COMMON SURGICAL PROCEDURES

In this section some of the more common surgical procedures are described. The operations discussed are organized by the system or region of the body with which they are concerned. The following areas are covered in this order:

• Male Reproductive System (For surgical procedures involving the female reproductive system, see under *Women's Health*, p. 988.

• Urinary Tract
• Abdominal Region
• Oral Cavity and Throat
• Ear Surgery
• Eye surgery
• Chest Region
• Vascular Surgery
• Orthopedic Surgery
• Neurosurgery

For *Plastic and Cosmetic Surgery*, see p. 976. *Uncommon Surgical Procedures*, including transplants, are discussed beginning on p. 982.

Many of the conditions treated in this chapter from a surgical point of view are also treated elsewhere, in the chapter devoted to diseases of the appropriate body system or organ; the reader is invited to turn to those chapters for additional information. For example, although heart surgery is discussed in this chapter, heart disease is treated in greater detail in Ch. 26, p. 1131. Likewise, many of the tumors described in this chapter are also discussed in Ch. 34, p. 1265.

Male Reproductive System

Surgical procedures of the prostate, testis, scrotum, and penis are considered in this section. Undescended testicles and vasectomy are also among the subjects discussed.

Prostate Surgery

The prostate gland is a small cone-shaped object that surrounds the male urethra, the tube that carries urine from the urinary bladder to the penis. It is normally about one-half inch long and weighs less than an ounce. Ejaculatory ducts empty through the prostate into the urethra and other ducts drain glandular secretions of the prostate into the urethra. Because of the intimate association of the prostate gland and the urinary tract, a disorder in one system can easily affect the other. A urinary infection can spread to the prostate and an abnormality of the prostate can interfere with the normal excretion of urine.

ENLARGEMENT OF THE PROSTATE: A relatively common problem is the tendency of the prostate to grow larger in middle-aged men. The gradual enlargement continues from the 40s on but the symptoms usually go unnoticed until the man is in his 60s. At that point in life, the prostate may have become so enlarged that it presses on the urethra and obstructs the flow of urine from the neighboring bladder. The older man may experience various difficulties in emptying his bladder. He may have to urinate more frequently, and suddenly find himself getting out of bed at night to go to the bathroom. He may not be able to develop a urine stream of the size and force he had in earlier years. He may have trouble getting the stream of urine started and it may end in a dribble.

In addition to the somewhat embarrassing inconveniences caused by prostate enlargement, the urinary bladder may not drain properly and can eventually lose its own muscle tone needed for emptying. Residual urine in the bladder can become a source of infection, and backflow into the ureters can gradually affect those tissues and the kidneys. It has been estimated that 20 percent of all older men may need treatment of some kind, including surgery, for correcting this problem of the prostate gland.

FACTORS INDICATING THE NEED FOR SURGERY: Factors that may decide in favor of surgical removal of the prostate include residual urine in the patient's bladder; blood in the urine, with evidence that the blood comes from the prostate; the severity of the inconveniences associated with irregular urination; and complications such as the presence or threat of failure of the wall of the urinary bladder, the formation of stones, and symptoms and signs of infection.

SURGICAL METHODS: There are sev-

eral methods of performing a *prostatectomy* (excision of all or part of the prostate) for relief of the symptoms of an enlarged prostate, a condition that may appear on the patient's medical records as *benign prostatic hyperplasia*. All of the methods are relatively safe and in none of the techniques is the entire prostate removed. One method, called *transurethral resection*, requires insertion of an instrument into the urethra through the penis. The instrument, a *resectoscope*, uses a high-frequency electric current to cut away the tissue inside the gland. This technique avoids open surgery and requires a postoperative hospital stay of only a few days.

OPEN SURGERY: The other techniques involve *open surgery,* that is, surgery in which an incision is made in the pelvic or rectal area to make the prostate gland accessible so that its inner tissues can be removed.

THE MALE REPRODUCTIVE SYSTEM

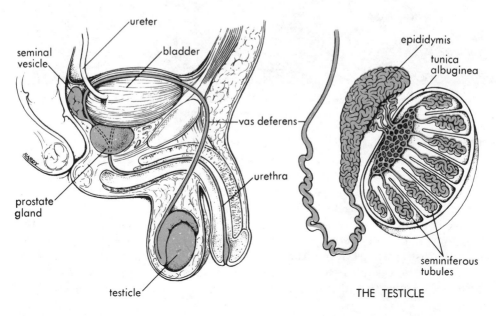

THE TESTICLE

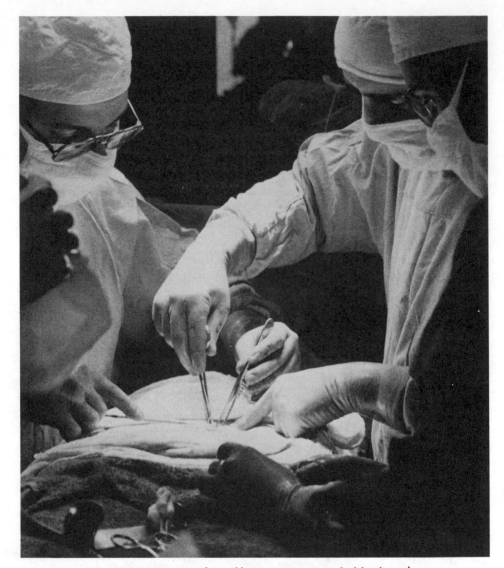

In a prostatectomy performed by open surgery, an incision is made
in the pelvic or rectal area to make the prostate gland accessible.

The differences in the various open surgery techniques depend upon such factors as where the incision should be made and the risks associated with the approaches. The incision is made either in the *perineum*, the region between the rectum and the testicles, or through the abdomen. Only a small percentage of patients experience complications or regrowth of the prostate tissues to produce a second enlargement problem. Impotence is usually not an aftereffect of the surgery, and libido is normal.

INFECTIONS OF THE PROSTATE: Infections of the prostate gland can involve obstruction of the urethra, but the problem usually can be resolved by the use of medications and techniques other than surgery. An abscess, however, may require an incision to drain the prostate. Surgery also may be recommended for the treatment of stones, or calculi, that develop in the prostate and cause obstruction or contribute to infections.

CANCER OF THE PROSTATE: Cancer of the prostate also may occur in older men, causing obstruction of the urinary flow or contributing to infection of the urinary tract. If examination including biopsy studies confirms the presence of cancer, the surgeon may recommend radical prostatectomy. In this procedure an incision is made either through the lower abdomen or through the perineum to remove the entire prostate gland and surrounding tissues such as the seminal vesicles. Hormonal therapy, chemotherapy, and radiation treatments also may be administered. See also p. 1280.

Tumors of the Testis

Tumors of the testis occur most frequently in younger men between the ages of 18 and 35. Such a tumor appears as a firm and enlarged testis and usually without pain unless bleeding is involved as a symptom. Testicular tumors generally are malignant and spread rapidly to other parts of the body, including the lungs. The onset of the disorder can be so insidious that the patient may seek medical advice for a more obvious secondary problem such as the apparent development of mammary glands on his chest, the result of disruption of his normal male hormonal balance.

Special laboratory tests and other examination techniques usually are required to determine which of several possible kinds of testicular tumors may be involved and the extent of metastasis of the cancer cells to other body areas. If cancer of a testicle is confirmed it is removed by an incision through the groin area, and neighboring lymph nodes also will be taken out. The surgical procedure usually is supplemented with chemotherapy and radiation. The prognosis, or chances for recovery, following surgical removal of a testicular tumor depends upon the particular kind of cancer involved and how far the disease had progressed before medical treatment was begun.

Tumors of the Scrotum and Penis

Tumors of the scrotum and penis are relatively uncommon but do occur. Cancer of the scrotum is usually associated with exposure to cancer-causing chemicals. Boys who worked as chimney sweeps a century ago tended to develop cancer of the scrotum from body contact with soot in coal-burning fireplaces. Cancer of the penis occurs usually in men who have not been circumcised. In either type of cancer, the treatment usually requires removal of the affected tissues. This can mean castration in the case of scrotal cancer or amputation of a part or all of the penis, depending upon the extent of the cancerous growth. Surgery that requires removal of a part of the reproductive system can have a devastating psychological effect on a man, but the alternative is likely to be early death from the spread of cancer.

Undescended Testicles

About ten percent of cases of tumors of the testis occur in men with an undescended testicle. Since the chances of a tumor developing in an undescended testicle are as much as 50 times greater than the incidence for the normal male population, the existence of an undescended testicle can warrant corrective surgery.

Ordinarily, the testicles descend from their fetal location in the abdomen into the scrotum about two months before birth. But in one case in 200 male births, a child is found with a failure of one or, less commonly, both testicles to descend properly into the scrotum. In addition to the risk of cancer, undescended testicles are associated with lack of fertility and other problems such as hernias.

CRYPTORCHIDISM: In male babies and small children, an undescended testicle sometimes can be encouraged to enter the scrotum by manipulation or administration of hormones. Many surgeons recommend that the developmental problem of undescended testicles, or *cryptorchidism*, be corrected before a child enters school, although the surgical procedure for correcting the situation can be postponed until adolescence or adulthood. The operation for correcting an undescended testicle is called *orchidopexy* and involves an incision in the groin to release the testicle and its attached cord from fibrous tissue holding it in the abdomen. The testicle may be brought directly down into the scrotum where it may be anchored temporarily with a suture. Or it may be brought down in stages in a series of operations to permit the growth and extension of blood supply to the testis. The original location of the undescended testicle determines which procedure is used.

Vasectomy

Vasectomy is a birth control technique that is intended to make a man permanently sterile. It does not involve the removal of any of the male reproductive system and does not result in a loss of potency or libido. A vasectomy is a relatively simple operation that can be performed in a doctor's office in less than 30 minutes and requires only a local anesthetic. The operation is similar to, but much less complicated, than the procedure in which a woman may be sterilized by cutting or tying her Fallopian tubes. A vasectomy requires no hospitalization, and the man is able to return to work or other normal activities after a day or two.

HOW THE PROCEDURE IS DONE: The vasectomy procedure requires a small incision, about one-half inch in length, on either side of the scrotum. The surgeon removes through the incision a short length of the *vas deferens*, the tube that carries spermatozoa from the testicles, and ties a piece of surgical thread at two points about an inch apart. Then a small piece of the vas deferens between the tied off points is snipped out of the tube. The procedure is done on each side. With the ducts of the vas deferens cut and tied, sperm from the testicles can no longer move through their normal paths to the prostate where they would become mixed with semen from the prostate and seminal vesicles and be ejaculated during sexual intercourse.

STERILITY IS USUALLY PERMANENT: A vasectomy does not immediately render a man sterile. Sperm already stored in the seminal "pipeline" can still be active for a period of a month to six weeks, and a woman who has intercourse with a vasectomized man during that period can become pregnant. On the other hand, a man who undergoes vasectomy should not expect that the severed ducts can be connected again should he want to become a father in the future. Sperm banks have been offered as a possible alternative for the man who might want to store some of his spermatozoa for future use, but there is little evidence that the sperm will remain fertile in a sperm bank for more than a year or 18 months. In rare cases, men who have undergone vasectomies have unintentionally become fertile again because of *canalization,* or creation of a new channel connecting the severed ends of the vas deferens; in one case the canalization occurred eight years after the vasectomy was performed.

The vasectomy is regarded as an extremely safe operation, and complications are infrequent. Some swelling and discomfort are reported by a small percentage of men undergoing the operation. Steroid hormone drugs are sometimes administered to control these aftereffects.

Urinary Tract

Surgical procedures involving urinary stones and tumors of the bladder, ureter, urethra, and kidney are considered in this section. Also dis-

THE FEMALE URINARY SYSTEM   THE MALE URINARY SYSTEM

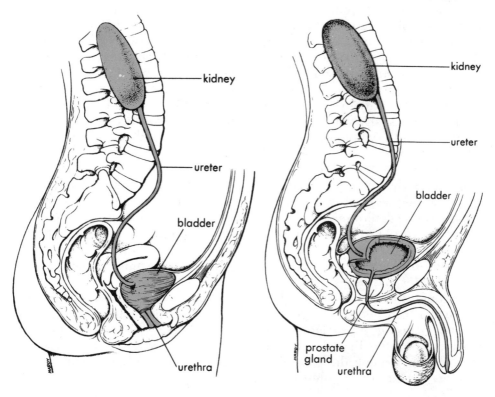

cussed are kidney cysts and conditions affecting the adrenal glands that might require surgery.

Urinary Stones

Most stones that occur in the urinary tract are formed in the kidneys, but kidney stones can travel to other areas such as the ureters and cause problems there. Various types of stones can develop in the kidneys from several different causes. A common cause is a metabolic disorder involving calcium, proteins, or uric acid. Other causes are infections or obstructions of the urinary tract, the use of certain drugs, such as diuretics, or vitamin deficiency.

SYMPTOMS: Kidney stones seldom cause problems while they are forming, but movement of the stones irritates the urinary tract and can cause severe pain; the irritation of the tissues may cause bleeding that will result in blood appearing in the urine. Other symptoms may indicate obstruction of the flow of urine and infection. In some cases obstruction of a ureter can lead to failure of the kidney. X-ray techniques can usually verify the cause of the patient's symptoms and locate the urinary stone. Most stones cast a shadow on X-ray film, and by injecting special dyes into the urinary system the degree of obstruction by a stone can be determined.

URETER STONES: Most stones released by the kidney are small enough to pass through a ureter to the bladder and be excreted while urinating. But if a stone is large enough it can become lodged in a ureter, causing excruciating pain that may be felt both in the back and the abdomen along the path of the ureter. Ureter stones often can be removed by manipulation, using catheter tubes that are inserted through the bladder. If the stuck stone cannot be manipulated from the ureter, an operation in a hospital is required. However, the surgical procedure is relatively simple and direct. An incision is made over the site of the stuck stone, the ureter is exposed and opened just far enough to permit removal of the stone. The operation is safe and requires perhaps a week in the hospital.

KIDNEY STONES: If the urinary stone is lodged in the kidney, the surgical procedure also is a relatively safe one although more complicated and requiring a longer hospital stay. The surgeon must work through skin and muscle layers to reach the kidney, then cut into the kidney if necessary to remove the stone. If the obstruction has been serious enough to impair normal kidney function or if infection has damaged the kidney tissue, the surgeon may elect to remove the affected kidney. Fortunately, the human body can get along fairly well with one good functioning kidney, so a *nephrectomy*, as the procedure is called, may not be as drastic a maneuver as the patient might imagine. If, on the other hand, the affected kidney has not been seriously damaged, the stone or stones can be removed with instruments or by the surgeon's fingers and the incision in the kidney sewed up so that it can resume its normal functions.

VESICAL STONES: Occasionally, urinary stones are found in the neck of the bladder or in the bladder itself. They are called *vesical stones* and, depending upon their size and other factors, may be removed by several techniques including use of a cystoscope inserted through the urethra. In some cases the stone can be broken into smaller pieces for removal. If it appears unlikely that the stone can be removed directly or by crushing it, the surgeon can make an incision directly to the bladder in a manner similar to the approach used in removing a stone from the ureter.

Bladder Tumors

About three-fourths of the tumors of the bladder occur in men past the age of 45. Although the specific cause of bladder tumors is unknown, doctors suspect that a cancer-producing chemical is involved. Several studies have found an association between the disease and cigarette smoking or occupations that require contact with organic chemicals used in making dyes. Tumors that appear in the female bladder are less likely to be cancerous than those that occur in the male bladder.

SYMPTOMS AND DIAGNOSIS: The first symptom of bladder tumor is blood in the urine. The tumor itself may cause no pain but an early complication could be an infection producing inflammation and discomfort in the region of the bladder. If the tumor blocks the normal flow of urine, the patient may feel pain or discomfort in the area of the kidneys; this condition is most likely to happen if the tumor is located at the opening of a ureter leading from a kidney to the bladder. An early examination of the bladder may fail to locate a small tumor, although X rays might show the growth as a bit of shadow on the film, and obstruction of a ureter could be seen. Nonetheless, exami-

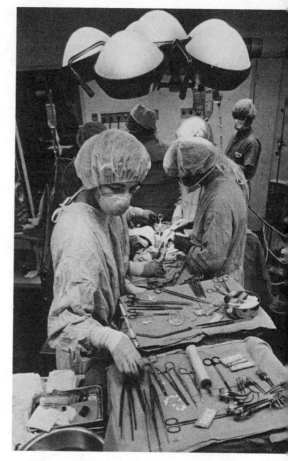

During a lengthy, complicated tumor operation, a scrub nurse must remain alert to the doctor's requests for forceps, clamps, and other instruments.

nation of the interior of the bladder by a cystoscope is necessary to confirm the presence of the tumor. A biopsy can be made by removing a few tissue cells from the area in a manner quite like the procedure for making a Pap smear test for possible cancer of the cervix in a female patient.

TREATMENT: Most early and simple cases of bladder tumor can be corrected by a procedure called *saucerization* by an instrument that removes the abnormal tissue, leaving a shallow wound that normally will grow over with healthy tissue cells. But a tumor that invades deeply into the wall of the bladder requires more radical therapy, such as surgery to cut away the part of the bladder that is affected by the growth. Radiation also may be employed to control the spread of tumor cells, particularly if laboratory tests indicate that the type of tumor cells involved are sensitive to radiation.

SURGICAL PROCEDURE: If it is necessary to cut away a part of the bladder, the surgeon simply shapes a new but smaller organ from the remaining tissues. If a total *cystectomy* is required to save the life of the patient, the entire bladder is removed, along with the prostate if the patient is a man. When the bladder is removed, a new path for the flow of urine is devised by the surgeons, usually to divert the urine into the lower end of the intestinal tract.

Tumors of the Ureter or Urethra

Tumors of the ureter, above the bladder, or of the urethra, below the bladder, may begin with symptoms resembling those of a bladder tumor, although X rays might show the growth as a bit of shadow on the normal flow of urine. Treatment also usually requires removal of the affected tissues with reconstructive surgery as needed to provide for a normal flow of urine from the kidneys.

Kidney Tumors

WILMS' TUMOR: Tumors of the kidney generally occur either in children before the age of eight years or in adults over the age of 25. The type of tumor that affects children usually is the Wilms' tumor, one of the most common kinds of cancer that can afflict a youngster. The tumor grows rapidly and may be painful even though there may be no obvious signs of urinary tract disorder in the child's urine. The tumor frequently becomes so large that it appears as an abdominal swelling. A Wilms' tumor usually occurs only on one side of the body, but in a small percentage of the cases the disorder can develop in both right and left kidneys. Kidney function may continue normally during growth of the tumor, but cancerous cells from the tumor may be carried by the bloodstream to other parts of the body, by metastasis, causing the problem to spread to the lungs and other vital organs.

Treatment usually requires surgical removal of the affected kidney and radiation therapy; the tumor cells responsible for the growth are sensitive to radiation. The younger the child and the earlier treatment is started, the better are the child's chances for recovery from a Wilms' tumor.

ADULT KIDNEY TUMOR: The adult type of kidney tumor, which is more likely to afflict men than women, may also appear as an enlarged abdominal mass. But unlike the Wilms' tumor, the adult kidney tumor presents as an early symptom blood in the urine. Bleeding from the kidney may be painless. X-ray studies may show an enlarged and sometimes distorted kidney. The patient may have symptoms indicating metastasis of the tumor cells to the lungs, bones, or other body systems. Adult kidney tumors are almost always malignant.

Treatment usually requires nephrectomy, or surgical removal of the diseased kidney. Radiation therapy may be provided in addition to the surgery, although the kind of tumor cells involved in the adult type of kidney tumor usually are resistant to radiation. Chemotherapy also may be offered. The chances for complete recovery from a kidney tumor depend upon several factors such as the location of the tumor in the kidney and the extent of metastasis of the cancerous cells to other organ systems.

Kidney Cysts

A *cyst* is a small pouch enclosed by a membrane; technically, the urinary bladder and gall bladder are cysts. But the cysts of medical disorders are small pouches or sacs filled with a fluid or viscous substance; they may appear on the skin, in the lungs, or in other body systems such as the kidneys.

SYMPTOMS: Kidney cysts produce symptoms that resemble the symptoms of cancer of the kidney; in a few cases kidney cysts are associated with tumors that cause bleeding into the cysts. In addition to the troublesome symptoms of flank pain and blood in the urine, untreated cysts can grow until they damage normal kidney tissue and impair the function of the organ's functions. Simple or solitary kidney cysts usually do not occur before the age of 40.

DIAGNOSIS: X-ray techniques are made to determine the exact nature of kidney cyst symptoms, but in some cases exploratory surgery is recommended to differentiate a cyst from a tumor. The cyst is excised, frequently by cutting away the exposed wall of the growth. The chances of the cyst re-forming are very slight.

POLYCYSTIC KIDNEY DISEASE: A different kind of kidney cyst disease, consisting of many small cysts, may be found in younger persons, including small children. The symptoms again may be flank pain and blood in the urine; examination may show some enlargement of the kidney. This form of the disease, sometimes called *polycystic kidney disease*, can be complicated by uremia and hypertension as the patient grows older. Treatment usually is medical unless the cysts interfere with urine flow by obstructing the upper end of the ureter. If the outlook for recovery through conservative treatment is poor, the surgeon may consider a kidney transplant operation. See p. 985.

Adrenal Glands

The adrenal glands are small hormone-producing organs that are located just above the kidneys. Although the combined weight of the two glands may be only one-fourth of an ounce, the adrenals affect a number of important body functions, including carbohydrate and protein metabolism and fluid balance. Surgery of the adrenal glands may be needed for the correction of various bodily disorders associated with oversecretion of the adrenal hormones; it may also be indicated to help control of cancer of the breast in women and cancer of prostate in men.

TUMORS OF THE ADRENAL GLANDS: Tumors of the adrenal glands produce a disorder known as *primary hyperaldosteronism*, which is marked by symptoms of muscle weakness, hypertension, abnor-

THE ADRENAL GLANDS

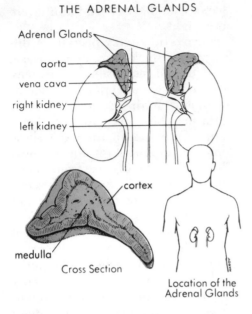

Adrenal Glands

aorta
vena cava
right kidney
left kidney

cortex

medulla
Cross Section

Location of the
Adrenal Glands

mones from other glands such as the pituitary, or master gland of the body, located at the base of the brain.

PRE-OPERATIVE TESTS: Before adrenal surgery for correction of a disorder is begun, the surgeon may ask for detailed laboratory tests and other diagnostic information. A radioactive scan to help locate and identify the kind of tumor more precisely may be ordered. Women patients who have been using oral contraceptives usually have to discontinue use of "the pill" for two months or more because the medication can interfere with laboratory studies of hormones in the bloodstream.

LONG-RANGE EFFECTS: Doctors handling the case also must evaluate the long-range effects of an adrenal gland operation because normal metabolism is likely to be disrupted by removal of the glands, if that should be necessary. Hormone medications usually are needed in such cases to replace the hormones normally secreted. An *adrenalectomy* (removal of an adrenal gland) sometimes is explained as the substitution of a controllable disease for a life-threatening disease that cannot be controlled by medical therapy. If only one of the adrenal glands must be removed, however, the patient may be able to recover and resume a normal life without the need for hormone medications.

SURGICAL PROCEDURE: The surgical approach to the adrenal glands is similar to that used in kidney operations. The incision may be made through the abdomen or through the flank. The surgery may be primarily exploratory, or the surgeon may excise a part of a gland, an entire

mally large outputs of urine, and excessive thirst. Another kind of tumor invasion of the adrenal glands can produce symptoms of hypertension with headaches, visual blurring, and severe sweating. Still another adrenal related disorder, called *Cushing's syndrome*, tends to affect women under the age of 40. The symptoms may range from hypertension and obesity to acne, easy bruising, and *amenorrhea* (cessation of menstruation). Adrenal tumors may also alter secondary sex characteristics of men and women; they may result in body hair and baldness in women and increased sex drive in men.

Despite the tiny size of the adrenal glands, they are complex organs and the varied disorders caused by tumors of the glands may depend upon the precise kind of tumor cells involved and the precise area of the glands affected by the tumor, as well as the interactions of the adrenal hormones with hor-

gland, or both glands, depending upon the extent of the disease, or upon other factors such as the need to control cancers in other parts of the body.

Abdominal Region

This section discusses the following procedures or conditions: appendicitis, peptic ulcers, hiatus hernia, adhesions, cancer of the stomach and of the intestines, gall bladder surgery, inguinal hernia, and hemorrhoids.

Appendicitis

Inflammation of the appendix is one of the most common causes of abdominal surgery today, particularly among children. But appendicitis was not recognized as a disease until 1886, leading some doctors to believe that this digestive tract infection may be related to a change in eating habits that occurred within the past century. The vermiform appendix, the site of the inflammation, is a short, wormlike (or *vermiform*) appendage at the junction of the small and large intestines. Its function in humans is unknown; plant-eating animals have an appendix but carnivorous animals, like cats, do not. Humans live quite well without an appendix, so it seems reasonable to have a diseased appendix removed.

THE ABDOMINAL REGION

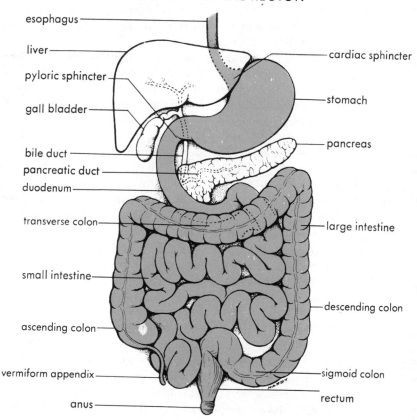

esophagus

liver

pyloric sphincter

gall bladder

bile duct

pancreatic duct

duodenum

transverse colon

small intestine

ascending colon

vermiform appendix

anus

cardiac sphincter

stomach

pancreas

large intestine

descending colon

sigmoid colon

rectum

SYMPTOMS: The appendix can cause trouble if it becomes obstructed by a foreign body, a tumor, an infection, or other cause of inflammation. Pain is a common symptom; there may be two kinds of pain at the same time: one, localized on the lower right side of the abdomen, near the site of the appendix; the other, more generalized and colicky, of the kind sometimes associated with gas in the intestine. Some patients experience diarrhea or a constant urge to defecate, an effect attributed to irritation of the bowel by the abnormal activity of the appendix. Frequently there is loss of appetite, nausea and vomiting, and a fever.

The symptoms of appendicitis may begin suddenly but frequently take from six to 18 hours to develop into a pattern typical of the disease, so most cases permit ample time for a doctor to examine the patient and make a diagnosis before the problem becomes critical. During the period that any symptoms suggest a possibility of appendicitis, the patient should avoid the use of any laxatives.

RUPTURED APPENDIX: A potentially serious complication of untreated appendicitis is rupture of the appendix, which can produce a slightly different set of symptoms because of the onset of *peritonitis*, a dangerous inflammation of tissues outside the intestinal tract. The contents of the ruptured appendix leak into the body cavity, spreading the bacterial infection and irritating the lining (peritoneum) of the abdominal cavity. Diarrhea and a fever of more than 101°F. are frequently associated with a perforated or ruptured appendix. The colicky pain

may disappear suddenly because the internal pressure ends with perforation of the wall of the appendix, but it is quickly replaced by the pain of peritonitis. The severe pain of peritonitis usually is made worse by any body movement, including the abdominal muscle movement required for coughing or sneezing.

Appendicitis with perforation is much more common in older persons, perhaps because the early symptoms of colicky pain that younger people notice are not felt by older people, so the disease is not detected until it has reached an advanced stage. Appendicitis also requires special attention in pregnant women because the enlarged uterus crowds and repositions segments of the intestinal tract and the potential threat grows more serious during the last trimester of pregnancy.

SURGICAL PROCEDURE: Laboratory tests usually are checked before surgery proceeds if there is no evidence of perforation. The usual symptoms of appendicitis can be produced by a number of other ailments, and the symptoms may diminish with bed rest, time, and medications. However, appendicitis must be considered in any case of acute abdominal complaints, and many doctors follow the rule of "When in doubt, operate." Surgery for appendicitis is fairly simple and safe if the appendix has not perforated. An incision is made in the lower right side of the abdomen, the connection between the end of the large intestine and appendix is tied off with surgical thread, and the appendix cut away from the stump. The actual operation, if uncomplicated by peritonitis or other factors, may require only a few minutes. A hospital stay of a few days is usually required while the diet is readjusted from nothing by mouth at first, to a liquid diet, then a soft diet, etc. Normal work activities usually can be resumed within two or three weeks following surgery. Complications other than those related to peritonitis are rare. In untreated cases involving peritonitis, however, the risk is very high.

Peptic Ulcers

The cause of peptic ulcers is still unknown, although the disease affects about ten percent of the population at some time in life. Men are four times as likely as women to develop ulcers; the incidence is highest in young and middle-aged men. Peptic ulcers may occur in the stomach, where they are called *gastric ulcers,* or in the duodenum, where they are called *duodenal ulcers.* Ninety percent of the ulcer cases that reach the doctor's office for treatment are in the duodenum, a short length of the small intestine just beyond the stomach. Autopsy studies indicate that gastric ulcers may be as common as duodenal ulcers, but are frequently not detected during the life of the individual.

CAUSES: The development of ulcers is associated with the possible action of gastric acid on the lining of the stomach and duodenum in people who may have inherited a sensitivity to the substances. Ulcers are also related to the use of certain drugs and exposure to severe burns, injury, emotional stress, and disease.

SYMPTOMS: A common symptom is a gnawing pain in the area of the stomach from 30 minutes to several hours after eating; the pain is relieved by food or antacid medications. The pain sometimes is described as heartburn and may be described as radiating from the abdomen to the back. Some patients report the discomfort is more like a feeling of hunger or cramps; they may be awakened from sleep by the feeling which is relieved by a midnight snack of milk or other foods. Attacks of ulcers may be seasonal, occurring in certain patients only in the spring and autumn. In severe cases there may be bleeding without any sensation of abdominal pain; bleeding occurs from erosion of the lining of the stomach or duodenum and penetration of blood vessels in those membranes.

Complications other than bleeding can include perforation of the wall of the stomach or duodenum by continued erosion, or inflammatory swelling and scarring by an ulcer at a narrow part of the digestive tract, causing an obstruction. A duodenal ulcer can erode into the head of the pancreas, which secretes its digestive juices into the small intestine in that area. The pain may then become more or less continuous regardless of efforts to palliate it with food or antacids.

Symptoms vary only slightly between duodenal and gastric ulcers. Gastric ulcer pain usually begins earlier after a meal, attacks generally last longer, and symptoms, including vomiting and loss of appetite, may be more severe than in duodenal ulcer. But because of the similarities, doctors usually rely on laboratory tests and X-ray studies to determine the precise location in the digestive tract of the peptic ulcer.

DUODENAL ULCERS: Duodenal ulcers nearly always occur within an inch of the pyloric valve separating the stomach from the small intestine. The pain or discomfort follows a cycle. The patient may experience no pain until after breakfast. The pain is relieved by the noon meal but returns in the afternoon and occurs again in the evening. Milk or other bland food or medications relieve the pain that may appear at various times in the cycle. The symptoms of duodenal ulcers also go through periods of remission and recurrence over periods of months or years. Most duodenal ulcers are treated with diet, drugs, and measures that encourage rest and relaxation.

SURGICAL PROCEDURES: Surgery for either duodenal or gastric ulcer is designed to reduce gastric acid secretion rather than simply to excise the ulcer from the normal digestive tract tissue. One surgical approach, called *subtotal gastrectomy*, involves cutting away a portion of the stomach in the area where it joins the duodenum. There are several variations of this technique, including one in which the remaining portion of the stomach is attached to the jejunum, a segment of the small intestine. The ulcerated portion of the duodenum may be removed during the reconstructive surgery of the digestive tract, or it may be left in the duodenal segment which is closed during the gastrectomy procedure.

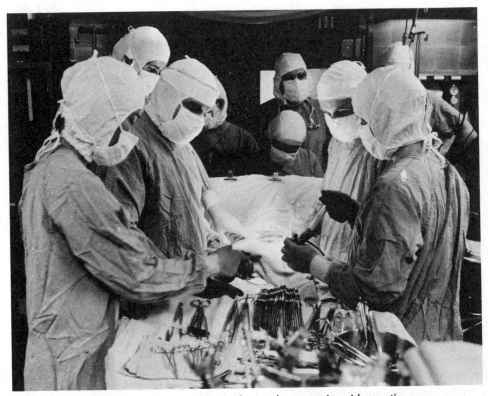

Surgery for ulcers is designed to reduce gastric acid secretion
rather than simply to excise the ulcer from the digestive tract tissue.

An interesting effect is that a duodenal ulcer usually heals, when left in place, after the gastric juices are routed into the intestine through the jejunum. The reconstructed stomach and stomach-to-intestine connection cause no serious problems in eating after the patient has recovered.

A second surgical approach, called a *vagotomy,* involves cutting a part of the vagus nerve trunk that controls the secretion of stomach acid. There are several variations of vagotomy, each technique affecting a different portion of the vagus nerve distribution to the stomach.

GASTRIC ULCERS: Stomach or gastric ulcers tend to develop in older persons more often than duodenal ulcers, and the problem seems to be less importantly related to the overproduction of gastric acid. The real hazard of stomach ulcers is that a significant percentage are found to be a kind of cancer and do not respond to the usual therapies for controlling peptic ulcer symptoms. If it is determined that a stomach ulcer is a malignant growth, a partial gastrectomy is performed in the same manner as an operation of that type for duodenal ulcers. The vagotomy approach is not used for treatment of a stomach ulcer unless the ulcer is excised at the same time.

Hiatus Hernia

The term *hiatus hernia* actually describes a diaphragmatic hernia or weakness in the diaphragm, the horizontal muscular wall separating the organs of the chest from the organs of the abdomen. A *hernia* is an abnormal protrusion of an organ or tissue through an opening. A *hiatus,* or opening, occurs naturally to permit the esophagus to carry food from the mouth to the stomach. Blood vessels and nerves also pass through the diaphragm. The diaphragm is an important group of muscles for contracting and expanding the lungs, forcing air in and out of the lung tissues.

Hiatus hernias are rare in children, but as people grow older there may be a weakening of the diaphragm muscles and associated tissues. Aided by a tendency toward obesity and the use of girdles and other tight garments, a portion of the stomach may be pushed through the opening designed by nature for use of the esophagus. Aside from the discomfort of having a part of the stomach in the chest, there are potential dangers of incarceration of the stomach, with obstruction, strangulation, and hemorrhage with erosion of the stomach lining. In severe complications, the entire stomach along with intestines and other abdominal organs may be forced through the hiatus hernia into the chest area.

The most common kind of hiatus hernia is sometimes called sliding hiatus hernia from the tendency of the stomach to slide in and out of the thorax, or chest cavity, when the patient changes body positions or as a result of the pressure of a big meal in the gastrointestinal tract. Sometimes the herniated stomach does not move at all but remains fixed, with a significant portion of the stomach above the diaphragm. Hiatus hernia causes heartburn symptoms, including regurgitation of digested food and gastric acid from the stomach, while lying down or when straining or stooping. The effect also may be noticeable in a woman during pregnancy.

NONSURGICAL TREATMENT: Many cases of hiatal hernia can be treated without surgery through a change of eating habits and the use of antacid medications. The patient may be advised to eat small amounts more frequently during the day with dietary emphasis on high-protein, low-fat foods. Some doctors recommend that patients use liquid antacid medications rather than antacid tablets or lozenges.

SURGICAL TREATMENT: When surgery is recommended to correct hiatus hernia, the repair may be performed either through the abdominal wall or through the chest. About three-fourths of the procedures are handled through abdominal incisions because doctors often find other abdominal problems that need to be corrected at the same time, such as peptic ulcers or gall bladder disease. The opening through the diaphragm is firmly closed with sutures to prevent upward movement of the stomach. The stomach and lower end of the esophagus may be anchored in place in the abdomen. The chances of recurrence are about one in ten, although some patients may continue to have a few of the symptoms of the disorder for a while after the hernia repair.

Adhesions

Adhesions may develop between various abdominal organs and the peritoneum, the membrane lining the abdominal cavity. The bowel may acquire adhesions that result in obstruction of the intestinal tract. Adhesions may form between the liver and the peritoneum or between the liver and the diaphragm. The symptoms may be pain or cramps in the area where tissues are literally stuck together; in more serious cases that involve bowel obstruction, symptoms may include constipation, vomiting, and distension of the abdomen. Adhesions do not show on X-ray film and can be difficult to diagnose unless the patient's medical history suggests a cause for the bands or filaments of tissues responsible for the adhesions.

CAUSES: The causes may be peritonitis, injury, infection, internal bleeding, or foreign objects. Adhesions occur after an operation, perhaps because of a bit of blood resulting from surgery or as a result of a speck of talc from the surgeon's glove or a fiber from a surgical drape that produces a foreign body reaction, much like an allergic reaction, when it comes in contact with the abdominal tissues. Disease organisms may enter the female abdominal cavity through the Fallopian tubes to produce adhesions, especially in the case of gonorrhea, which can escape early detection in women because of the lack of obvious symptoms.

COMPLICATIONS: Adhesions can cause complications such as changing the position of the intestinal tract through twisting or otherwise distorting its path so that bowel movements are obstructed. If the involved portion of the intestine becomes seriously damaged so that it no longer functions properly, the surgeon may have to remove that section. Generally, when the surgeon is correcting the problem of adhesions, a relatively simple procedure of cutting away the tissue bands or filaments holding organs in abnormal ways, he inspects the organs to determine if they appear to be in good working order. That part of the operation may add 15 or 20 minutes to the time spent on an operating table but it helps insure that the patient will not have to be returned soon for further surgery.

Cancer of the Stomach

There are several possible types of stomach tumors but one kind, called *adenocarcinoma,* is one of the greatest killers of men over the age of 45. Although the incidence of stomach cancer in the United States has declined considerably since the end of World War II, the death rate from this problem in the U.S. alone is about 15,000 per year. In central and eastern Europe the incidence of stomach cancer is about four times, and in Japan seven times, that of the United States. Almost two-thirds of the stomach cancers develop near the pylorus, the opening from the stomach into the small intestine; only five percent involve the entire stomach area.

SYMPTOMS: Symptoms include a feeling of heaviness rather than pain following a meal. The patient in many cases mysteriously loses his appetite for meat and begins to lose weight. There may be vague symptoms of an upset stomach, with some vomiting, especially if the tumor begins to obstruct the pylorus so that stomach contents cannot be emptied into the intestine. The vomitus usually is the color of coffee grounds, suggesting a loss of blood from the stomach lining because of the tumor, and the patient's stools also may be dark in coloration because of internal bleeding. The doctor frequently can confirm his suspicions about the cause of the

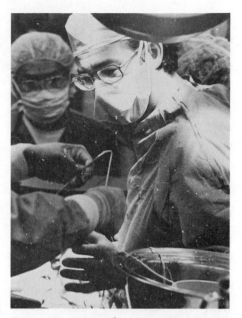

A surgeon necessarily must possess intense powers of concentration to bring to his work—as this doctor, who is performing abdominal surgery—clearly does.

symptoms by laboratory analysis of a specimen of cells from the stomach, by X-ray studies of the stomach, or by an examination with a gastroscope that permits a direct view of the interior of the stomach. In some cases the doctor will be able to feel an abnormal mass in the stomach by palpating the stomach area of the abdomen with his hands.

TREATMENT: Treatment is by cutting away the tumor and surrounding tissues that may be involved, including parts of neighboring organs. The lymph nodes in the region of the stomach are also removed. The remaining part of the stomach is used to build a new digestive organ, as in a case of partial gastrectomy for correcting a peptic ulcer problem. However, before beginning reconstructive surgery the doctor usually orders biopsy tests of the remaining tissues to make sure the new stomach will not be made of tissues in which tumor cells have spread. If the edges of the remaining stomach wall are found to contain tumor cells, the surgeon simply extends the area to be removed. As in subtotal gastrectomy for peptic ulcers, the remaining portion of the stomach may be connected directly to the upper portion of the small intestine, at the duodenum or the jejunum.

Meals are provided in the form of intravenous feedings for the first few days following surgery. Sips of water may be permitted on the second or third day after the operation with the amounts gradually increased to one or two ounces of water per hour as the new digestive system adjusts to fluid intake. Then soft or bland foods can gradually be taken orally in a half-dozen small feedings each day. It may take three or four months for the new stomach to distend and adjust to normal eating habits of the patient.

POST-OPERATIVE EFFECTS: Some patients may experience a variety of symptoms ranging from nausea to cramps and diarrhea while recovering from stomach surgery. The symptoms form what is known as the dumping syndrome which occurs within a half hour after a meal, presumably by rapid distention of the upper portion of the small intestine as fluid rushes, or is dumped, into that part of the digestive tract from the new stomach. The effects can be controlled by a change of diet to eliminate starches and sugars, by delaying the intake of fluids until after the meal, by medications, and by training the patient to lie in a recumbent or semirecumbent position to lessen discomfort following a meal. The symptoms occur in only a small proportion of stomach surgery patients, and they usually diminish gradually during the period of recovery.

Cancer of the Intestines

SMALL INTESTINE: Tumors of the small intestine are not common but they also are not rare. It has been estimated that less than five percent of all tumors of the gastrointestinal tract occur in the small intestine. Of tumors that do develop in this portion of the gastrointestinal tract, about 90 percent are benign, or noncancerous, growths. The symptoms of small intestine tumors may include bleeding, obstruction, and perforation of the intestinal wall. However, most tumors of the small intestine produce no symptoms at all. When tumors are found in the small intestine they usually are found at the same time in other parts of the body, and usually in a patient over 40 years of age, although the more malignant growths can occur in younger persons. Treatment of a cancer of the small bowel is by removing the affected section and administration of radiation therapy for certain kinds of cancerous tumors.

LARGE INTESTINE: Tumors of the large intestine, unlike those of the small bowel, account for a large proportion of cancers of the human body and for most of the malignant growths of the entire gastrointestinal tract. Over 40,000 deaths each year in the United States are due to cancers of the colon and rectum portions of the large bowel. And about three-fourths of all large-intestine tumors develop near the rectal portion of the bowel where, ironically, they should be easily available for detection during physical examination.

Tumors of the large intestine can be found in persons of any age, but they occur most frequently in patients who are of middle age or older, reaching a peak of incidence around the age of 65. Men are more likely to develop cancer of the rectum, but women are more frequently affected by cancer of the colon. While cancer of the large intestine tends to occur among members of the same families at a rate that is two or three times the normal incidence, it is believed that family environment factors, such as life style and diet, are the causative influences rather than hereditary factors. People who develop cancer of the large intestine usually eat foods that are low in cellulose and high in animal fats and refined carbohydrates.

Bowel cancers appear to grow in size at a very slow rate, doubling about once every 20 months, so a number of years may elapse between the start of a bowel tumor and the appearance of signs or symptoms of cancer.

SYMPTOMS: The location of the growth can influence the type of symptoms experienced. Cancer in the right colon may be found as an abnormal mass during a physical examination by a physician after complaints of fatigue and weakness and signs of anemia. The tumor can develop to a rather large size without producing signs of blood in the stools. Cancer in the left colon, by contrast, may be found after complaints of alternate periods of constipation and frequent urge to defecate, pain in the abdomen, and stools marked by dark or bright red blood. When the cancer is in the rectum, the patient may find blood mixed with the bowel movements but experience no pain in the early stages. Other symptoms of cancer of the large intestine may mimic those of appendicitis, hemorrhoids, peptic ulcer, or gall bladder disease.

As noted above, most cancers of the large bowel are close enough to the end of the intestinal tract to be observed directly by palpation or the use of fiberoptic instruments such as a sigmoidoscope or colonoscope that can be inserted into the rectum or colon. Biopsy samples can be removed for study and X-ray pictures taken after a barium enema has coated the bowel membrane so that abnormal surfaces are marked in black-and-white contrast.

SURGICAL PROCEDURES: Surgical procedures for treatment of cancer of the large intestine vary somewhat according to the location of the growth, but the objective is the same: to remove the affected portion and reconstruct the bowel so that normal digestive functions can resume. Radiation therapy and chemotherapy may be used in the treatment of certain advanced cases. When surgical treatment is begun soon after the first symptoms are diagnosed, the chances of curing cancer of the large bowel are very good.

If there are complications, such as obstruction of the portion of the large intestine, the surgery may be conducted in a series of stages over a period of several weeks. The several stages involve a colostomy procedure in which an opening is made in the wall of the abdomen to permit a portion of the intestinal tract to be brought to the surface of the body.

After the complicating problem is treated and resection of the cancerous segment is completed, the colostomy is closed by sewing the open end of the bowel to the remaining portion and closing the opening in the abdomen.

PRE-OPERATIVE STEPS: Some special pre-operative measures are ordered for patients awaiting surgery for treatment of bowel cancer. They consist primarily of several days of liquid diets, laxatives, and enemas to make the interior of the intestinal tract as clean as possible. Other measures will be directed toward correction of anemia and compensation for possible loss of blood resulting from the cancer's invasion of bowel tissues.

Gall Bladder Surgery

Gall bladder disease is one of the most common medical disorders in the United States. It has been esti-mated that more than 15 million Americans are affected by the disease and about 6,000 deaths a year are associated with it. The incidence increases at middle age; one of every five women over the age of 50 and one of every 20 men can expect to be treated for gall bladder symptoms. Approximately 1,000 people in the United States enter operating rooms each day for removal of gallstones, a primary cause of the symptoms of the disorder.

GALLSTONES: Gallstones generally are formed from crystals of cholesterol that gradually increase in size in the gall bladder; some, however, are formed from other substances such as bile salts and breakdown products of old red blood cells. Because they are very small in size, the stones may produce no symptoms at first. But as they grow in size they become more threatening and eventually can block the normal flow of

A surgeon sews up his patient's incision at the close of a gall bladder operation—an extremely common type of surgery in the U.S.

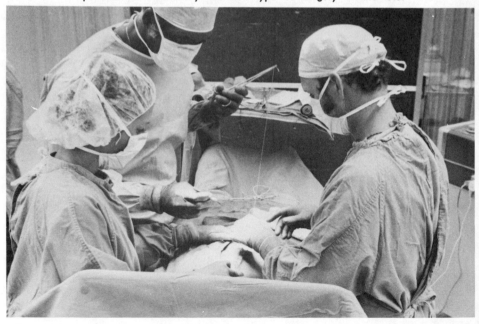

bile from one of the bile ducts emptying into the intestine. Bile contains substances needed by the body to digest fats in the diet.

SYMPTOMS: A common symptom of *chronic cholecystitis*, or gallstone disease, is a pain that appears suddenly in the upper abdomen and subsides slowly over a period of several minutes to several hours. The pain may occur after a meal or with no apparent relationship to meals. There can be tenderness in the upper right side of the body, with pain extending to the shoulder. The pain also can appear on the left side or near the center of the upper abdomen, producing misleading symptoms suggesting a heart attack. Nausea, heartburn, gas, indigestion, and intolerance of fatty foods are among other possible symptoms. The gall bladder attacks may occur frequently or there may be remissions (periods without symptoms) lasting for several months or years.

A careful and extensive physical examination, including X-ray studies of the gall bladder area, may be needed to confirm the presence of gallstones. Until recently, the most commonly used test was the oral cholecystogram (OCG), in which the patient swallowed an iodine-based "dye," or contrast agent. X rays taken about 12 hours after administration of the dye might or might not provide useful "pictures" of the gallstones. As a result, ultrasound has largely replaced X rays as a primary test for suspected gallstones.

ACUTE CHOLECYSTITIS: About three-fourths of the cases of acute cholecystitis are patients who have had previous attacks of gallstone disease. In the acute phase there is persistent pain and abdominal tenderness, along with nausea and vomiting in many cases and a mild fever. Complications may include perforation, or rupture, of the gall bladder, leading to peritonitis, or development of adhesions to neighboring organs such as the stomach or intestine.

TREATMENT: Surgical treatment of chronic or acute cholecystitis is basically an elective procedure that can be scheduled at a time convenient to the patient. But acute cases with complications may require emergency operations. The patient can usually be maintained after surgery on intravenous fluids and pain-killing medications.

A number of alternatives to surgery have been developed. A gastroenterologist may use an endoscope on older patients or those in poor health. The endoscope, a tube inserted through the chest wall, enables the physician to view the gall bladder's duct area and to widen its opening so that small gallstones can slip through the small intestine. Using a small basket on the endoscope, the physician can sometimes catch and withdraw or crush the stones.

In gallstone surgery, the abdomen is opened so that the surgeon can examine the gall bladder and the ducts leading from it for stones. The gall bladder may be freed of stones and a temporary drainage tube inserted, with an opening to the outside of the upper abdomen. But usually the surgeon removes the entire gall bladder in an operation called a *cholecystectomy*. The bile duct, which remains as a link between the liver and the small intestine, gradually replaces the gall bladder in function. Most patients require no more than ten days to two weeks of hospitalization, and can resume normal work activities in a month to six weeks.

Other nonsurgical treatments include chemical preparations. Chenodeoxycholic acid or chenodiol has been given orally to dissolve smaller, floating cholesterol stones. But the drug has little effect against pigment stones or stones with a high calcium content, and can cause diarrhea as a side effect. Researchers have worked experimentally with ursodeoxycholic acid and other drugs that have been found to dissolve gallstones in both animals and humans.

Among the most advanced techniques is *choledocholithotripsy,* a nonsurgical method using shock waves to destroy gallstones. Already in use as a method of shattering kidney stones, lithotripsy requires only a local anesthetic and the recovery period lasts only a few days. The physician uses a hollow tool—the lithotripter—that is inserted through the patient's chest until it approaches the stones. With a foot switch, the physician then triggers a jolt of high-voltage, low-current electricity that shatters the stones.

Inguinal Hernia

An inguinal hernia (hernia of the groin) can develop in either men or women at almost any age from infancy to late adult years. But the incidence of inguinal hernia is much more common in males. An inguinal hernia is one in which the intestinal tract protrudes through the opening of one of the inguinal rings on either side of the groin. In males, the inguinal rings are temporary openings through which the testicles descend

into the scrotum before birth; in females, the openings permit the passage of a ligament supporting the ovary.

CAUSES: Normally, the inguinal rings are closed after the birth of the child. However, they may fail to close completely or the muscles and connective tissues may become stretched or weakened in later years to permit a portion of the abdominal contents, usually part of the intestine, to protrude. A number of factors can contribute to the development of a hernia, including physical strain from exercise or lifting, straining over a bowel movement, coughing spells, pregnancy, pressure of abdominal organs, or obesity.

REDUCIBLE AND IRREDUCIBLE HERNIAS: The hernia may be *reducible,* that is, the bulge in the abdominal wall may disappear when the body position is changed, as in lying down, only to reappear upon stand-

INGUINAL HERNIA

muscular wall of abdomen
intestine
bladder
inguinal canal
vas deferens
loop of intestine in scrotum

In this type of indirect hernia, a loop of small intestine has pushed through the weakened inguinal canal in the abdominal wall and descended into the scrotal sac.

ing. An *irreducible* hernia does not allow the hernia sac contents to return to the abdominal cavity; an irreducible hernia also may be called *incarcerated*, a term aptly describing the hernia as being trapped. A serious complication is strangulation of the hernia contents, which usually involves obstruction of normal blood flow and resulting damage or destruction of the incarcerated intestines. A strangulated hernia may be life-threatening because of the possibility of gangrene in body tissues damaged by incarceration.

SURGICAL PROCEDURE: Some hernias are called direct, some indirect, for purposes of medical records. These terms indicate to the surgeon specific layers of muscle and connective tissue that have been breached and are of no real significance to the patient because the surgical repair procedures are essentially the same for either type. In the absence of complications, the operation is fairly simple and usually can be performed with either a general or local anesthetic. An incision is made in the lower abdomen in the area of the hernia, the protruding organ is returned to its normal position, and the weakened or ruptured layers of muscle and connective tissue are repaired and reinforced to provide a strong internal wall that will hold the abdominal contents in place. In some cases the surgeon will use available tissues from the patient's own body in building a new wall against future hernias. The surgeon also may use a variety of materials including silk, catgut, stainless steel, tantalum mesh gauze, or mesh screens made of plastics in building a new barrier.

RECOVERY: The hospital stay for hernia repair is relatively brief, usually from three days to a week; some healthy children undergo surgery early in the morning and return home in the evening of the same day. The patient usually is instructed to avoid exercise or exertion for a couple of weeks and can return to work in a month to six weeks, depending upon the work load expected. Hernias tend to recur in only a small percentage of cases among adults and very rarely in children.

Femoral Hernia

About five percent of all hernias of the groin area are femoral hernias, with the hernia bulge appearing along the thigh. Femoral hernias occur about four times as frequently among women and usually appear in middle age. While a femoral hernia is not necessarily limited to obese patients, it is more likely to be associated with being overweight and the movement of a bowel segment or the urinary bladder into the hernia frequently is preceded by a fat pad—a mass of fatty tissue. Femoral hernias are more prone to incarceration and strangulation than inguinal hernias. The surgical treatment of femoral hernias is similar to that used in the repair of inguinal hernias, although the incision may be made through the thigh in a few cases.

Hemorrhoids

Hemorrhoid, a term derived from Greek words meaning "blood flowing," refers to a system of arteries and veins that serve the rectal area. The medical problem known as *hemorrhoids*, or *piles*, is a tortuous enlargement of the hemorrhoidal veins, a problem similar to the varicose veins of the legs. Causes of the varicosities of the hemorrhoidal veins include the human peculiarity of standing and walking in an erect posture—animals that walk on all fours do not get hemorrhoids.

Women during pregnancies are particularly subject to hemorrhoidal problems because of the pressure on the veins of the lower body area. Other causes are constipation and straining at stool; diseases of the digestive tract resulting in anal infection; and cirrhosis of the liver, which obstructs blood flow and puts increased pressure on the hemorrhoidal veins.

SYMPTOMS: Symptoms usually include bleeding, which may stain the patient's clothing; irritation and discomfort, including itching, in the anal region; and occasionally pain with inflammation. Because rectal bleeding also can be a sign of a number of other diseases, the doctor usually makes a thorough examination to rule out other possible causes, such as cancer or ulcerative colitis.

TREATMENT: If the hemorrhoids do not warrant surgery, medical treatments may be prescribed. *Prolapsed hemorrhoids* (veins that protrude from the anus) can be reduced by gentle pressure. Bed rest, warm baths, and medications are also a part of medical treatments. A type of injection chemotherapy sometimes is used to control bleeding and eliminate the varicosed veins.

Surgery can be used to excise all the affected tissues, and the disorder also can be treated by cryosurgery in which the hemorrhoids are destroyed by a probe containing supercold liquid nitrogen or carbon dioxide. The patient usually is able to recover and return to work within one or two weeks after surgical removal of the hemorrhoidal tissues.

Oral Cavity and Throat

This section discusses oral cancers, tonsils and adenoids, and surgery of the thyroid. For a discussion of cosmetic surgery of the face area, see pp. 976–982.

Oral Cancers

There are many potential problems of the mouth, or oral cavity, besides an occasional toothache. Surgical treatment frequently is needed to correct a disorder or to prevent a life-threatening situation from developing. Cancers of the lips, tongue, hard and soft palate, and other areas of the mouth, for example, affect about 25,000 people in the United States each year. Elsewhere in the world, the incidence varies considerably according to sex and location; the rate in Hong Kong for men is three times the figure for women, and the incidence of oral cancer for women in Hong Kong is nearly 10 times as high as that of women in Japan. Environmental factors such as tobacco and contact with chemical and physical agents have been suggested as causes, although one form of oral cancer, known as *Burkitt's lymphoma,* is believed to be transmitted by a mosquito-borne virus.

CANCER OF THE LIP: Oral cancers tend to occur after the age of 45. Some types of oral cancer, particularly when the lips are affected, are found most frequently in persons exposed to a great deal of sunlight. Farmers, sailors, and other outdoor

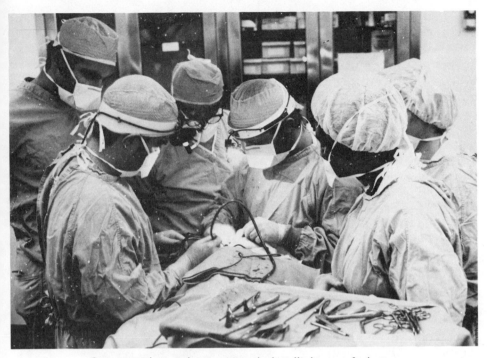

Surgery on the nasal cavity. Note the headlights worn for better visualization. The surgeon at the left applies a speculum to enlarge the nasal opening and aspirates fluids with the tube.

workers develop such tumors around the age of 60, with the lesion appearing on the lower lip. Like other cancers, cancer of the lip may begin as a tiny growth but if untreated can spread through neighboring tissues and eventually destroy part of the chin. Treatment may include both radiation therapy and surgical excision of the growth; if surgery is performed when the tumor is small the scar is likewise small. Obviously, the larger the tumor is allowed to grow, the more difficult the treatment.

CANCER OF THE CHEEK: Similarly, cancers that develop on the inner surface of the cheek usually can be excised and the wound closed with simple surgery if treatment is started early. If the cancer is allowed to grow before treatment, the surgery becomes more complicated with removal of tissues extending to the outer skin layers and repair of the wound with skin grafts. Radiation therapy also may be used to augment the surgical repair.

CANCER OF THE MOUTH: Cancer of the floor of the mouth may be second only to lip cancer in rate of occurrence of oral cavity tumors; together they may account for half of the oral cavity cancers in the United States. A tumor of the floor of the mouth may involve the under surface of the tongue, the lower jawbone, and other tissues of the area. A small lesion detected early can be controlled in most cases by excision of the growth and radiation therapy.

CANCER OF THE TONGUE: The tongue may be the site of cancerous growths beginning in the 30s of the patient's life, particularly if the individual is a heavy user of tobacco and alcohol and has been neglectful of proper oral hygiene, such as brushing the teeth regularly. If the growth is at the tip of the tongue rather than underneath or along the sides, the operation is easier and there is less chance that the normal function of the tongue will be impaired by removing the growth and surrounding tissue cells. Radiation therapy for cancer of the tongue sometimes involves the implantation of needles containing radium into the tongue. The procedure is done while the patient is under a general anesthetic. Tumors at the base of the tongue, as well as some growths on the floor of the mouth, sometimes are approached through an incision in the neck.

OTHER SURGERY: Apart from cancers, surgery of the oral cavity may be needed to treat genetic defects, such as cleft lip and cleft palate, damage to tissues from injuries, and noncancerous tumors of the soft tissues, such as cysts. For information on cleft lip and cleft palate, see p. 463. For a discussion of cosmetic surgery of the face, see p. 976.

Tonsils and Adenoids

Tonsils and adenoids are glands of lymphoid tissue lying along the walls near the top of the throat. The tonsils are located on the sides of the pharynx, or throat, near the base of the tongue. Unless an adult's tonsils are inflamed, they may not be easily visible to a doctor or other person looking into the throat, but when inflamed and swollen they can be seen without difficulty. The adenoids are located higher in the pharynx and cannot be seen by look-

ing into the back of the mouth without special instruments because the palate, or roof of the mouth, blocks the view.

TONSILLITIS: The function of the tonsils and adenoids apparently is that of trapping infectious organisms that enter the body through the nose and mouth. But sometimes the glands do such a good job of collecting infections that they lose their effectiveness, becoming enlarged and inflamed, a condition known as *tonsillitis*. The patient develops fever and sore throat and the breathing passages become obstructed. The infections can spread through the nearby Eustachian tubes to the ears, causing *otitis*

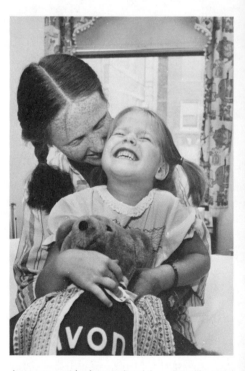

A young patient hospitalized for a tonsillectomy gets some loving comfort from her mother before the operation. Tonsillectomies are no longer routinely performed on young sore-throat victims.

media (inflammation of the middle ear), resulting in deafness. Disease organisms also can spread from the tonsils and adenoids to the kidneys, joints, heart, eyes, and other body areas. Many youngsters survive occasional bouts of tonsillitis and the infections can be treated with antibiotics and medications to relieve pain and fever symptoms. But many surgeons recommend that the tonsils and adenoids be removed if tonsillitis occurs repeatedly.

TONSILLECTOMY: A *tonsillectomy* (removal of the tonsils) is not a complicated operation but it usually is performed under a general anesthetic if the patient is a child. A local anesthetic may be used for an adult. The adenoids usually are removed at the same time; they consist of the same type of lymphoid tissue in the same general area, and adenoids develop similar problems from the same kind of infectious agents. An overnight stay in the hospital may be required or it may be possible for the patient to have the tonsils and adenoids removed in the morning and be released from the hospital in the evening of the same day, after a few hours of post-operative rest under medical observation.

PRE-OPERATIVE AND POST-OPERATIVE CARE: The patient may receive antibiotic medications two or three days prior to surgery and is instructed to avoid eating foods or drinking fluids for at least 12 hours before the operation. If the patient has a cold or other viral infection, the surgery may be delayed or postponed. Some surgeons also prefer to avoid tonsillectomy operations during the hay fever season. If there is any evidence of bleeding after the patient is released, such as spitting blood, he is

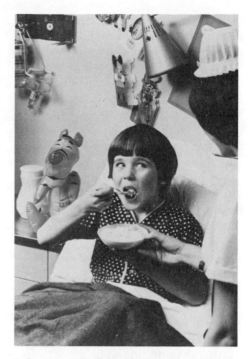

Following a tonsillectomy, the young patient is fed bland liquid or semi-liquid foods such as ice cream, pudding, and milk. This staves off irritation of sensitive throat tissue.

returned to the hospital and the surgeon is notified; the bleeding usually can be controlled without difficulty. The patient also returns for checkups a couple of weeks after the operation and again about six months later.

ADENOIDECTOMY: In some cases, a doctor may recommend an *adenoidectomy* (removal of the adenoids) without a tonsillectomy. This is particularly true when the patient suffers from recurrent ear infections and hearing loss. An adenoidectomy is a relatively simple operation performed under a local anesthetic when the patient is an adult or older teen-ager; a general anesthetic is preferred for younger patients.

The surgeon can reach the adenoid mass through the open mouth of the patient. The tissue grows on a palate ledge near the point where the nasal passage enters the back of the mouth cavity. Using a special instrument, the surgeon cuts away the adenoid tissue within a few minutes. A medicated pack is inserted into the postnasal area to help control bleeding and the patient is moved to a recovery room. The only aftereffects in most cases are a soreness in the postnasal area for a few days and, occasionally, a temporary voice change that is marked by a nasal tone while the wound heals.

Thyroid Surgery

The thyroid gland lies along the trachea, or windpipe, at a point just below the Adam's apple. Secretions of the thyroid gland are vital for metabolic activities of the body, and the gland's functions are closely orchestrated with those of other endocrine glands of the body. When the thyroid is less active than normal, mental and physical functions are slow and the patient gains weight. When the gland is overly active, body functions operate at an abnormally fast pace, with symptoms of weight loss, irritability, heart palpitations, and bulging eyes. Occasionally, lumps develop on the thyroid, requiring medical or surgical treatment. A lump on the thyroid gland may be a nodular, or nontoxic, goiter. Or it could be a tumor. A nodular goiter poses several threats: it can make the thyroid gland become overactive, it can press on the windpipe and cause hoarseness, or it can develop into a cancer. Some growths of the thyroid gland can be treated effectively with medications, radiation, or a combination such as radioactive iodine. However, when conservative forms of therapy no longer appear to control the condition, or when it is suspected that a thyroid growth may be a malignant cancer, surgical removal of the affected area is advised promptly.

SURGICAL PROCEDURE: The operation itself is fairly simple. An incision is made through the skin folds of the neck, neck muscles beneath the skin are separated, and the affected portion of the gland is cut away. The neck and throat area may be sore and painful for a few days after the operation; within a few weeks the patient can resume normal activities. A thin scar remains at the line of incision but it is usually partly concealed by skin folds of the neck.

Ear Surgery

Surgical treatment of the ear usually is directed toward restoring the function of normal hearing which may have been lost or impaired by disease or injury. The eardrum, or tympanic membrane, can be perforated or ruptured by direct injury, by the shock waves of an explosion, or by an infection of the middle ear. Infection or injury also can disrupt hearing function by damaging the

THE THYROID GLAND

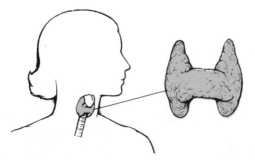

THE EAR

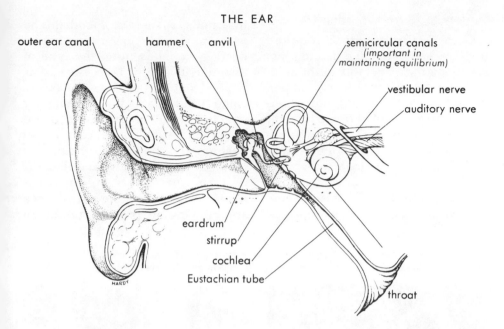

ossicles, a chain of tiny bones that transmit sound waves from the eardrum to the inner ear. Disease, aging effects, and exposure to loud noises can cause hearing loss or impairment.

Surgery of the ear usually involves working with the middle ear, the compartment between the eardrum and the inner ear, which contains the nerve endings that carry impulses to the auditory centers of the brain. The middle ear contains three ossicles, known by their common names of *hammer, anvil,* and *stirrup*—terms that suggest their functions in translating movements of air molecules into the vibrations the brain understands as sounds.

Otitis Media

One common disease of the middle ear is otitis media, which can occur by infection from a number of different kinds of organisms. Otitis media also can develop from secre-

tions or fluids such as milk being forced into the ear through the Eustachian tube, particularly in infants that are fed while they are in a reclining position. The symptoms of otitis media are pain in the ear, fever, and loss of hearing; a small child may indicate the symptoms by crying and tugging at the ear.

SURGICAL PROCEDURE: Many cases of otitis media respond to medical treatment, such as the use of antibiotics, but for patients who suffer severe pain or who have middle ears filled with pus a surgical procedure called *myringotomy* is performed. Myringotomy means simply perforating the eardrum. But the operation usually is performed in a hospital, under a local anesthetic, and with great care to avoid disturbing the ossicles or other ear structures beyond the eardrum. The middle ear is drained and the eardrum either heals spontaneously or can be subsequently repaired with a graft from the patient's own tissues.

Surgery to Correct Hearing Loss

Occasionally surgery is required to correct a conductive hearing loss involving the structures of the middle ear. Such problems happen more frequently among older persons due to abnormal tissue growths that in effect "freeze" the ossicles so they no longer work with their normal flexibility. Ossicular disorders also can occur in younger persons, including children, because of congenital defects, injury, or repeated infections, as of otitis media. The exact procedure for restoration of hearing depends upon the type of disorder. If one of the ossicles has slipped out of position or has become rigidly attached to another structure like the tympanic membrane, the tiny bones can be repositioned or freed from the tissues that may have immobilized them. It is not unusual for the surgeon, working in a space about the size of a pea and viewing his progress through a

Microsurgery, which makes use of a microscope and often of tiny and delicate instruments, is particularly helpful in treating eyes and ears.

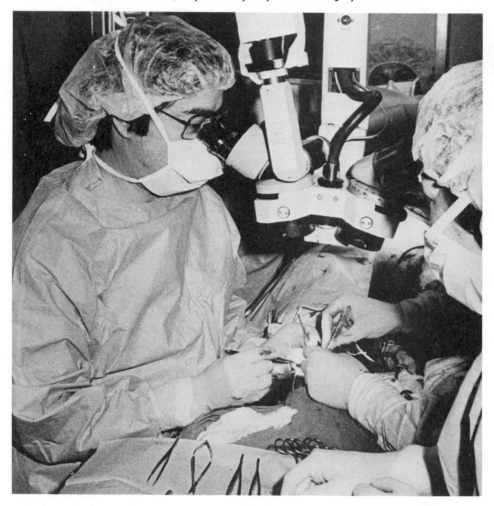

microscope, to literally take the middle ear structures apart, rebuild the organ with bits of plastic or metal shaped like the ossicles, and reconstruct the eardrum with tissue grafts. This kind of surgery is called *microsurgery*.

Inner Ear Disturbances

Disorders of the inner ear usually are treated with medications. Surgery in that area is seldom performed unless there is a great risk to the life of the patient. Little can be done to restore hearing loss due to nerve deafness except with hearing aids; these are designed to pick up sounds on the affected side of the head and route the sounds by electronic circuitry to an area where they can be picked up by remaining functional auditory nerves. See p. 981 for a discussion of plastic surgery on the ears.

Eye Surgery

Among common types of eye surgery are procedures for correcting eye muscles, glaucoma, cataracts, cornea, and retina disorders. Operations on the eye muscles are intended to correct crossed eyes or similar problems in which the two eyes fail to work together.

Crossed Eyes

The condition technically known as *strabismus*, in which one eye drifts so that its position is not parallel with the other, is caused by a congenitally weak muscle. Infants often appear to have crossed eyes, but in most cases the drifting corrects itself by the time the baby is six months old. If the condition persists beyond that time, a doctor should be consulted. He may recommend the use of an eye patch over the stronger eye so that the weaker one will be exercised. If this does not achieve the desired result, he may prescribe special glasses and eye exercises as the child gets older so that there is no impairment of vision.

CORRECTIVE SURGERY: If corrective surgery proves necessary after these measures, it is usually done before the child enters school. The opera-

THE EYE

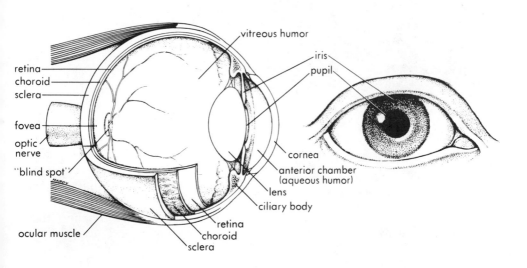

retina
choroid
sclera
fovea
optic nerve
"blind spot"
ocular muscle
vitreous humor
iris
pupil
cornea
anterior chamber (aqueous humor)
lens
ciliary body
retina
choroid
sclera

tion is a simple one involving the muscle and not the inside of the eye itself. Each eye has six *extraocular* muscles—muscles originating outside the eyeball—to move the eye up, down, left, right, etc.; the surgeon lengthens or shortens these muscles, as may be required, to coordinate the eye movements. The operation is safe and requires only a brief hospital stay.

AMBLYOPIA: If the lack of eye coordination is not corrected a kind of blindness called *amblyopia* can result in one of the eyes. This condition occurs particularly in young children who depend upon the vision of one good eye; the function of the other eye is allowed to deteriorate. It has been estimated that about two million Americans have lost a part of their vision in this manner. Crossed eyes should receive professional attention early enough to prevent a permanent visual handicap.

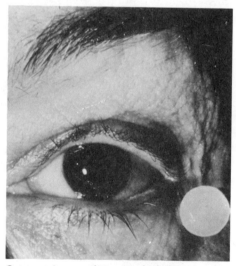

Cataract is a condition in which there is a loss of transparency of the lenses of the eyes. The picture above shows a normal eye and a cataract (opaque lens) outside the eye.

Cataract

Cataract is a condition in which there is a loss of transparency of the lenses of the eyes. Each lens is made up of layers of cells naturally formed to focus a visual image on the retina at the rear of the eyeball. As a result of aging, or because of an injury to the eye, the lens may develop cloudy or opaque areas, or *cataracts*, that result in a blurring of vision. About five percent of the population of the United States has cataracts. Some doctors claim that anyone who lives long enough can expect to have cataracts, although age is not the only determining factor.

SURGICAL CORRECTION: The condition can be corrected rather easily by several different kinds of surgical procedures. Among these, a relatively simple, advanced technique involves a microsurgery procedure called extracapsular extraction followed by implantation of a new lens. Using this method, the surgeon first makes a tiny incision in the cornea. Reaching through that incision, the surgeon then makes a circle of tiny cuts in the lens. The lens and its cataract are then drawn through the opening in the cornea. The back part of the lens remains in place to support the implant lens.

Extracapsular extraction has begun to replace older techniques. These include dissolving the tissues holding the lens in place with a liquid enzyme, freezing the lens with a supercold probe, and grinding the lens tissue with a high-speed instrument. Extracapsular extraction requires only a local anesthetic injected into the facial muscles. Because the sutures are tiny, healing time can be as short as a few weeks.

The timing of cataract surgery presents the patient with a difficult decision. To help you make up your mind, the doctor may use a potential acuity meter (PAM) to show what kind of vision you should have after a cataract is removed. The PAM projects a light beam that flashes a standard eye chart through tiny clear areas in the cataract. Because the beam hits your retina directly, you can read the chart without interference.

Lens implants normally effect greatly improved vision. But for optimum results most patients need to wear eyeglasses or contact lenses after the operation. Because implanted lenses cannot focus as your eye's natural lens does, you will probably need reading glasses. The artificial lenses may require some adjustments to compensate for visual illusions as to distances and shapes, but the blurring of progressive blindness will have been eliminated.

Sometimes after cataract operations, patients notice that the rear part of the lens left in to support the implant has begun to cloud. In such a case a surgeon may use a laser beam to punch a tiny hole in the clouded area. The hole lets light rays reach the retina unimpeded.

Cornea Transplant

The cornea of the eye is a clear window of several cells in thickness at the very front of the eye. While it is protected by the constant sweeping of the corneal surface by the eyelid and the washing of the surface by tears, it is vulnerable to injury and infection, allergies, and metabolic disorders. The simple habit of rubbing the eyes can distort the shape of the cornea, changing the normal round shape to a cone shape. Eventually, a cornea may degenerate from wear and tear and become clouded so that the patient can no longer see clearly, if at all. It is possible, however—and has been since the 1930s—to replace a clouded cornea with an undamaged cornea from a deceased person. Corneas are contributed by donors and stored in eye banks.

SURGICAL PROCEDURE: When only a portion of the cornea needs to be replaced, as is often the case, a disk encompassing the damaged cornea is carefully cut out and a piece of new cornea of precisely the same size and shape is sewn into the remaining tissue of the old cornea. The reconstructed cornea is treated with an-

(Left) A severely burned and damaged cornea requiring plastic surgery. *(Right)* A cornea transplanted to the damaged eye. After being stored for several days in a preserving medium, the cornea is clear 24 hours after the operation. The white arc is a reflection from a slit lamp biomicroscope.

tibiotics and bandaged for several weeks. More than three-fourths of the cornea transplants are successful; the chances of success depend upon many factors, including the health of the remaining tissues of the original cornea.

Glaucoma

Glaucoma, a leading cause of blindness, is a disease caused by a failure of the fluid produced inside the eye to drain properly. The fluid, or *aqueous humor,* is produced in the anterior chamber of the eye, between the cornea and the lens. In a normal eye it drains through a duct at the base of the cornea at the same rate at which it is produced. But if the drainage system is obstructed, fluid buildup creates pressure backwards through the eye. If untreated, such pressure can cause gradual blindness by crushing the nerves at the back of the eye.

TREATMENT: Some cases of glaucoma can be treated with medications that control the rates of fluid production and drainage. But when medications are no longer effective or when an acute attack occurs, with symptoms of severe eye pain sometimes accompanied by abdominal pain, nausea, and vomiting, surgery within a matter of hours is recommended. Several surgical procedures for the treatment of glaucoma are available; all are designed to release the fluid pressure in the eye. One common procedure involves cutting a small opening in the iris. Another technique is to insert a fine wire into the duct that normally drains the fluid and literally ream it open.

An estimated ten million people in

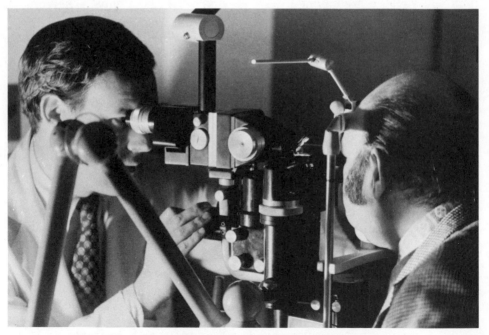

A patient being treated by laser beam. This form of therapy is used in some cases of retinal bleeding associated with diabetic retinopathy.

the world are afflicted by glaucoma, and the chances of it developing increase with age. Women are twice as likely to develop the disease as men, and there is some evidence that the risk is hereditary. However, it also is easily preventable and controllable, since glaucoma usually develops slowly and can be detected during routine eye examinations in its early stages.

Retinal Detachment or Disease

Retinal detachment can occur from bleeding in the retinal area, an injury, a change in the shape of the eyeball, or other causes. The surgical treatment to correct the problem usually is related to the specific cause. For example, if fluid or blood has accumulated behind the retina, it is drained away. Alternatively, pressure may be directed within the eyeball to push the retina back into its proper position. For some cases, such as those associated with *diabetic retinopathy,* a kind of retinal bleeding in diabetes patients, a laser beam is used to seal the blood vessels responsible for the tiny hemorrhages in the eye.

Chest Region

This section deals with surgery of the lungs and heart. For a discussion of cosmetic surgery of the chest area, as of the breast, see p. 979.

The Lungs

Before the era of modern drugs such as antibiotics, lung disorders were the leading cause of death in the United States. Lung diseases are still common enough. With every breath taken in, the lungs are vulner-

able to damage from disease organisms, chemicals, and air pollutants, many of which did not exist 50 years ago when pneumonia and tuberculosis were among the greatest threats to human life. Because the lungs are not as sensitive to pain as some other organs, a respiratory disorder may develop insidiously with few or no symptoms. When pain is felt in the chest area, the source of the pain may be the chest wall, the esophagus, or the bronchial tubes that branch from the trachea into smaller units that distribute air through the lung tissues. Other symptoms of respiratory disease may be coughing, shortness of breath, or sputum that contains blood.

TUBERCULOSIS: Any of the above signs or symptoms could be associated with tuberculosis, which also can cause loss of appetite, weight loss, lethargy, and heavy perspiration, especially during the night. Tuberculosis is still one of the most common causes of death in the world, and new cases are found in the United States each year at a rate of 18 per 100,000 population. In addition, an estimated 35 million Americans are tuberculin-positive, indicating they have been in contact with the infectious organism but have developed an immune response to it. For an explanation of how tuberculosis is spread and of tests devised to check its spread, see pp. 1187-1190.

SURGICAL TREATMENT OF TUBERCULOSIS: A dozen different drugs are available for medical treatment of tuberculosis and several types may be taken in combination by a patient. Intensive treatment may require a hospital stay of several months and use of the drugs for at least 18

THE RESPIRATORY SYSTEM

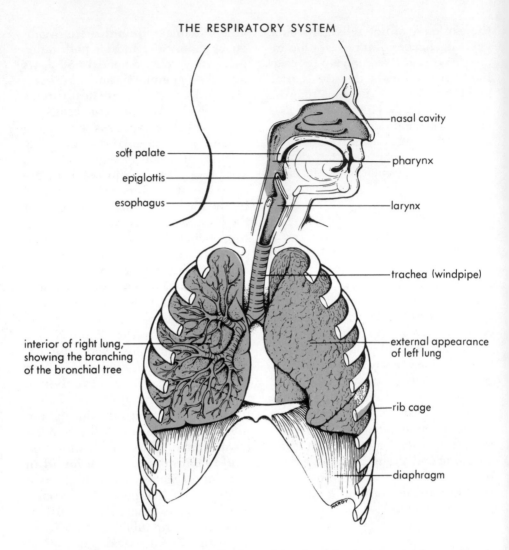

soft palate

epiglottis

esophagus

interior of right lung, showing the branching of the bronchial tree

nasal cavity

pharynx

larynx

trachea (windpipe)

external appearance of left lung

rib cage

diaphragm

months. However, because of adverse side effects of drugs, resistance of the bacterium to the drugs, and other reasons, surgery may be required. If one of the five lobes of lung tissue—the right lung has three lobes, the left lung two—has been severely damaged by tuberculosis, it may be removed by surgeons. In some instances, doctors may recommend that surgery be undertaken to allow one of the lungs to rest while it recovers from the infection. This is accomplished by crushing

the phrenic nerve, under a local anesthetic, creating a partial paralysis of the diaphragm. Partial lung collapse also can be accomplished by removing parts of the ribs over the affected lung.

LUNG CANCER: Cancer of the lung may appear with early symptoms of coughing, wheezing, or the appearance of blood in sputum; in about ten percent of cases there is chest pain or shortness of breath. However, it is not unusual for the lung-cancer patient to have no complaints of illness. Chest X-rays during a routine physical examination may reveal the disease. In many cases, the cancer develops from metasases of cancers that have spread from other body systems. Medical therapy for lung cancer patients, including the use of radiation, is primarily for the purpose of relieving pain or other symptoms. The only effective cure is surgical excision of the affected lung tissue along with the nearby lymph nodes. Surgical treatment is most effective in young adults when the tumor has not invaded neighboring tissues, although the five-year survival rate for lung cancer is still poor.

Chest surgery may require several specialists, in addition to a general surgeon—for example, an oncologist (cancer specialist) and cardiologist.

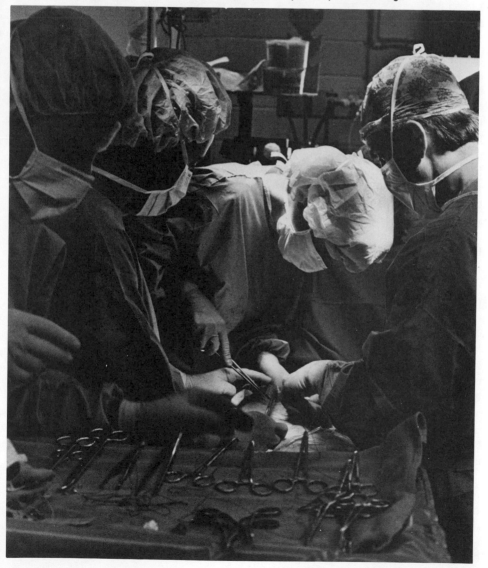

Heart Surgery

Heart surgery procedures that are routine in many hospitals today were unheard of a generation ago. Since World War II techniques have been devised to permit attachment of a heart-lung machine to the human body so that the patient's blood can be circulated and refreshed with oxygen while the heart itself is stopped temporarily for surgery.

HEART VALVE REPAIR: While the blood flow is shunted away from the heart, surgeons can replace a diseased heart valve which may have become calcified with deposits that keep it from closing normally. An artificial valve made of metal and plastic may be used to replace the patient's diseased mitral valve that no longer effectively controls the flow of blood from the left atrium to the left ventricle of the heart. Artificial valves also can be installed between the right chambers of the heart. In some cases, a diseased valve leaf may be repaired with a graft of tissue from the patient's body.

Installation of artificial heart valves has had a remarkably good record of success; some surgeons recommend the procedure over other techniques for treatment of heart valve diseases and report the operation has been well tolerated by patients more than 70 years of age. Life expectancy is increased for most patients, and while some activities may be restricted, they are able to have comfortable and more normal lives after such operations.

SEPTAL DEFECT: Another kind of heart surgery is used to correct a septal defect. The right and left atria of the heart are separated by a septum, a wall of muscular tissue. A similar but much thicker septum separates

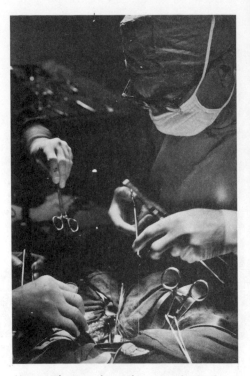

Many advances have been made in heart surgery since World War II, including a whole range of sophisticated repairs of existing parts and the implanting of artificial parts.

the left and right ventricles. Occasionally, usually because of a birth defect, the septum does not close completely and blood flows from one side to the other through the opening in the heart wall. The problem is solved by putting the patient on a heart-lung machine while the heart is opened and the septum closed either by sewing the opening or by stitching into the septum a patch of plastic material. See the illustrations on p. 965.

COARCTATION OF THE AORTA: An equally dramatic bit of heart surgery is used to correct a defect called *coarctation*, or narrowing, of the aorta, the main artery leading from the heart. This short, pinched section interferes with normal blood

THE HEART

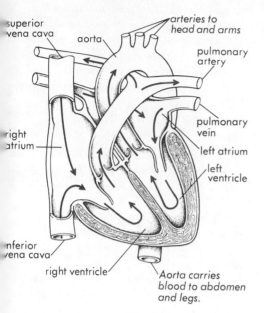

superior vena cava

aorta

arteries to head and arms

pulmonary artery

right atrium

pulmonary vein

left atrium

left ventricle

inferior vena cava

right ventricle

Aorta carries blood to abdomen and legs.

flow. If untreated, the patient may die of a ruptured aorta or heart failure. Treatment requires an operation in which the narrowed section of the aorta is cut away and the two normal-sized ends sewed together. In some cases, a piece of plastic material is sewed into the reconstructed aorta to replace the coarctated section.

AORTAL-PULMONARY ARTERY SHUNT: A comparatively simple bit of heart surgery is employed to correct a defect that occurs in some newborn children. Before birth, when the lungs are not needed because fresh blood is supplied from the placenta via the umbilical cord, the aorta is connected by a shunt to the pulmo-

SEPTAL DEFECTS

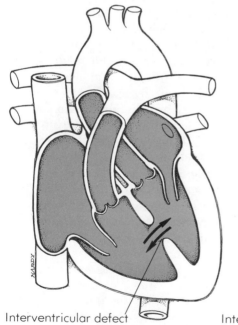

Interventricular defect   Interatrial defect

A normal heart in cross section *(top)*, showing the circulation of the blood. An interventricular defect *(bottom left)* allows blood to pass directly between the left and right ventricles. An interatrial defect *(bottom right)*, with the aorta seen in cross section over the left atrium, allows blood to pass freely between the two atria. Any septal defect interferes with the effectiveness of the pumping action of the heart.

nary artery. After birth the shunt closes in most cases so the pulmonary artery can carry the blood from the heart to the lungs for oxygenation. In some children this shunt fails to close. To correct the defect and prevent heart failure, the surgeon opens the child's chest, ties off the open shunt, and cuts the ligated connection.

Vascular Surgery

This section consists of discussions of aneurysms, varicose veins, phlebitis, and intermittent claudication.

Aneurysm

When a blood vessel develops a balloonlike malformation the defect is called an aneurysm. A common complication of the aneurysm is that it may rupture if not treated. A ruptured aneurysm of a large blood vessel, or of a small blood vessel in a critical area such as the brain, can be fatal or severely disabling.

SURGICAL PROCEDURES: If the aneurysm develops at a vital site such as the aorta, heroic surgical measures may be required to correct the problem. Before the important artery can be clamped off, the patient may have to be attached to a heart-lung machine and the body temperature lowered so as to reduce normal body functions to a minimum. After the aneurysm is removed, that section of the aorta may have to be replaced with a piece of plastic artery. Not all aneurysms require such complicated methods of repair; if the ballooning section of artery develops as a saclike appendage, it frequently can be tied off and removed while the relatively small opening between the blood vessel and the sac is sewed closed.

Surgical removal of an aneurysm is the only available treatment for the disorder. The surgery is much less complicated if the abnormal section of the blood vessel is replaced before it ruptures than after. When the patient has recovered from correction of the aneurysm he can resume a rather active, normal life style.

Varicose Veins

Varicose veins can develop in many parts of the body. But they are most obvious and commonly a problem when they appear in the legs, especially in the *saphenous veins,* large veins that lie close to the surface of the skin.

CAUSES: The cause of varicose veins is a failure of tiny valves in the blood vessels to function properly so that venous blood destined for the heart flows backwards and forms pools which can make the veins distended, tortuous, and painful. Varicose veins are related to the erect posture of humans; the heart pumps blood through arteries to the extremities but the return flow must fight the pull of gravity. Ordinarily, venous blood gets a boost up the legs by a pumping action of leg muscle contractions. Valves in the legs are designed to let the blood move upward but are supposed to block any backward flow. People whose jobs require them to stand all day are among those likely to suffer from a breakdown of the normal functioning of the valves. Women who have had multiple pregnancies and obese individuals are also apt to develop varicose veins.

ULCERATION: Varicose veins can cause ulcers in the lower leg near the ankle that bleed through the skin after an injury to the area.

THE SAPHENOUS VEINS

femoral

great
(or internal)
saphenous

small
(or external)
saphenous

The saphenous veins of the leg, which lie close to the surface of the skin, are those most likely to become varicosed. Although the external saphenous is sometimes called "small" to distinguish it from the internal saphenous, both are large veins.

TREATMENT: One kind of surgical treatment of the varicosed vein is *ligation,* which means tying or binding. An incision is made in the leg, usually in the area of the groin. The diseased saphenous vein is severed from its connection with the larger femoral vein and is tied off. The function of a ligated vein is taken over by other veins in the leg. An alternate kind of surgery for varicose veins, sometimes called *stripping,* requires either a series of small incisions along the path of the vein, from the groin to the ankle, or an internal stripping by use of a special, long, threadlike instrument. The diseased

vein is then removed and any connections with other veins ligated.

Varicose vein surgery is used for treatment of the *superficial* veins— those that are close to the skin. The operation is simple and can be performed under a local anesthetic in many cases. When multiple varicose veins are on both legs, all of the problem veins can be stripped and ligated at the same time. A hospital stay of several days may be required, and dressings are needed on the treated legs for two or three weeks after the operation.

Phlebitis

A problem related to varicose veins is *phlebitis,* a disease that usually involves the larger, deep veins of the legs with inflammation, pain, and swelling. Phlebitis is much more serious than varicose veins because a large vein is involved and a clot usually forms, obstructing return blood flow of the limb. The danger is that the clot will break loose— that is, become an *embolus*—and travel to the lungs where it can obstruct a vital blood vessel, with serious or even fatal results. The obstructing clot is called an *embolism.*

CAUSES AND TREATMENT: Causes of phlebitis can be injury, infection, poor circulation, or simply sitting for long periods of time. Medical therapy may include wet dressings and medications, especially anticoagulant drugs to thin the blood and reduce the chances of clot formations. Supportive bandages, leg exercises, and elevation of the legs may also be recommended.

SURGICAL PROCEDURE: Surgery is reserved usually for cases in which medical therapy fails to control the risk of emboli forming. The surgical procedure is directed toward treatment of the deep vein that is the source of the phlebitis symptoms. The surgeon may open the vein to remove the clot, or a device can be inserted in the vein to strain out any clots that may form in the vein and travel toward the lungs. In some cases the surgeon may block the upward flow of blood from the affected vein, allowing other veins in the leg to assume that function. However, if other veins already have been stripped or ligated in the treatment of varicose veins it is unlikely that a surgeon would occlude or block the flow of blood in a deep leg vein.

Intermittent Claudication

Intermittent claudication is a disorder of blood circulation of the legs involving the arteries. It is primarily a disease of aging, with gradual, progressive narrowing of the lumen (interior space) of the arteries by atherosclerosis. Atherosclerosis of the arteries occurs in other parts of the body, including the arms. Intermittent claudication is marked by muscle fatigue and pain when the leg muscles are used, as in walking. The symptoms are relieved by rest. The condition can be relieved by drugs, particularly medications that help dilate the arteries, but in severe cases surgery to reconstruct the leg arteries is the solution.

SURGICAL PROCEDURE: The surgeon may build a bypass artery by grafting a length of plastic tubing into the affected blood vessel and around the area blocked by atherosclerotic narrowing. Sometimes surgeons will use a piece of a vein from the patient's body to make a bypass artery; for example, a vein from the arm may be transformed into an artery for the leg. Another procedure involves simply removing the portion of the artery blocking the normal flow of blood.

Orthopedic Surgery

Orthopedics originally was the name given the subject of treating deformities of children; the original Greek term could be translated as "normal child." But the medical world now uses the word to describe treatment of the bones, muscles, joints, and associated tissues of the body's locomotion apparatus. Orthopedic surgery, therefore, might involve repair of a broken big toe as well as treatment of a whiplash injury to the neck.

This section discusses disorders of the spine, including herniated (or "slipped") disk, fractures, and torn ligaments.

Slipped Disk

The spinal column of 33 stacked vertebrae is a common source of painful problems that require orthopedic treatment. In addition to helping support the weight of the body above the hips, the vertebrae are subjected to a variety of twists, turns, and strains during a typical day. Much of the nearly continuous shock exerted on the spinal column is absorbed by the gel-like disks between the vertebrae.

SYMPTOMS: Eventually, one of the disks may *herniate,* or slip out of place, causing pressure on a spinal nerve. The result can be severe pain that radiates along the pathway of the nerve as far as the lower leg. The pain may be accompanied by muscular weakness and loss of reflexes, even perhaps by a loss of feeling in part of the leg affected by a pinched or squeezed nerve. This condition, known popularly as a slipped disk, has symptoms of low back pain or leg pain that are similar to those of other disorders such as intermittent claudication, arthritis, strained muscles, and prostatitis. Also, a herniated disk can occur near the top of the spinal column with symptoms of head and neck-area pains. But more than 90 percent of herniated disk cases involve the lumbar region of the spinal column, in the lower back.

DIAGNOSIS: Doctors usually can confirm a herniated disk problem by a technique called *myelography*, in which a dye is injected into the spinal canal and X-ray pictures taken. Another procedure, called *electromyography*, can help determine which nerve root is involved.

TREATMENT: Conservative measures generally are used at first to reduce the pain and other symptoms. They include bed rest on a hard mattress, medications, and sometimes the use of traction and back braces. If conservative therapy fails to correct the problem and the diagnosis has been well established by a myelogram, surgery may be advised to remove the herniated disk.

SPINAL FUSION: The surgeon may recommend a procedure called spinal fusion, in which the edges of several of the vertebrae are roughened and a piece of bone from the pelvis grafted onto the roughened edges. The bone graft will fuse with the vertebrae and in effect make the several vertebrae a single bone. However, the fused vertebrae will not interfere noticeably with body movements after the fusion is completed, which takes about six months. The operation requires a hospital stay of

from one to two weeks and the patient must wear a body cast for the first few weeks and then use a back brace for a period of possibly several months. The patient usually can return to work and resume some normal activities within a couple of months after the operation. Strenuous activity, however, is usually restricted after an operation on the spinal column.

Other Spinal Disorders

SPONDYLOLISTHESIS: Spinal fusion surgery also may be used to correct two other kinds of spinal disorders. One disorder is known as *spondylolisthesis*, a condition in which one of the vertebrae slips out of alignment. Spondylolisthesis usually occurs at the bottom of the group of lumbar vertebrae, where that section of the spinal column rests on the sacrum.

SCOLIOSIS: The other disorder is *scoliosis*, or abnormal curvature of the spinal column. If the case of scoliosis is mild and causes no severe symptoms, it may be treated with conservative measures such as braces and special exercises. Surgical treatment of scoliosis may involve not only spinal fusion but reinforcement of the spinal column with metal rods attached to the vertebrae to hold them in proper alignment.

Disorders of the cervical portion of the spinal column, in the area of the neck, may cause symptoms similar to those of a herniated disk in the lower back. But there is pain in the neck and shoulders and weakness in the arms. Surgical treatment also is similar, with removal of a herniated disk portion or fusion of cervical vertebrae when conservative therapy, with bed rest, neck braces, and medications, does not prove helpful.

Fractures

Many fractures of the spinal column also are treated by fusion operations, use of casts or braces, bed rest, or traction, in addition to therapy directed toward the specific problem. Spinal fractures frequently are compression fractures of vertebrae caused by falling in a sitting or standing position or mishaps in which a bony process of a vertebra is broken. Spinal fractures that result in permanent damage to the spinal cord, with resulting paralysis, are relatively uncommon.

REDUCTION OF FRACTURES: Fractures of the long bones of the arms and legs are treated by a method called *reduction*, the technique of aligning the broken ends of the bones properly so the healing process will not result in a deformity. Reduction also requires that the muscles and surrounding tissues be aligned and held in place by immobilizing them as the break heals.

If the break is simple enough, the limb can be immobilized by putting a plaster cast around the part of the limb involved after the fractured ends of the bone and associated tissues have been realigned. In complicated cases with a number of bone fragments resulting from the fracture and surrounding tissues in some disarray, the patient usually is given a general anesthetic while the surgeon reorganizes the shattered limb like a player assembling pieces of a jigsaw puzzle. If some of the needed pieces are missing, the surgeon may fill in the gaps with bone from a bone bank, although bone

bank materials usually are not as effective in the healing process as pieces of the patient's own bones.

USE OF INTERNAL APPLIANCES: A common technique of modern fracture surgery is the application of wires, screws, pins, metal plates, and other devices to provide internal fixation of a broken long bone during the healing process. Nails and pins may be used to fasten the fractured neck of a femur, the long bone of the upper leg, to the shaft of that bone. A steel rod may be driven through the shaft of a long bone to align the broken sections. Screws may be used to hold together bone ends of a fracture in which the break runs diagonally across the shaft. Screws also may be employed to hold a metal plate or strip of bone from the patient's own body across the break. The screws, nails, and other devices generally are well tolerated by the body and may be left in the bones indefinitely if they do not cause adverse reactions after the healing process is completed. See the illustration on p. 971.

TRACTION: Traction frequently is employed to hold a limb in alignment while a fracture is healing. A clamp sometimes is placed at one end of the fractured limb and a weight attached by wires over a pulley is connected to the clamp. Depending upon the kind of fracture and type of traction prescribed, a system of several weights and pulleys may be rigged around the bed of a patient to fix the bone and related tissues in correct positions.

Torn Cartilage

Joints of the body can be vulnerable to damage from sudden twisting

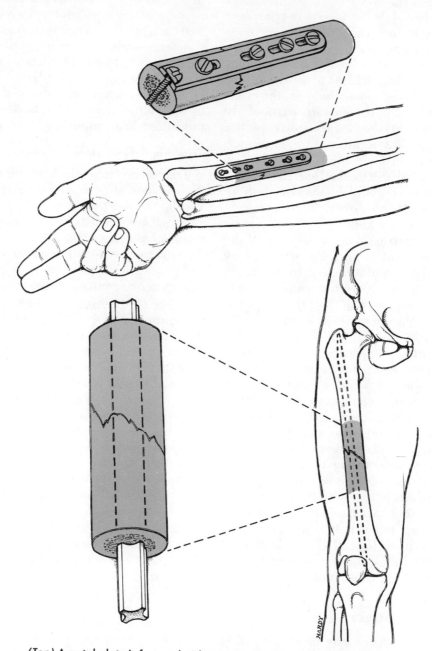

(Top) A metal plate is fastened with screws to secure a fractured bone in the arm (the radius). The enlarged portion shown in cross section in color is also shown as it appears in the patient's arm. *(Bottom)* A steel rod has been driven through the center of the femur of the leg to hold the jagged ends of the fractured bone in proper alignment. Such appliances are sometimes left in place indefinitely when there are no adverse reactions.

and turning actions, particularly when the force of the individual's body weight is added to the pressure on the joint. The effect of such forces on the knee joint can result in tearing of the half-moon-shaped cartilages that cushion friction of the upper and lower leg bones where they are joined. Sports fans are particularly aware of the vulnerability of the knee joint because of the high incidence of knee injuries to athletes, especially in football and basketball. Obese individuals are also particularly liable to develop cartilage problems in the knee.

SYMPTOMS: When a cartilage of the knee joint is torn, the patient may feel pain and weakness in the area of the injury. Swelling usually occurs and in more than half the cases the knee cannot be straightened because it has become "locked" by the cartilage. There may be a remission of symptoms, but surgery frequently is required sooner or later.

SURGICAL PROCEDURE: The surgeon makes an incision in the area of the kneecap and cuts away the torn cartilage. Full recovery takes several weeks after the first few post-operative days, during which the patient remains in bed with the affected leg elevated. Special exercises are required to overcome muscle weakness in the leg and to help the patient learn to use the leg with part of the cartilage cushion missing.

Neurosurgery

Neurosurgery may be employed to treat a wide assortment of disorders involving the nervous system, from the brain to nerve endings in the fingers and toes. Neurosurgery may involve treatment of epilepsy, Par-

kinson's disease and psychiatric disorders, as well as herniated disks of the spinal column and aneurysms that affect the nervous system. Causes of neurosurgical problems can be injury, tumors, infectious diseases, or congenital disorders.

This section includes discussions of trigeminal neuralgia, brain tumors, and head injuries.

Trigeminal Neuralgia

Trigeminal neuralgia is one of many types of pain that sometimes can be treated by surgery. The disorder, also known as *tic douloureux* or *facial neuralgia,* tends to develop in persons between 40 and 60 years of age, causing attacks of acute pain and muscular twitching in the area of the face containing branches of the trigeminal nerve. The painful attacks occur with no apparent reason but seem to be associated with certain stimuli such as touch or temperature changes at points around the face and mouth. During periods of attacks, the patient may avoid eating, shaving, or any other activity that might trigger a spasm of severe pain. But the pain attacks also may cease, with or without treatment, for three or four months, only to resume for weeks or months.

TREATMENT: Alcohol injections and medications may offer relief of symptoms, but when symptoms continue surgery frequently is recommended. The operation consists of an incision to reach the root of the nerve and cut the divisions that appear to be involved with the painful symptoms. However, cutting the nerve can result in loss of feeling for the entire side of the face, including the cornea of the eye, so that the patient must wear special glasses to

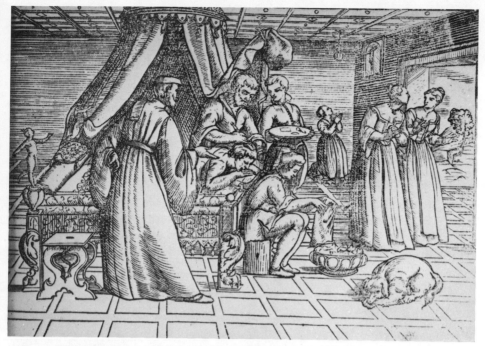

This 16th-century Venetian woodcut shows a surgeon working on a patient's skull with a trephine, a drill specially designed for such an operation.

protect the cornea. An alternative procedure that is not always effective involves exposing the nerve root and rubbing it, a technique that seems to produce a temporary loss of sensation in the nerve fibers.

Brain Tumor

Brain tumors are popularly associated with neurosurgery skills. And while brain surgery requires great skill and knowledge of brain anatomy, which in itself is quite complicated, most brain tumor operations are conducted safely and successfully. Diagnosing, locating, and identifying a brain tumor are challenges faced by the doctor before surgery begins. There are a dozen major types of brain tumors plus some minor types. The types of tumors tend to vary according to the age of the patient; the patient's age and the type of tumor may suggest where it develops.

SYMPTOMS: Because brain tumors can cause organic mental changes in the patient, the symptoms of changed behavior can be mistaken for neurotic or psychotic disorders with the result that a patient may spend valuable time receiving psychiatric treatment rather than surgical treatment; autopsies of a significant number of patients who die in mental hospitals reveal the presence of brain tumors. In addition to mental changes, the person suffering from a brain tumor may complain of headaches, experience convulsions, or display signs of neurological function loss such as abnormal vision.

DIAGNOSIS: The specific signs and symptoms along with X-ray studies, electroencephalograms, and other tests help the doctors determine the site and extent of growth of a brain tumor. A recently developed technique called *CAT scanning* (for *computerized axial tomography*) aids the neurosurgeon by producing a series of X-ray pictures of the interior of the skull as if they were "slices" of the brain taken in thicknesses of about two-thirds of an inch. The detailed anatomical portrait of the patient's brain helps pinpoint the disorder and indicate whether it is a tumor or another kind of abnormality.

SURGICAL PROCEDURE: The usual method of removing a brain tumor after it has been diagnosed and located is a procedure called a *craniotomy*. The entire head is shaved and cleaned to eliminate the possibility that a stray bit of hair might fall into the incision that is made in the scalp. After the scalp has been opened, a series of holes are drilled in a pattern outlining the working area for the surgeon; a wire saw is used to cut the skull between the drilled holes.

Removing the tumor is a delicate operation, not only because of the need to avoid damage to healthy brain tissue but because accidental severing of a blood vessel in the brain could produce a critical hemorrhage. The surgeon tries to remove the entire tumor, or as much of the tumor as appears possible without damaging vital brain tissues or blood vessels. All of the various types of brain tumors are considered dangerous, whether malignant or benign, because within the rigid confines of the skull there is no opportunity for outward release of pressure. Therefore any growth may compress or destroy vital brain tissues if left untreated.

After the tumor is removed, the piece of skull removed at the start of the operation is replaced and the scalp flap is sewed in place. Radiation therapy may be administered for a month to six weeks after surgery to destroy any tumor tissue left behind or tumor cells that may have drifted into the spinal canal. Some tumors near the base of the brain may be treated effectively with radiation alone if the tumor cells are radiosensitive. Tumors of the pineal gland and the pituitary gland also may be treated with radiation.

Head Injuries

BRAIN HEMORRHAGE: Head injuries, such as a blow to the head, can produce massive hemorrhages within the skull. As in the case of brain tumors, the expanding pool of blood within the skull gradually compresses the brain tissue and can result in death unless the problem is corrected. The damage of a brain hemorrhage can be insidious, with no immediate signs or symptoms of the problem until irreversible changes have occurred in the brain tissue. The patient may receive what may appear to be a minor head injury, for example, and not lose consciousness. Or he may be unconscious for a brief period, then recover and appear very alert. But gradually, over a period of hours or even days, neurological signs of disintegrating brain function appear.

TREATMENT: The treatment requires a procedure similar to that used for removing brain tumors. An opening is made in the skull to remove the blood or blood clot and relieve pressure on the brain tissues.

The chances for full recovery depend somewhat on the extent of brain damage caused by the hemorrhage before treatment.

SKULL FRACTURE: Surgical treatment for a skull fracture may combine techniques of various other methods for fractures and brain injuries. The scalp is shaved and cleaned carefully so the surgeon can determine the extent of the injury and its location with respect to vital tissues under the skull. With the help of X rays and signs of neurological damage, the surgeon frequently can tell how severe the fracture may be and whether there is bleeding beneath the skull.

TREATMENT: If the skull appears to be intact but there are signs of a brain hemorrhage, the skull is opened to remove the blood or blood clot and relieve pressure on the brain. If the skull fracture is compound and depressed, or with skull fragments in the brain tissue, efforts also must be made to elevate the depressed bone section so it does not press on vital brain areas and to remove bits of bone or other foreign materials that

The location and size of a brain aneurysm can be identified by X-ray pictures after an opaque dye has been injected into the bloodstream.

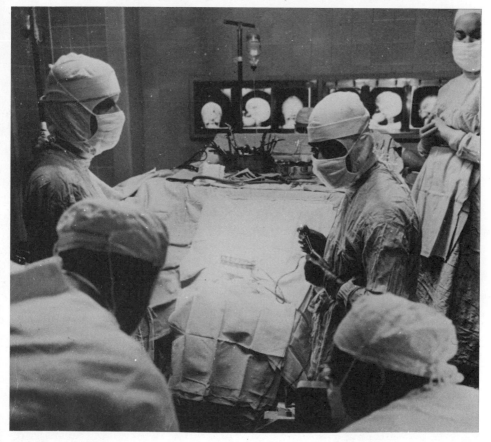

may have entered the brain.

Surgeons frequently can rebuild a fractured skull by replacing missing bits of bone or adding appropriate synthetic materials such as a piece of metal plate. Full recovery depends upon such factors as the age of the patient and the severity of damage before treatment was started. Younger patients generally respond better to the repair procedures, but full recovery from a severe skull fracture may take as long as a year.

ANEURYSM IN THE BRAIN: Aneurysms can develop in blood vessels of the brain, and like aneurysms in other parts of the body they can be corrected surgically. A ruptured aneurysm produces a brain hemorrhage. The condition is most likely to develop in people over the age of 30; in patients over 40, women are more likely than men to be victims of the disorder. The approach to repair of an intracranial aneurysm depends upon the condition of the patient and the location and size of the aneurysm, which frequently can be identified by X-ray pictures after an opaque dye has been injected into the bloodstream. The diseased blood vessel may be ligated, reinforced, or repaired, depending upon the conditions found by the surgeon after the aneurysm has been exposed and examined.

PLASTIC AND COSMETIC SURGERY

The use of surgical techniques for the correction of physical deformities is by no means a modern development. The practice goes back to ancient India, where as early as the sixth century B.C. Hindu specialists were reconstructing noses, reshaping ears, and grafting skin for reducing scar tissue.

Through the centuries, improvements in procedure and new types of operations became part of the common fund of information. During World War I, great technical advances were made when the Medical Corps of the United States Army created a special division of *plastic surgery* to treat the deformities caused by battle injuries. Today's plastic surgery is based on many of the procedures perfected then and during World War II.

In recent years, attention has been focused not only on birth and injury deformities, but on lesser irregularities as well. Surgeons in the field of *cosmetic surgery* perform such procedures as nose reconstruction, face lifting, reshaping of breasts, removal of fatty tissue from upper arms and legs, and the transplanting of hair to correct baldness.

There is no longer any reason for someone to suffer from the emotional and professional problems caused by abnormalities in appearance. No child should be expected to live with the disability of a cleft lip or crossed eyes. A young woman tormented by what she considers to be a grotesque nose can have it recontoured to her liking. An older woman who finds wrinkles a social liability can have them removed. Anyone interested in undergoing any form of cosmetic surgery should stay away from so-called beauty experts, and deal only with a reputable surgeon or physician.

Some surgical specialists, called *plastic surgeons,* perform cosmetic or plastic surgery exclusively. Other surgeons and physicians, including general surgeons, dermatologists, ophthalmologists, and others are qualified to do some kinds of plastic surgery, usually the techniques related to their particular specialties. The kind of surgery desired should first be discussed with the family doctor, who can then evaluate the problem and recommend a qualified surgeon to deal with it.

Before undergoing any kind of plastic surgery, the prospective patient should realize that it is neither inexpensive nor totally painless. Most cosmetic surgery is performed in hospitals, which means that in addition to the surgeon's fees there can be a bill for the anesthetist, use of the operating and recovery rooms, and for the hospital stay itself. Also, because cosmetic surgery is often optional surgery, surgery not needed to ensure the patient's physical health, it may not be covered by a health-insurance policy. Getting one's nose fixed, for example, may cost between $500 and $1,500.

Reshaping the Nose

Known technically as a *rhinoplasty,* the operation for the reconstruction of the nose is not only one of the oldest, but also one of the most common forms of cosmetic surgery. Depending on the demands of facial symmetry and individual taste, the nose can be shortened, straightened, narrowed, or even lengthened. If a nose

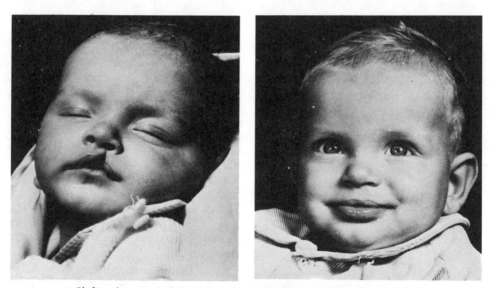

Cleft palate and cleft lip interfere with the infant's ability to suck and, if uncorrected, would later cause speech impairment. These pictures show how surgery can correct the disfigurement.

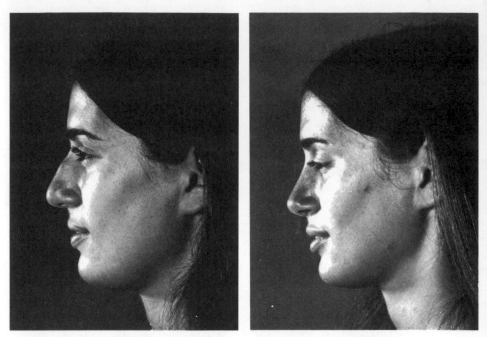

Pictures taken before and after rhinoplasty. Reconstruction of the nose is done through the nostrils so that there is no scarring of facial tissue. The surgery is performed under local anesthesia in a hospital.

deformity has caused breathing problems, the surgeon will take the correction of this into account in planning the reconstruction.

Barring accidents, most children's noses are perfectly adequate until they enter their teens, when the facial bones begin to take on the contours determined by inheritance. Teen-agers are especially sensitive about their looks. If nose surgery seems advisable, therefore, it is usually undertaken when the child is between 14 and 16 years of age, though the operation is also performed on adults.

In many cases, parents agree with the youngster about the need for surgery. In some families, however, the parent who has lived with a nose very similar to the one which the child finds so objectionable may take a negative view of the need for correction. If a serious disagreement results, it may be necessary to seek family counseling from a professional source to resolve it.

SURGICAL PROCEDURES: When a nose reconstruction is being planned, the surgeon requires photographs of both the left and right profiles as well as front and under views of the nose. Transparent paper is placed on top of the photos, and the recommended changes are drawn over the original nose structure. The patient's preferences are always taken into account, but the surgeon has a final say in determining the suitability of the new shape in terms of appearance and function. In some cases, facial surgery to build up an underdeveloped chin, called a *mentoplasty,* is recommended so that better balance of the features is achieved.

The surgery itself is performed under local anesthesia in a hospital. It is done through the nostrils so that there is no scarring of facial tissue. The skin is loosened from the bone and cartilage, and these are reshaped to the desired specifications. The skin then resettles on its new frame, and the new shape is retained by packing the nostrils and splinting the nose.

THE HEALING PROCESS: The packing is left in place for about three to five days or until it can be removed without sticking. The total dressing stays on for about a week. During the healing period, the nose is cleaned with cotton swabs. All swelling in the area vanishes in about a month, and within a year the reconstructed nose is as strong if not stronger than its original counterpart.

Cosmetic Breast Surgery

INVERTED NIPPLES: The condition in which the nipples are turned back into the breasts rather than projecting from them can be corrected by a simple operation. The breast tissue is cut to release the nipple so that it can be pulled outward to the normal position. This surgical procedure is sometimes recommended to facilitate the nursing of a newborn baby.

BREAST LIFTING: Breasts that sag even though they are not too large can be lifted to a more attractive contour by an operation that consolidates the tissue. The surgical procedure consists of removing strips of skin from the base of the breasts and bringing the rest of the skin together under tension so that it is tight

enough to support the tissue in an upward position.

BREAST REDUCTION: In spite of all the publicity given to breast augmentation, most cosmetic surgery involving the breasts is concerned with reducing rather than enlarging them. Breast reduction is frequently undertaken not only to improve appearance, but also for purposes of health and comfort.

The operation, called a *mastoplasty*, is performed under general anesthesia and consists in cutting out fatty tissue and skin. Although the incision may be large, the resulting scars are no thicker than a hairline and are hidden in the fold below the breasts.

The most remarkable thing about this type of surgery—and the reason for its being considerably more complicated than breast enlargement—is the repositioning of the nipples so that they are properly placed relative to the newly proportioned breast contours.

BREAST ENLARGEMENT: The techniques used in this operation, called a *mammoplasty*, have changed over the years. Early operations to augment the size of the breasts involved the injection of paraffin, but this was soon abandoned as unsatisfactory. Considerable experimentation with the use of various synthetics as well as with the use of fatty tissue taken from the buttocks didn't provide good results either.

Silicone—a form of man-made plastic material of great versatility—was first used in this connection in the form of sponges, and later was injected in liquid form directly into the tissue. However, the federal Food and Drug Administration has

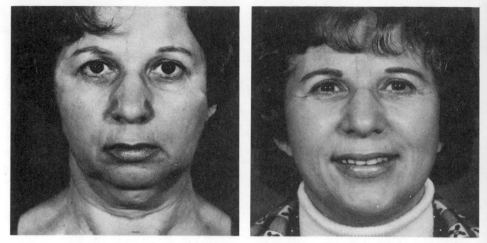

This patient underwent rhytidoplasty (face lift) and mentoplasty (chin buildup). Face lift removes wrinkles by tightening facial skin and removing the excess. Scars are hidden under hair and behind the ears.

ruled that the use of liquid silicone is unsafe and illegal, since its presence would mask signs of malignancy. Another problem with liquid silicone is that it has a tendency to drift to other parts of the body.

In the latest techniques of breast augmentation, a silicone gel or saline solution is placed in a flexible silicone bag shaped to resemble the breast. The bags are inserted through incisions under the breast tissue, and to date appear to be the safest and most satisfactory solution to the problem of breast enlargement.

Face Lift

Face lifting, or *rhytidoplasty,* is a form of cosmetic surgery designed to eliminate as far as possible signs of aging such as wrinkles, pouches under the chin and eyes, and sagging tissue generally. About 7,000 such operations are performed each year with satisfactory results.

In deciding on the advisability of a face lift, a reputable surgeon will take into account the person's age, emotional stability, and physical condition. The main procedure involves tightening the skin after the surplus has been removed. The resulting scars are usually hidden in the hair and behind the ears. Those directly in front of the ears are visible only under very close scrutiny. Even after a face lift, however, the same wrinkles will eventually reappear because of the characteristic use of the individual's facial muscles.

Body Lift

Recently, interest has grown in the application of cosmetic surgery to the problem of removing surplus fat from various parts of the body. Once considered controversial, the operation is being performed by many plastic surgeons. But these specialists emphasize that each person with a problem of surplus fat requires individual consultation and treatment.

Traditionally, to reduce the size of

the upper arms or legs, the abdomen, or the buttocks, an incision was made in a natural fold of the body area in question. The surrounding skin was loosened, the surplus fat and the excess skin removed, and the remaining skin was stretched tight and sutured. The procedure usually left a long scar.

In *suction lipectomy*, a new, alternative procedure, the surgeon does not make a long incision. Instead, the specialist makes a series of tiny, half-inch-long incisions. A suction device called a blunt cannula (which looks like a long straw) is inserted into the incisions. The cannula suctions out, or "vacuums" out, the excess fat. The operation can be performed on the stomach, buttocks, chin, calf, and ankle areas.

Suction lipectomy, also called *lipolysis*, involves normal surgical risks. The skin in the area of the operation may acquire a rippling effect. Some damage could be done to nerves and blood vessels. Bruising could last for several weeks. The patient may have to wear supportive clothing for four to six weeks. Plastic surgeons stress that the procedure is not a weight-reduction technique for the obese, but a contouring operation.

Eyelids

The shape and size of the eyelids can be changed by an operation called a *blepharoplasty*. In this procedure, an incision is made in the fold of the upper eyelid, and excess skin and fat are removed. The technique can be used to correct congenital deformities such as hanging upper eyelids that do not fully open. When a comparable incision is made below the lash line on the lower lid, the surgeon can remove the fat which causes bags under the eyes.

Ears

Surgery to correct protruding or overlarge ears is called *otoplasty*. Though it can be performed on adults, it is usually performed on children before they enter school to prevent the psychological problems that often result from teasing. In the procedure, an incision is made behind the ear, cartilage is cut, and the ear is repositioned closer to the

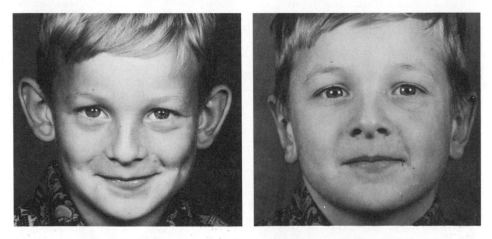

Surgery to correct protruding or overlarge ears is called otoplasty. It is usually performed on children before they enter school to prevent the psychological problems that often result from teasing.

skull. Otoplasty can also build up or replace an ear missing because of a birth defect or accident.

Scar Reduction

Unsightly scars that are the result of a birth defect or an injury can usually be reduced by plastic surgery to thin hairlines. The procedure is effective only if there has been no extensive damage to surrounding areas of underlying tissue, as sometimes occurs in severe burns. The operation involves the removal of the old scar tissue, undermining the surrounding skin, and pulling it together with very fine stitches.

Hair Transplant

A comparatively new solution to the problem of baldness is the technique called hair transplantation. This involves the surgical grafting of hair-bearing skin taken from the back part and sides of the scalp onto the bald areas of the head. The transplanting is usually done in the surgeon's office with the patient receiving a local anesthetic. The surgeon can make anywhere from 10 to 60 transplants in an hour's session.

Within about a month, the hairs in the grafted skin fall out, but the roots remain, and most of these eventually produce new hair. The areas from which the grafts are taken remain hairless, but since each transplant is very small, about 150 or 200 graftings can be done without creating any conspicuous bald spots. Transplanted hair has the same thickness and appearance that it had in its former location.

UNCOMMON SURGICAL PROCEDURES

Organ Transplants

The notion of man's ability to rebuild human bodies from parts of other humans or from artificial organs probably is as old as the dreams that men might some day fly like birds or travel to the moon. Some of the oldest documents, thousands of years old, tell of medical efforts to transplant organs, limbs, and other tissues to save lives or enable disabled persons to pursue normal activities. In recent decades, medical scientists have discovered how to overcome some of the obstacles to organ transplanting, just as other scientists have learned to fly higher and faster than birds and travel beyond the moon.

Tissue Compatibility

A major obstacle to organ transplants has been one of *histoincompatibility* (*histo* means "tissue"): the tissues of the person receiving the transplant tend to reject the tissues of the transplanted organ. The problem is quite similar to that of allergies or the body's reaction to foreign bodies, including infectious organisms. Each individual has a set of antigens that are peculiar to that person, because of genetic variations among different persons. The histoincompatible antigens are on the surfaces of the tissue cells. But in most cases the antigens on the cells of the transplanted organ do not match those of the person receiving the transplant, so the recipient's body in effect refuses to accept the transplant.

The major exception to this rule is found in identical twins, who are born with the same sets of antigens. The organs of one twin can be transplanted to the body of the other twin with a minimum risk of rejection. Antigens on the tissue cells of brothers and sisters and of the parents will be similar, because of the biological relationship, but they will not be as compatible as those of identical twins. Even less compatible are antigens of people who are not related.

TYPES OF GRAFTS: There is virtually no problem in transferring tissues from one area to another of the same patient. Skin grafts, bone grafts, and blood-vessel transplants are commonly made with a patient's own tissues, which have the same antigens, as in spinal fusions, repair of diseased leg arteries, and so on. Tissue transplants within an individual's body are called *autografts.* Transplants of tissues or organs from one human to another are called *homografts. Heterografts* are tissues from one species that are transplanted to another; they offer the greatest risk of histoincompatibility and are used mainly as a temporary measure, such as covering a severely burned area of a person with specially treated pieces of pigskin. The heterograft will be rejected but it will provide some protection during the recovery period.

Much of the experience of surgeons in handling tissue transplants between humans came from early experiments in skin grafting. It was found that histoincompatibility in transplants of skin appeared to sensitize the recipient tissues in the same way that allergy sensitivity rises. Thus, when a second skin graft from the same donor is attempted, the graft is rejected more rapidly than the first graft because of the buildup of antibodies from the first rejection. The same sort of rejection reaction can occur in transplants of kidneys, hearts, and other organs unless the problem of histoincompatibility is overcome.

IMMUNOSUPPRESSIVE CHEMICALS: In order to make the host body more receptive to an organ transplant, *immunosuppressive* chemicals are injected into the recipient's tissues to suppress their natural tendency to reject the foreign tissue. However, the technique of suppressing the immune response of the host tissues is not without hazards. By suppressing the natural rejection phenomenon, the transplant recipient is made vulnerable to other diseases. It has been found, for example, that persons who receive the immune response suppression chemicals as part of transplant surgery develop cancers at a rate that is 15 times that of the general population. Transplant patients also can become extremely vulnerable to infections, such as pneumonia.

ANTIGEN MATCHING: The breakthrough in human organ transplantation was helped by the development of a system of matching antigens related to lymphocytes—a type of white blood cell—of the donor and recipient. At least a dozen lymphocyte antigens have been identified, and it is possible to match them by a process similar to matching blood factors of patients before making a blood transfusion. If all or most of the antigens of the donor tissue and the

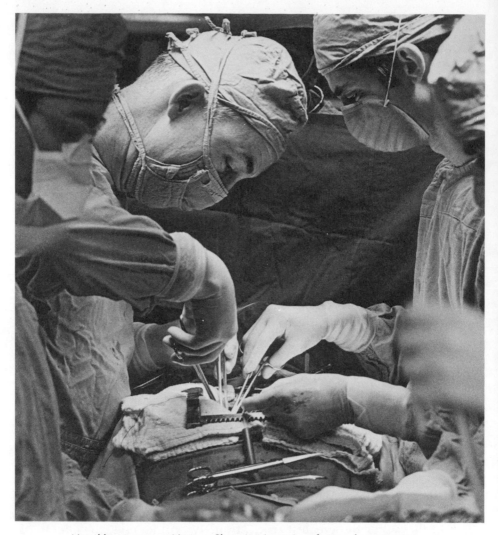

Noted heart surgeon Norman Shumway (center) performs a heart transplant operation. This type of surgery is still highly experimental.

recipient match, the chances for a successful transplanting procedure are greatly enhanced.

Antigen matching is less important in some kinds of homografts, such as replacing the cornea of the eye. The cornea is a unique kind of tissue with no blood vessels, and therefore is unlikely to be invaded by antibodies of the recipient. Pieces of human bone also may be used in homografts with a minimum risk of rejection, although surgeons usually prefer to use bone from the patient's own body in repairing fractures and other orthopedic procedures.

Types of Transplants

CORNEA TRANSPLANT: Cornea transplants helped to pioneer the art of homografts. The first successful cornea transplants were made during the 1930s. In addition to the absence of rejection problems because of incompatible antigens, cornea transplants probably succeeded in the early days of homografts because only small pieces of the tissue were used. See p. 959.

KIDNEY TRANSPLANT: Kidney transplants began in the 1950s. Antigen typing was unknown at that time, but doctors had learned of the genetic factors of blood groups and found from experience that although kidney transplants from siblings and parents could eventually be rejected, the rejection phenomenon was delayed. The first truly successful kidney transplant operation was performed in Boston in 1954 between twin brothers; doctors had tested the tissue compatibility of the twins first by making a small skin transplant to see if it would be rejected. Knowledge acquired later of immunosuppressive drugs enabled surgeons to make kidney transplants between persons who were not twins.

More than 5,000 kidney-transplant operations have been performed with an 82 percent survival rate of two years or more when the donor was related to the recipient. When a cadaver kidney was transplanted, the two-year survival rate was 65 percent. It has been estimated that as many as 10,000 kidney-disease patients each year could benefit from a transplanted organ, but a lack of available kidneys in satisfactory condition restricts the number of transplants. An alternative for some kidney patients awaiting an organ transplant is hemodialysis, a process which performs as an artificial kidney. See p. 1251 for further information on dialysis.

Cross-species transplants—animal hearts implanted in humans—seemed also to hold out hope for persons suffering from serious heart impairments.

HEART TRANSPLANT: The first successful human heart transplant was performed by Dr. Christiaan Barnard in Cape Town, South Africa, in 1968. The patient survived more than 18 months and led a relatively active life until the second heart failed because of a rejection reaction. Many heart transplant operations have been performed since 1968, with varying success, sometimes leading to complete recovery and sometimes to recovery for long periods of time. Heart transplants were found to be more difficult than some other organ transplants, such as of the kidney, because the heart must be taken from the donor at virtually the moment of death and immediately placed in the body of the recipient. Because of concern about determining the moment of death, the medical profession has offered guidelines for answering this complex ethical and legal question.

Success of a heart transplant operation may depend on the health of other organ systems in the patient's body; persons in need of heart transplants usually have medical problems involving the lungs and kidneys as a result of the diseased heart. And heart transplant patients frequently seem less able to tolerate the use of immunosuppressive drugs that must be administered after surgery. The introduction of cyclosporine as an immunosuppressant in the early 1980s changed the picture substantially, however. Medical evidence indicated that cyclosporine would lead to a five-year survival rate among heart transplant patients of 50 percent or more. Because cyclosporine speeds rehabilitation after an operation, average hospital stays for patients receiving the immunosuppressant have been reduced from 72 to 42 days.

Conducted before cyclosporine came into common use, one study of a group of transplant patients showed that fewer than 40 percent survived beyond the first year. Several lived more than two years after the operation.

BONE-MARROW TRANSPLANT: Limited success has been reported in efforts to perform bone-marrow transplants. Bone-marrow transplants are performed to supply patients with active leukocytes to fight cancer and other diseases. The successful early cases have involved transplants between sisters and brothers who had been typed for tissue compatibility.

OTHER KINDS OF TRANSPLANTS: Surgeons also have experimented with varying success with human transplants of livers, lungs, and pancreas tissue. Lung transplant efforts have been hampered by infection, rejection, and hemorrhage. Because the lungs are exposed to pathogenic organisms in the environment they are especially vulnerable to infections when the host tissues have been treated with immunosuppressive chemicals. Liver transplants are difficult to perform because of a lack of satisfactory donor organs and the complex circuitry of arteries, veins, and bile duct that must be connected to the recipient before the liver can begin to function.

Most major organ transplants are considered only in terms of a "last ditch" effort to prolong the life of a patient who is critically ill. While homografts are not always a perfect success and may lengthen a patient's life by only a few years, remarkable strides in these surgical techniques have been made over a relatively short period of time. Surgeons who specialize in organ transplants state that even greater progress could be made if a greater supply of donor organs were available.

Reattachment of Severed Members

Because an individual's tissues present no histocompatibility problem with other parts of his own body, severed fingers and other members can be rejoined to the rest of the body if vital parts are not damaged beyond repair. Children sometimes suffer amputation of a part of a finger during play or in accidents at home. For example, a finger tip can be severed when caught in a closed door of an automobile. If the severed part of the finger is saved and the patient is given immediate medical care, the finger usually can be rejoined and sutured in place with a very good chance of survival of the graft.

Rejoining a Severed Limb

One of the most dramatic cases of a rejoined limb in American medical annals involved a 12-year-old whose right arm was severed at the shoulder when he was crushed between a train and a tunnel wall in 1962. Railroad workers called an ambulance, and the boy, his severed arm still encased in his sleeve, was rushed to a hospital. The boy was given plasma by doctors who packed the severed arm in ice and flushed out the blood vessels of the arm with anticoagulant drugs and antibiotics. During three hours of surgery, the major veins and artery of the arm were carefully stitched to the vessels at the shoulder. For the next five hours, doctors joined the bones, located the main nerve trunks and connected them to the nerve ends in the shoulder, and repaired the muscles. The boy was released from the hospital three weeks after the accident but returned for additional operations to connect various nerve fibers. That operation was a success, but similar attempts to rejoin severed arms of middle-aged men have failed despite heroic attempts by surgeons to restore the limbs as functioning parts of the body.

A Chinese factory worker suffered accidental amputation of his right hand when it was caught in a metal-punching machine, and was rushed to a hospital in Shanghai. Chinese medical reports of the case indicate that a procedure similar to the one used on the American boy was followed. Blood vessels were rejoined first to permit the flow of blood to tissues. This was followed by surgery to connect the tendons and main nerve trunks. The bones of the forearm, where the amputation occurred, were joined and held in place with metal plates and screws. Doctors reported that the graft was successful, and the patient, a 27-year-old man, was able to move his fingers again within three weeks after the accident.

Medical records indicate that major reattachments of severed limbs are still rare, although rejoined finger tips, ears, and other parts not involving main arteries, veins, or nerve trunks are not as uncommon.

CHAPTER 21

Women's Health

The special health matters that are related to a woman's reproductive system belong to the branch of medicine known as *gynecology*. *Obstetrics* is a closely related specialty associated with pregnancy and childbirth. The distinction is something of a technicality for most patients, since obstetricians usually are quite capable of handling gynecological cases and vice versa. The practice of obstetrics and gynecology is commonly combined in a medical service identified by the contraction *Ob-Gyn*. However, there are medical matters that are specifically concerned with female reproductive organs and related tissues but have little to do with obstetrics. For a discussion of obstetrics, see *Infertility, Pregnancy, and Childbirth*, p. 570.

The Gynecological Examination

What should a woman expect on her first visit to a gynecologist? First, the gynecologist will interview her, asking about her family, her medical history, and any fears or apprehensions she may have about her personal health. The woman's answers and comments are written into her medical records for future reference. The information can contain important clues that may help in diagnosing any present or future disorders.

A sample of urine and a sample of blood are usually obtained for laboratory tests. During the ensuing physical examination, the woman lies on a special examination table with her feet in metal stirrups and

988

her knees apart. A nurse will be present to assist the doctor. While lying in the *lithotomy position,* the woman's abdomen will be palpated for lumps or other abnormalities. The breasts also will be palpated for possible lumps. Then an external inspection of the vulva and surrounding areas is made by the doctor, followed by internal inspection, in which a speculum is used to spread apart the sides of the vagina so that the cervix is exposed. A digital examination (using the fingers) is made of the walls of the vagina and rectum and the neighboring tissue areas, in a search for possible growths or other abnormal conditions. And a sample of cells and secretions from the cervix is taken for a Pap smear test (described in detail on p. 1020).

In addition to the examination of the breasts and reproductive system, the gynecologist usually conducts a general physical examination, recording information about height,

weight, blood pressure, heart and lung condition, and so on. The routine physical examination, like the medical history, provides additional clues which, when added to the results of the examination of the breasts and reproductive system, will give a complete picture of the patient's gynecological health.

Following the examination, the gynecologist discusses his appraisal of the woman's condition and answers questions. He will discuss whatever treatment she needs. Medications can be explained at this time, including reasons why certain drugs can or should not be taken. If any surgery or further testing is recommended, those aspects of the health picture also should be discussed in some detail. Any important information that might be misunderstood or forgotten should be jotted down for future reference.

Results of some laboratory tests and the Pap smear are not usually available for several days. But the

DES, a synthetic hormone, was given to thousands of pregnant women in the 1950s, apparently causing many of their daughters to get cancer.

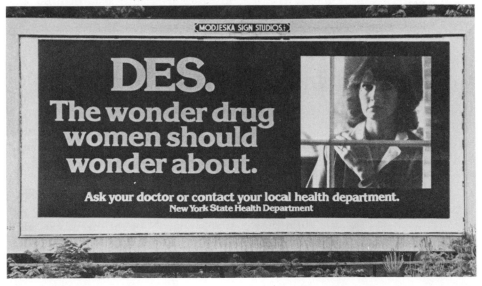

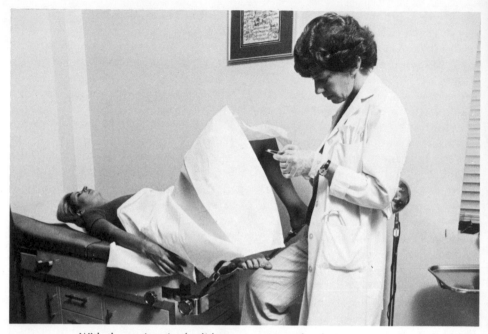

With the patient in the lithotomy position, the doctor prepares a slide with cells taken from the patient's cervix for the Pap smear test.

doctor or nurse will contact the patient when the results are available and advise if she should return in the near future for follow-up testing. The woman also should discuss arrangements for future checkups or Pap smear tests rather than wait until signs or symptoms of a serious disor- der warrant an immediate visit. In the event of some possible future physical complaint, the fact that the woman has established some basic medical records with her gynecolo- gist will be of help in making a prop- er diagnosis and establishing the best course of treatment.

MENSTRUAL DISORDERS

Among the health concerns of wom- en that specifically belong to gyne- cology are menstrual disorders. Nor- mally, the first menstrual period (menarche) occurs about age 12 or 13, or sometimes earlier or later. Periods are generally irregular for the first year or two, and then they tend to recur at intervals of 24 to 32 days. Each period begins about two weeks after ovulation, or the release of an egg cell (ovum) from the ovary —unless, of course, the ovum hap- pens to be fertilized in the interval and pregnancy interrupts the whole process.

The menstrual flow, which lasts from three to seven days, is com- posed mainly of serum, mucus, and dead cells shed from the lining (en- dometrium) of the uterus. The loss of blood is minimal, usually from two to four ounces. The volume of flow, as well as the time schedule, tends to be fairly regular for most women. When one's menstrual pattern varies noticeably from the expected pattern, and in the absence of pregnancy, it may be a sign of a physical or emotional disorder.

Amenorrhea

Failure to menstruate is called *amenorrhea.* Amenorrhea is a natural effect of pregnancy and of nursing a baby. In an older woman, it may be a sign of menopause. But if a nonpregnant or nonnursing woman after menarche and before menopause (say between the ages of 17 or 18 and 52) fails to menstruate for two or more periods, she should bring it to the attention of a doctor —unless, of course, she has undergone a hysterectomy or other surgical or medical treatment that eliminates menstruation.

Primary Amenorrhea

When menarche has not occurred by the age of 16 or 17, the absence of menstruation is called *primary amenorrhea.* In such a case, a physical examination may show that an imperforate hymen or a closed cervix is obstructing the flow of menses, or a congenital defect may be interfering with menstruation. In almost all cases, menarche can be started with a bit of minor surgery, by treatment of any existing systemic disease, or by the injection of sex hormones; or it will start spontaneously later.

Secondary Amenorrhea

When menstrual periods cease after menarche, the condition is known as *secondary,* or *acquired,* *amenorrhea.* Secondary amenorrhea may involve missing a single menstrual period or many periods in consecutive months. Among possible causes of interrupted menstruation are certain medications, drugs of abuse, emotional stress, normal fluctuations in ovarian activity in the first few years after menarche, and a number of organic diseases. Medicines that can disrupt normal menstrual activity include tranquilizers and other psychotropic (mind-affecting) drugs that apparently influence hormonal activity in the brain centers, amphetamines, and oral contraceptives. When a particular medication is found to be the cause of amenorrhea, the medical treatment may be judged to be more important than maintaining normal menstrual cycles. When the use of oral contraceptives is followed by amenorrhea for six or more months, normal menstrual activity may resume eventually, but it can often be started sooner by a prescribed medication. Among drugs of abuse known to cause amenorrhea are alcohol and opium-based drugs.

Just as the mind-altering effects of psychotropic drugs involve the hypothalamus and pituitary glands in the brain, which control the hormones that regulate menstrual functions, emotional stress seems to have a parallel influence on the incidence of amenorrhea. *Anorexia nervosa,* a disorder associated with emaciation due to an emotional disturbance, also can result in an interruption of menstruation.

Other factors contributing to secondary amenorrhea are measles, mumps, and other infections; cysts and tumors of the ovaries; changes in the tissues lining the vagina or uterus; premature aging of the ovaries; diabetes; obesity; anemia; leukemia; and Hodgkin's disease. In many cases, normal or near-normal menstrual function can be restored by medical treatment, such as administration of hormones, or by surgery, or both. In one type of amenorrhea, marked by adhesion of the walls of the uterus, curettage (scraping of the uterus) is followed by insertion of an intrauterine contraceptive device (IUD) to help hold the uterine walls apart.

Menorrhagia

Almost the opposite of amenorrhea is *menorrhagia*, an excessive menstrual flow. The causes of menorrhagia are as varied as those associated with amenorrhea. They include influenza and other infectious diseases, emotional stress, polyps of the cervical or uterine tissues (see p. 1016), hypertension, congestive heart failure, leukemia, and blood coagulation disorders. Menorrhagia may occur during the early stages of a young woman's reproductive life soon after reaching puberty, and medical treatment may be necessary to control the excessive loss of blood. In some cases, dilation and curettage is recommended in addition to the administration of hormones and other medications, such as iron tablets to correct anemia resulting from the loss of red blood cells.

DILATION AND CURETTAGE: *Dilation and curettage*, generally referred to as *D and C*, is a procedure in which the cervix is dilated and the cavity of the uterus is cleaned out by a scooplike instrument, a curette. The same procedure is sometimes used to abort an embryo or to remove a tumor or a polyp.

Although it takes only a few minutes to perform a D and C, the procedure is done in a hospital while the patient is anesthetized. There is no afterpain, only a dull discomfort in the lower pelvic region similar to menstrual awareness.

A physical examination is usually made to determine if there are tumors anywhere in the reproductive organs. Except where tumors are found to be a causative factor, most women will resume normal menstrual cycles after treatment of menorrhagia with medications and D and C. For women beyond the age of 40, the doctor may recommend a hysterectomy to prevent recurrence of excessive menstrual blood loss.

Polymenorrhea and Metrorrhagia

These medical terms refer to two other ways in which menstrual peri-

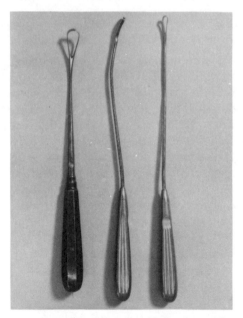

Two types of curettes are shown above. The middle and right instruments are the same, seen from different angles.

ods may depart from typical patterns. *Polymenorrhea* is abnormally frequent menstruation, so that menstrual periods occur at intervals of less than 21 days. This short interval may be the natural established pattern for some women. If it is not, the cause may be physical or emotional stress. *Metrorrhagia* is marked by menstrual bleeding that occurs erratically at unpredictable times. It may be the result of a cyst in the lining of the uterus, a tumor in the reproductive tract, polyps, or some hormonal imbalance, including a disorder of the thyroid gland.

Dysmenorrhea

Abdominal or pelvic pain occurring just before or along with the onset of menstruation is known as *dysmenorrhea*. The symptoms include severe colicky abdominal cramps, backache, headache, and, in some cases, nausea and vomiting. As with amenorrhea, there are two general types of dysmenorrhea, primary and secondary.

Primary Dysmenorrhea

This type includes all cases in which no organic disorder is associated with the symptoms, which are presumed to be due to uterine contractions and emotional factors. More than 75 percent of all cases are of this type. Primary dysmenorrhea generally begins before age 25, but it may appear at any time from menarche to menopause. It frequently ends with the birth of the first child.

Since primary dysmenorrhea by definition occurs in the absence of organic disease, the diagnosis can be made only after a careful medical history is compiled and a special study of the reproductive organs is made to insure that no disorder has been overlooked. In some cases, oral contraceptives may be prescribed because of the effect such drugs have in suppressing ovulation; the contraceptives prevent the natural production of the hormone progesterone, which is responsible for certain tissue changes associated with the discomfort of dysmenorrhea. Analgesic drugs to relieve pain and medications that help to relax muscles may be prescribed. However, medication is often less beneficial than emotional support—including the easing of any stress at home, school, or work, and reassurance about the worries sometimes associated with menstruation.

Secondary Dysmenorrhea

This condition comprises all menstrual pain that is due to or associated with an organic disease of the reproductive organs, such as endometriosis (see p. 1018) to cite just one example. Secondary dysmenorrhea can occur at any age.

Edema and Premenstrual Tension

Primary dysmenorrhea is often associated with fluid accumulation in the tissues (edema) and sensations of bloating and pelvic heaviness that increase with physical activity. But those symptoms subside after the menstrual flow begins. Although physical activity may aggravate some cases of dysmenorrhea, exercise can be helpful for other patients. Simple exercises that include twisting and bending the trunk often produce beneficial results if performed two or three times a day. During menstrual periods, most women are able to work, play, bathe, swim, and carry on as usual with all their physical activities.

Premenstrual fluid retention and premenstrual tension very often co-exist. Premenstrual tension produces greater discomfort in some women than menstruation itself. About half of all women experience the effects at some time during their reproductive years, particularly after the age of thirty. Typical symptoms are anxiety, agitation, insomnia, and depression. A women may appear irritable, sometimes moody or sullen, or aggressive for about a week or ten days before the start of a menstrual period. Some women experience headaches, a bloated feeling, nausea and vomiting, and diarrhea or constipation. Seemingly unrelated conditions, ranging from mental illness to obesity, tend to be aggravated at this time. Many women develop unusual appetites, and weight gain can be as much as eight pounds, due mostly, however, to fluid retention in the tissues. This fluid is quickly lost through urination once the menstrual flow has begun.

Treatment of premenstrual tension is similar to that recommended for dysmenorrhea. In order to alleviate edema, the doctor may recommend a low-salt diet and a diuretic, particularly for the days between ovulation and the beginning of a menstrual period. The woman may also be encouraged to divide her daily food intake into numerous small meals rather than three square meals a day. A greater proportion of the calorie allowance might be shifted to proteins instead of carbohydrates. Oral contraceptives that suppress ovulation may be pre-scribed. Although tranquilizers may be prescribed for a woman who displays agitation as an effect of premenstrual tension, women who show signs of depression and self-pity would benefit more from stimulants and encouragement toward a more active life style.

Minor Menstrual Problems

BLOOD CLOTS: There is not usually any cause for alarm if blood clots are expelled during menstruation. Ordinarily, the menstrual flow is completely liquefied, but a few clots tend to appear when the flow is profuse. However, if many clots appear and the flow seems excessive, medical advice is recommended, since these conditions may be a sign of fibroid tumors in the uterus. See p. 1017.

ORAL CONTRACEPTIVES: Women on combination birth-control pills can expect to see a changed menstrual pattern. The flow becomes slighter than before and very regular. For a discussion of oral contraceptives, see Birth Control, p. 605.

ODOR: The menstrual flow of a healthy woman generally has a mild odor which develops when it is exposed to the air or to the vulva. Some women are concerned about this odor, although it usually is not offensive. When it is, it tends to be associated with inadequate bathing. Detergents are added to some commercial tampons and pad products, and special deodorants have been developed to mask the odor. However, such materials produce allergic reactions in some women, and they can have the unfortunate effect of masking an odor that may be the sign of an abnormal condition.

ONSET OF MENOPAUSE: Menstrual irregularities almost always precede the natural cessation of menstrual function. For a full discussion of menopause, see p. 632.

Postmenopausal Bleeding

Bleeding that occurs after the final cessation of menstrual activity should be seen as an urgent signal to seek medical advice. The bleeding may be painless or painful and may range from occasional spotting that is brownish or bright red to rather profuse bleeding that continues for several days or more. The various signs and symptoms should be noted carefully because they can help suggest to the doctor the possible cause of bleeding. Bleeding after the menopause is often a sign of cancer of the cervix or the lining of the uterus, but there is a wide variety of other possible causes, including polyps, ulcers, hypertensive heart disease, an ovarian tumor, or infection. In many cases, the problem can be treated by dilation and curettage or withdrawal of any hormone medications, such as estrogens prescribed for menopausal symptoms, or both. In these cases, if D and C and treatment and discontinuance of hormone therapy fail, the doctor may advise a hysterectomy.

INFECTIONS OF THE REPRODUCTIVE TRACT

Vaginal and other reproductive tract infections are among the most common gynecological problems, and among the most stubborn to treat successfully.

Leukorrhea

A whitish, somewhat viscid discharge from the vagina, which is known medically as *leukorrhea,* may be quite normal, especially if it is not continual but occurs only intermittently—prior to menstruation, for example, or associated with sexual excitation. It may also be increased when oral contraceptives are used.

Constant leukorrhea, on the other hand, often is a sign and symptom of an abnormality. Leukorrhea due to disease can occur at any age. It is generally associated with an infection of the lower reproductive tract. The discharge may occur without any discomfort, but in some cases there is itching, irritation, and *dyspareunia* — the medical term for painful intercourse (see p. 1018).

Laboratory tests of vaginal secretions may be needed to help identify the precise cause of the discharge. Leukorrhea can result from vaginal ulcers; a tumor of the vagina, uterus, or Fallopian tubes; gonorrhea; or infection by any of various disease organisms of the vulva, vagina, cervix, uterus, or tubes. It may also be due to an abnormality of menstrual function, or even emotional stress.

Treatment, of course, depends on the cause. If the discharge is due to an infection, care must be taken to avoid being reinfected or transmitting the disease organism through sexual contact or possibly contaminated underclothing, etc. The condition may be particularly difficult to control if the woman is pregnant or suffers from some chronic disorder, such as diabetes.

THE FEMALE REPRODUCTIVE SYSTEM

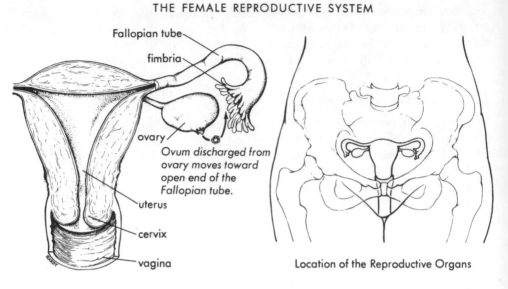

Location of the Reproductive Organs

Moniliasis

Moniliasis, also known as *candidiasis,* is an infection by a yeastlike fungus that is capable of invading mucous membrane and sometimes skin in various parts of the body. Inside the mouth, the organism causes thrush, most commonly in babies. When the organism invades the vaginal area it causes a scant white discharge of a thick consistency resembling that of cottage cheese. There is itching, burning, and swelling of the labial and vulvar areas. The symptoms tend to worsen just before the menstrual period. The occurrence of the disease is thought by some to be enhanced by oral contraceptives. Antibiotic therapy, too, generally favors the moniliasis organism, which is unaffected by the antibiotics that destroy many of the benign organisms that regularly share the same environment.

Moniliasis is treated with suppositories, creams, and other medications. The woman's partner should be treated at the same time to prevent a cycle of infection and reinfection of both partners, because the fungus will otherwise spread to the genital tissues of the man.

Trichomoniasis

A type of leukorrhea that consists of a copious yellow to green frothy and fetid discharge is caused by infection by the *trichomonas* organism. The organism causes an irritating itching condition that tends to set in or worsen just after a menstrual period. The condition is diagnosed by a test similar to a Pap smear, made with a specimen taken from the vagina. Trichomonas organisms, if present, are easy to identify under a microscope; they are pear-shaped protozoa with three to five whiplike tails.

The organism favors warm moist areas, such as genital tissues, but it can also survive in damp towels and wash cloths, around toilet seats, and on beaches and the perimeters of swimming pools. Thus it can spread from one member of a family to other members and from one woman to other women. *Trichomoniasis* is not technically a venereal disease, but it can be transmitted by sexual contact. When one partner is infected with trichomoniasis, both must be treated at the same time and a condom must be worn during intercourse.

Several drugs are available for treating trichomoniasis, including tablets taken orally and suppositories inserted in the vagina. The tablets usually are taken three times daily for ten days, after which an examination is made to determine if any trichomonas organisms are still present. The oral medication may be continued for several months if the infection resists the drug— some studies show that the organism appears to survive in about ten percent of treated cases. There are douches available in drugstores for removing the discharge, but women are advised to consult their physi-

cians before experimenting with home remedies or over-the-counter products that may be offered as douche treatments for trichomoniasis. The substances contained in some douches can aggravate the condition or irritate the vaginal tissues.

Herpes Simplex Virus Type 2

In recent years, doctors have become aware of a viral infection that is acquired by contact with the mucous membranes of an infected person. The mucous membrane of the mouth and lips, the genitals, or the rectum may be affected. The causative agent is known as *Herpes simplex virus Type 2*, or *HSV-2*. It is similar to but not the same as the virus that causes fever blisters, or cold sores, which is Type 1 (HSV-1). Information about the incidence of Type 2 is not well documented. The virus is associated with some spontaneous abortions,

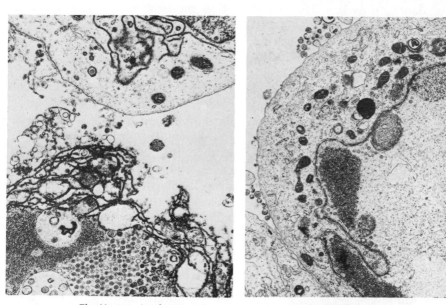

The Herpes simplex virus Type 2, greatly magnified under an electron microscope. This virus can cause serious damage to a newborn baby if the mother is infected with it at the time of delivery.

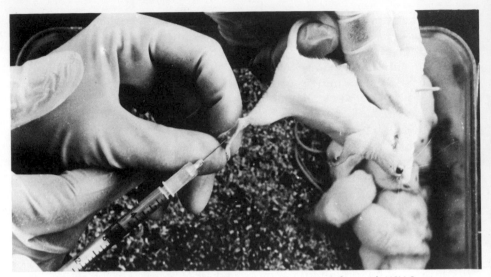

In a laboratory study, a researcher injects a mouse's foot with HSV-2 virus, which will remain in a latent state in the animal's nervous system.

stillbirths, and deaths of newborn babies. If the mother is infected at the time of delivery, the virus can be transmitted to the baby as it passes through the vagina. The central nervous system, including the brain, may be damaged by the virus if the baby becomes infected. To avoid exposure to the virus, a Caesarian delivery is recommended when the mother is infected.

SYMPTOMS: Patients with their first HSV-2 infection usually complain of intense itching, painful blisterlike eruptions, and ulcerated patches with a discharge. Other symptoms may include genital pain and vaginal bleeding. Fever, swelling, difficult urination, and a general feeling of ill health and lack of appetite may accompany the infection. Diagnosis of HSV-2 is verified through biopsies and smears examined microscopically, cultures, and the presence of HSV-2 antibodies.

Symptoms may subside after a few weeks but recurrences are common,

though they are less painful and of shorter duration. There is no known cure for the viral infection.

TREATMENT: Treatment was once limited to applications of anesthetic creams, steroid ointments, and other medications to relieve symptoms. No drug has been found to attack the viruses while they are "hibernating" in cells at the base of the spine. But one antiviral drug, *acyclovir*, has been found to reduce recurrent outbreaks and to block flareups for up to several months.

Taken orally in pill form, acyclovir in tests has brought relief, but not cures, to hundreds of subjects. The drug is ingested daily. Researchers have discovered that the capsules kill or neutralize the herpes viruses only when they are active. Because of evidence that the virus may be related to the subsequent development of cervical cancer, women sufferers should have Pap smear tests at intervals of six months instead of the usual twelve.

VENEREAL DISEASES

The name of Venus, the goddess of love, is preserved in the term *venereal disease* in recognition of the fact that the venereal diseases are commonly transmitted by sexual contact during intercourse. Although the term can be applied to any infection that is transmissible through sexual activity, such as moniliasis or trichomoniasis, *venereal disease* is usually confined to syphilis, gonorrhea, and three lesser infections that are of concern to public health authorities and are reportable by law in the United States—lymphogranuloma venereum, chancroid, and granuloma inguinale. Although doctors are required to report all infectious cases that come to their attention, there are no reliable figures on the number of people who are in urgent need of treatment but fail to seek it, either through indifference or ignorance. It is generally agreed that the number is very high. See also p. 1261 for additional information about venereal diseases.

Syphilis

Potentially the most devastating of the venereal diseases, syphilis was once known as the great pox, so-called in comparison with the less-dreaded scourge, smallpox. Its gravity was greatly lessened by the discovery of penicillin, which provided the first quick and effective cure for the early stages of the disease. At the time of the introduction of antibiotics, more than 100,000 new cases of syphilis were reported each year. The incidence then dropped dramatically to about 6,000 cases a year, but the rate began rising during the 1960s and 1970s. A partial explanation for the increased incidence may be that the widespread use of oral contraceptives led to a reduced use of the condom during intercourse. There also is some evidence that oral contraceptives subtly alter vaginal secretions, thereby providing a climate that allows the organisms to thrive. Nearly 25,000 infectious syphilis cases were reported in the United States in the mid-1970s, leaving an untreated reservoir, according to the American Social Health Association, of probably more than 450,000 persons.

Primary Syphilis

Syphilis is caused by a spirally shaped bacterium belonging to a group of spiral organisms known as *spirochetes*. Sexual intercourse is the usual path of transmission, since the organism is too fragile to survive long exposure on contaminated objects. It is killed by heat, dryness, ordinary antiseptics, and soap, but it can tolerate cold and survive freezing. It is thought to be capable of penetrating intact mucous membrane, such as the inner surface of the mouth, or skin that may be intact but is more commonly marked by a lesion.

Once inside the body, the spirochetes can spread to almost any organ, producing inflammation and tissue destruction. Syphilis sometimes is called the great imitator of diseases because it produces signs and symptoms resembling a wide variety of organic disorders. Even the initial manifestation of syphilis can be misleading. The first sign is a painless chancre, or ulcer, which

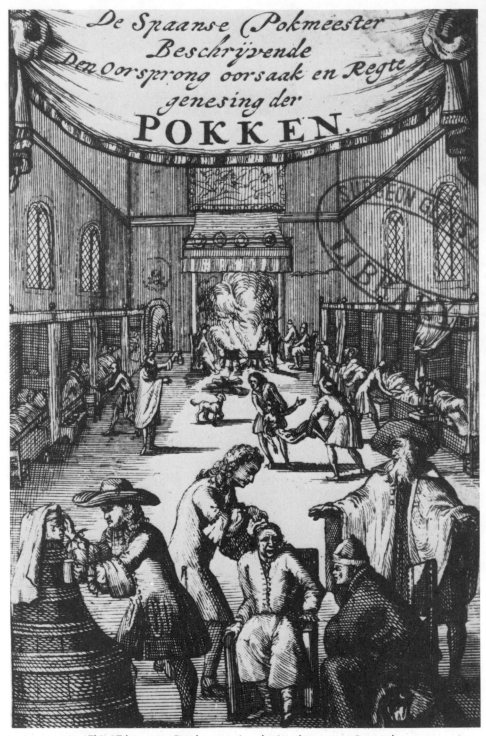

This 17th-century Dutch engraving depicts doctors treating syphilis in a venereal-disease ward. ("Pokken" means "pox" in Dutch.)

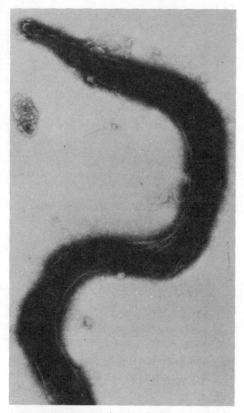

A *Treponema* spirochete, which causes syphilis, enlarged about 40,000 times. Note the spiral shape of the organism.

may be small, single or multiple, and look like almost any other ulcer. Syphilitic chancres in women occur mostly on the external genital areas, in the vagina, or on the cervix, but they may appear on the breasts, lips, or in the mouth. Ordinarily, chancres heal completely and leave no scar. This primary stage, the first sign of infection, may occur at any time from about ten days to three months after a communicable contact with an infected person or object. The usual interval is about three weeks.

Secondary and Latent Stages

About six weeks after the appearance of the chancre, whether or not the patient was aware of it, secondary-stage lesions develop in most untreated cases. These secondary lesions take the form of a rash or almost any other kind of skin eruption. The skin lesions may appear on the trunk of the body, on the face, the arms and legs, or the palms of the hands and soles of the feet. The lesions may or may not cause itching. It is possible for a patient to develop a primary chancre without the later appearance of the secondary-stage skin symptoms.

A latent phase of many years' duration follows untreated secondary syphilis. The only clue to the presence of syphilis in the body during the latent period is the presence of the organism responsible as revealed by a blood test.

Tertiary Syphilis

If syphilis is not treated during the primary, secondary, or latent stages, it can progress to late syphilis, which usually involves chronic destructive effects in the central nervous system, the heart, bones, liver, stomach, or other tissues. The skin, mucous membranes, and other organs may develop rubbery tumors called *gummas*. A gumma lesion can occur in the throat and affect the larynx or the respiratory tract. The gummas frequently have the appearance of malignant tumors; biopsies are needed to determine whether the growths are caused by cancer or by syphilis.

One of the most dangerous effects of untreated syphilis is an invasion of the circulatory system, resulting in an aneurysm (dilated part) of the aorta just above the heart, with damage to the aortic valve that causes a decrease in blood flow to the coronary arteries. A ruptured aneurysm can produce a fatal hemorrhage. While gummas may respond to antibiotic treatment in the late stage of syphilis, damage to the heart valve and arteries may not be reversible.

GENERAL PARESIS: Similarly, permanent tissue damage to the brain and nerves can result from syphilitic invasion of the central nervous system—the chronic, progressive form of syphilis known as *general paresis*. The damage evolves in an insidious manner, and early symptoms may include headaches, a tendency to forget things, or difficulty in concentrating. Mental effects may progress from memory loss to psychotic symptoms of delusions of grandeur.

TABES DORSALIS: Syphilis involving deterioration of the sheaths of spinal nerves (demyelination) and other destructive changes in the spinal cord is known as *tabes dorsalis*. The patient may become incoordinated in movement. Tremors of the hands and fingers may be noticed, as well as tremors of the lips and tongue. Vision may be affected, and sensory effects can range from sharp sudden pains to a loss of feeling. The patient may lose control of bladder function or the ability to walk.

Congenital Syphilis

The latent syphilitic condition is not uncommon, and it is a period of great danger to the fetus if an infected woman, especially a recently infected woman, becomes pregnant at this time. The fetus can acquire syphilis through the placenta and be born with congenital syphilis. Or it can be stillborn or die shortly after birth. Some of the signs of syphilis in an infant born with the congenital form of the disease are similar to those of secondary syphilis. Others are very different, more closely resembling tertiary syphilis. Because of the hazards to the child, most doctors test the mother's blood for the presence of the spirochete during the first three months of pregnancy and again during the last three months; syphilis acquired during pregnancy is especially likely to affect the fetus. Treatment of the mother has the added benefit of treating the fetus. Treatment begun before the eighteenth week of pregnancy prevents syphilis from developing; treatment begun after the eighteenth week cures the fetus of syphilis.

Treatment of Syphilis and Public Health

Therapy for primary or secondary syphilis usually consists of injections of penicillin, or an alternative antibiotic if the patient is allergic to penicillin. The dosage of penicillin may vary according to the stage of the disease. A single injection might be administered for a patient in the primary or secondary stage, while the patient having latent syphilis might require daily doses of antibiotics for one to two weeks.

Patients are usually interviewed regarding their past contacts with other individuals, who may have become infected. If they can be located, they may be advised to receive a penicillin injection or other antibiotic as a protective measure, regardless of whether or not blood tests reveal the presence of the syphilis spirochete. Further blood tests at regular intervals thereafter are also recommended for exposed as well as infected persons to assess their status.

VD CLINICS: Free venereal disease (VD) clinics are available to both men and women in many parts of the United States. Any person who has become infected with syphilis, who thinks he or she may have been exposed to syphilis, or who has signs or symptoms of syphilis can receive a checkup to determine if there is cause for concern. The clinics make blood tests on a small sample of blood taken from a pricked finger. This blood test sometimes is called a Wasserman test, an STS (for serological test for syphilis), or by other names, depending upon the screening technique used. A positive test reaction would be followed by a more detailed series of tests and examinations. A screening test for syphilis is required in most of the United States in order to obtain a marriage license.

Information about the nearest VD clinic can usually be obtained from a county medical society, a local health department, or a local hospital. Many towns have a "hot line" available for persons who want to obtain venereal-disease information by telephone. A toll-free number, 800-523-1885, has been established to permit persons anywhere in the United States to get information about nearby venereal disease clinics.

Gonorrhea

Of the estimated total of nearly three million cases of venereal disease treated each year in the United States, more than half involve

gonorrhea. Gonorrhea is a primary infection of the lining of the urinogenital tract, rectum, and pharynx caused by a spherical pus-producing bacterium called a gonococcus. The common vernacular name for the disease is *clap* or *GC*.

Like syphilis, gonorrhea is not invariably acquired through sexual contact. One example is the spread of the gonococcus germ to the eyes of a baby born to an infected mother. However, the usual route of transmission of gonorrhea is by sexual contact. The several strains of the gonococcus organism differ in virulence. Unlike its response to many other kinds of infectious diseases, the human body apparently does not produce antibodies after exposure to gonorrhea; therefore, a person does not acquire a natural protection from the disease organism after being infected.

Women often carry the disease without symptoms and transmit it to others. In fact, women without symptoms have been described as the major reservoir of gonorrhea. Women quite frequently learn of their infection only because of the development of symptoms in the male partner or because an infected man has reported the identities of women with whom he has had sexual contact.

Symptoms and Complications

In men, the symptoms may begin suddenly with a profuse puslike discharge from the penis, accompanied by a frequent urge to urinate, though urination is painful. The gonococcus germ may spread into the prostate gland, the seminal vesicles, and the epididymis, a portion of the seminal ducts just above the testis. In a woman a gonorrheal infection is much more insidious, often without any symptoms.

However, some women do have symptoms of gonorrhea. They may include irritation or inflammation of the urethra, a vaginal discharge, and possibly serious complications such as pelvic inflammatory disease, with lower abdominal pain, nausea and vomiting, chills, fever, and involvement of the Fallopian tubes. If untreated at an early stage, the gonorrheal infection can result in scarring and sealing of the Fallopian tubes. This complication, called *salpingitis*, can be caused by other infections as well. It was more commonly a result of gonorrhea before the development of effective antibiotic medications; it was also, and still is, a cause of female sterility.

Because of changing sexual attitudes in recent years, gonorrheal infections and complications that were once associated with young heterosexual adults now occur frequently in young teen-agers and male homosexuals. Prepubertal girls —girls who have not begun to menstruate—may acquire gonorrhea through sexual activity but, because of their immature reproductive systems, they seldom develop the complications of salpingitis or pelvic inflammatory disease that affect mature women who are not treated at an early stage.

GONORRHEAL ARTHRITIS: *Gonorrheal arthritis*, once a complication associated mainly with untreated male patients, is now reported to be more common in women than in men. It is also found more frequently now than in past years among male homosexuals. Gonorrheal arthritis may be marked at the onset by fever, pains in one or more joints of the body, and, in many cases, a rash about the hands and feet. The knee joint is most commonly involved, but the pain may be felt in the wrists, ankles, elbows, hips, or shoulders. In more than half the cases, the inflammation also affects the tendons. If untreated, the arthritis of gonorrhea can destroy the joints, resulting in permanent disability.

Diagnosis and Treatment

Most cases of gonorrhea can be treated effectively with penicillin or other antibiotics. A single injection of penicillin is the recommended therapy for most cases, but when complications occur larger doses may have to be given for a period of from one to two weeks. Penicillin is the treatment used to eradicate gonococcal infection of the eyes, a problem that once accounted for more than ten percent of the cases of blindness in children. The spread of gonorrhea to the eyes is possible, although unlikely, in adults. The main symptom is a puslike discharge accompanying inflammation of the cornea.

Since there are no blood tests for gonorrhea infections, diagnosis depends on testing samples of the puslike discharge or other body fluids. For most men, it is a fairly simple procedure to obtain a sample of a suspicious discharge from the penis, place it on a microscope slide, stain it, and examine it for the presence of gonococci. It is more difficult to obtain a reliable sample of an infected secretion from most women. The doctor or clinic technician may take a sample of the secretions in the vagina and culture them in a special way.

Sometimes the diagnosis is made from a culture taken from the rectum, urethra, or pharynx, where the disease organism may be found. Because syphilis and gonorrhea are sometimes acquired at the same time, doctors treating patients for gonorrhea frequently take a blood sample to test for the syphilis spirochete.

Even if the gonococcus is identified, antibiotic treatment is not a surefire guarantee of a cure, because some gonococci may not be reached by the antibiotic medication; also, some strains of the disease have in recent years shown an immunity to the antibiotics used. The recommended personal controls are the use of a condom by the man during intercourse and the use of penicillin medication immediately following any suspected exposure to the disease. Other prophylactic measures that are effective in lessening the risk of one partner's contracting gonorrhea from the other include, for both partners, bathing before intercourse and urinating both before and afterwards. Abstinence in the presence of a penile discharge and during menstruation are also recommended.

Lymphogranuloma Venereum

This disease, also known as *LGV* and *lymphogranuloma inguinale*, is a venereal disease that produces a primary lesion like a small blister, which ruptures to form a small ulcer. It is caused by a virus that is spread by sexual intercourse, although sexual contact is not necessary for transmission of the disease. It can be acquired by contact with the fluid excreted by a lesion.

The primary lesion usually appears in the genital area within one to three weeks after contact with an infected person. It may appear only briefly or be so small as to go unnoticed. But the disease spreads to neighboring lymph nodes, where the next sign of the disorder appears ten days to a month later. The swelling of the lymph nodes (forming *buboes*) is often the first symptom to be noted by the patient; the lymph nodes become matted together and hard, forming channels (or *fistulas*) through which pus drains to the surface of the skin. Enlargement of the lymph nodes may produce painful swelling of the external genitalia. The lymph-node involvement may spread to the anal region, leading to rectal constriction and painful bowel movements.

Since the lesions of lymphogranuloma venereum may resemble those of syphilis, chancroid, or certain nonvenereal diseases, doctors usually make a number of tests to determine whether or not the condition is, in fact, LGV. Therapy includes administration of antibiotics and sulfa drugs for a period of about a week up to a month, depending on the severity of the infection.

Chancroid

Chancroid, or *soft chancre,* is a venereal disease transmitted by a bacterium that causes a tender, painful ulcer. The ulcer, which may erode deeply into the tissues, follows the formation of a primary pustule at the site of infection. The pustule appears within five days after contact with an infected person. While essentially a venereal disease, like other venereal diseases it is transmissible without sexual intercourse. Doctors, for example, have been known to develop a soft chancre on a finger after examining an infected patient. Doctors usually do tests to make sure that the lesion is not a syphilitic chancre. Although the disease can spread from the genital region to other parts of the body, the soft chancre generally is self-limiting. Therapy consists of administration of sulfa drugs or tetracycline.

Granuloma Inguinale

Granuloma inguinale, also called *granuloma venereum,* is not the same, in spite of the similarity in name, as lymphogranuloma venereum. It is an insidious, chronic venereal disease that produces lesions on the skin or mucuous membrane of the genital or anal regions. The first sign of the infection may be a painless papule or nodule that leaves an ulcer with a reddish granular base. If untreated, the lesions tend to spread to the lower abdomen and thighs. In time, the sores produce a sour, pungent odor. Antibiotics such as streptomycin and tetracycline are prescribed. Relapses may occur and cure may be slow, especially in cases of long standing.

EXTERNAL VENEREAL MALADIES

The three conditions described below—two of them related to viruses and the third a parasitic infestation—may generally be considered sources of discomfort and disfigurement rather than threats to general health. All three are transmissible by other means besides sexual contact.

Warts

Venereal warts, known medically as *condyloma acuminatum,* are caused by a virus that proliferates in the warmth and moisture of the anal and genital regions. They occur within the vagina and rectum as well as externally about body openings and on the external genitalia of both men and women. Although generally harmless, venereal warts may be contagious and cause varying amounts of discomfort. Syphilitic lesions or other disorders of the genital region may simulate the warts, so it is important that the necessary tests be made to rule out more serious disorders. Discharges, as from gonorrhea or other infections, tend to aggravate the discomfort of venereal warts and encourage their spread.

In some cases, drugs may be used to remove the warts. They also may be removed by *cryosurgery,* a technique employing liquid nitrogen to freeze and destroy the virus-affected cells forming a wart. However, removing the wart may not completely remove the virus, which can be the "seed" of additional warts at the same site. Many doctors recommend that venereal warts be left alone unless they are a source of discomfort to the patient.

Molluscum Contagiosum

Another viral disease transmitted during sexual intercourse is known

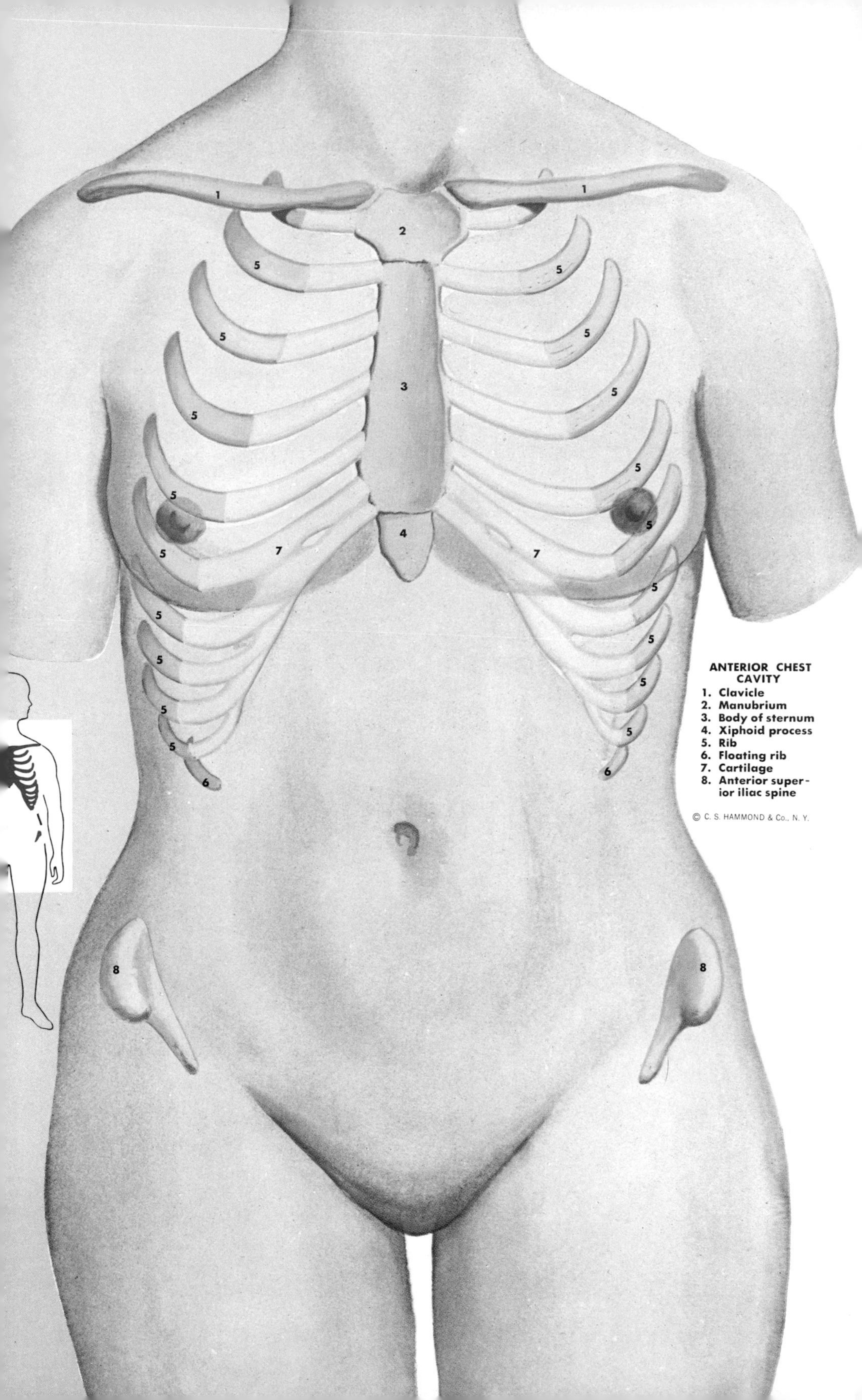

ANTERIOR CHEST CAVITY

1. Clavicle
2. Manubrium
3. Body of sternum
4. Xiphoid process
5. Rib
6. Floating rib
7. Cartilage
8. Anterior super-
   ior iliac spine

© C. S. HAMMOND & Co., N. Y.

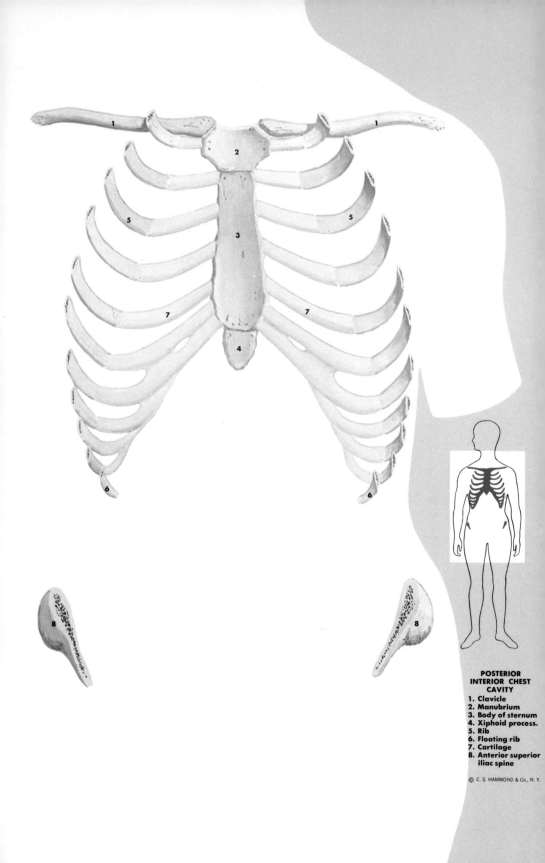

**POSTERIOR
INTERIOR CHEST
CAVITY**
1. Clavicle
2. Manubrium
3. Body of sternum
4. Xiphoid process.
5. Rib
6. Floating rib
7. Cartilage
8. Anterior superior
   iliac spine

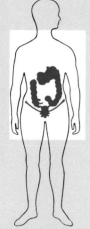

ANTERIOR STOMACH, COLON, AND ORGANS OF REPRODUCTION

23. Esophagus
24. Stomach (cardia)
25. Stomach (fundus)
26. Stomach (body)
27. Stomach (pylorus)
28. Duodenum
31. Ileum
32. Ileocolic junction
33. Caecum
34. Ascending colon
36. Descending colon
37. Sigmoid colon
39. Vermiform appendix
40. Taenia coli
45. Spleen
49. Superior mesenteric artery
50. Superior mesenteric vein
51. Pancreas (head)
52. Pancreas (tail)
80. Bladder
81. Urachus
82. Pubic symphysis
83. Inguinal ligament
100. Uterus
102. Vagina (cross section)
103. Fallopian tube
104. Ostium of fallopian tube
105. Ovary

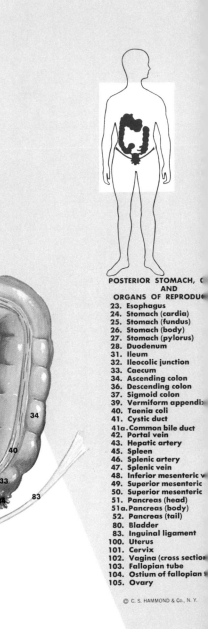

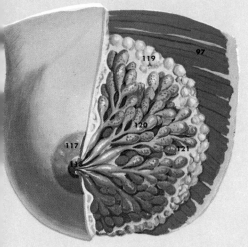

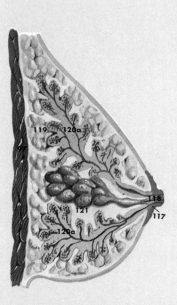

LACTATING BREAST

97. Pectoralis major muscle
117. Areola
118. Nipple
119. Fat
120. Lactiferous (milk producing)
     glands and ducts
120a. Cross section of gland and duct
121. Tissue separating and supporting
     glandular tissue

STRUCTURE OF THE MAMMARY GLANDS

The mammary glands are composed of three major elements:
1. Their skin covering and special structures (nipple, areola).
2. The lactiferous glands or functional units of the breast.
3. The supporting structures, the connective tissue "ligaments" and the fat tissue that makes up the mass of the breast.

The breast is supported by the "suspensory ligaments." These are anchored to the sheet of connective tissue surrounding the pectoralis major muscle, and extend in a complex network separated by the fat tissue outward to the skin. The lactiferous glands are buried in the supporting tissues and empty outward onto the surface of the nipple. These glands at first are very small and clustered just beneath the nipple and areola. In pregnancy they enlarge and push downward into the mass of the breast causing it to enlarge in turn. The enlargement continues through the period of breast feeding, following which the glands gradually grow smaller and the entire breast returns to normal size.

HAMMOND & Co., N. Y.

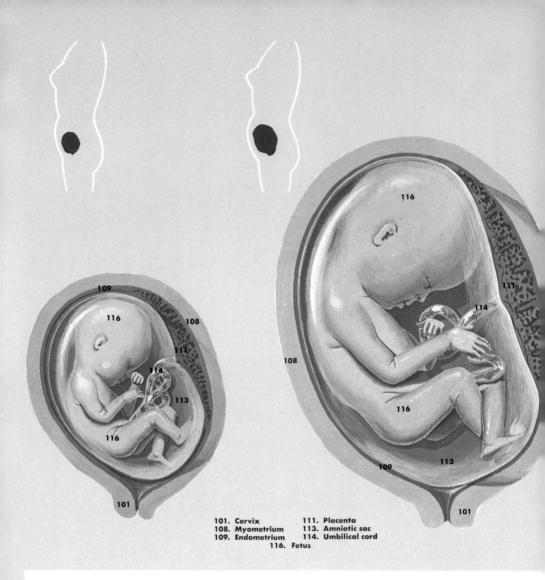

101. Cervix
108. Myometrium
109. Endometrium
111. Placenta
113. Amniotic sac
114. Umbilical cord
116. Fetus

THE FETUS AT 3 1/2 AND 6 MONTHS

Most of the definitive development of the fetus occurs during the first 3½ months, and the remaining 5½ months is primarily concerned with gradual increase in size and maturation of organs already begun. The fetus receives all of its nourishment through the placenta and umbilical cord. There is no direct contact between fetal and maternal blood in the placenta. During its entire development, the fetus floats in a fluid (amniotic fluid) contained within a sac (the amniotic sac) attached to the placenta. This sac is in turn surrounded by the uterine cavity, the endometrium and the muscle or myometrium of the uterus.

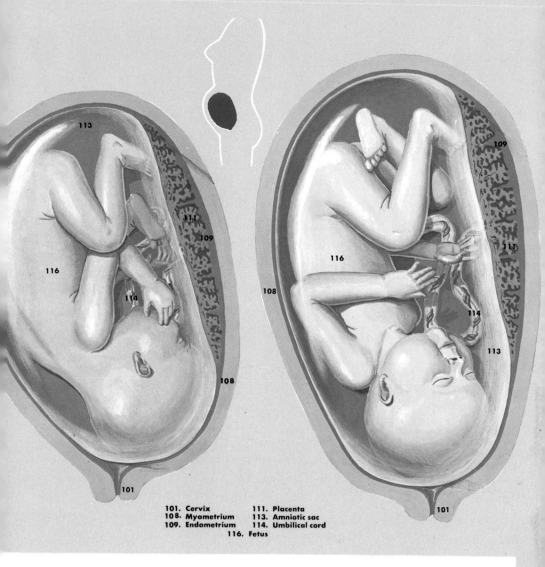

101. Cervix
108. Myometrium
109. Endometrium

111. Placenta
113. Amniotic sac
114. Umbilical cord

116. Fetus

THE FETUS AT 8 AND 9 MONTHS

Until birth, the fetus is surrounded by the amniotic sac and fluid, and at-tached to the placenta by the umbilical cord. The fetus continues to increase in size and the uterus stretches to accommodate it. Usually before the eighth month the fetus assumes a head-downward position. At birth, the amniotic sac ruptures, the fluid escapes, and the child is slowly pushed out of the uterine cavity by the contractions of the myometrium. Shortly after birth of the child, the placenta is similarly expelled having been detached from the endometrium.

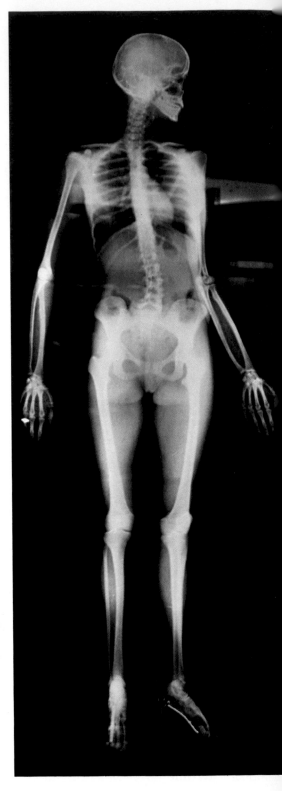

X-RAY OF THE HUMAN BODY
SHOWING THE
BONE STRUCTURE

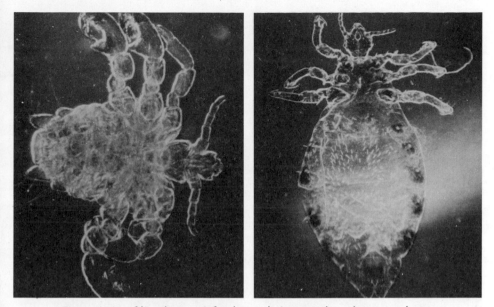

Two varieties of lice that can infest human beings are shown here greatly enlarged. The crab louse *(left)* lives primarily in pubic hair and is transmitted by sexual contact; the head louse *(right)* can live in scalp or pubic hair.

by the medical term *molluscum contagiosum.* The disease can also be transmitted by ordinary person-to-person contact, as between members of a family or children in a classroom. The virus causes raised lesions containing a waxy, white material. The lesions, which may be very small or as large as an inch in diameter, occur on the skin or mucous membranes, commonly in the anal or genital area but sometimes on the face or torso. The lesions may last for several months or several years, then disappear spontaneously, or they may be removed by medications or surgery.

Pubic Lice

Infestations of pubic lice constitute a unique kind of venereal disease. Pubic lice, known popularly as *crabs,* are a species somewhat larger than body and head lice but still almost invisible to the naked eye.

These whitish, oval parasites usually remain in the hair of the anal and genital regions, but they may sometimes be found attached to the skin at the base of any body hair, including the eyelashes and scalp. A very few pubic lice in the anal and genital areas can cause intense irritation and itching. The itching results in scratching which, in turn, produces abrasions of the skin. The lice may also produce patches of bluish spots on the skin of the inner thighs and lower abdomen. Another sign of their presence is the appearance of tiny brown specks deposited by the lice on the inside of undergarments.

Pubic lice are commonly spread by sexual contact, but they can be acquired from toilet seats, clothing, towels, bedclothes, combs, or any article of intimate use. Creams or ointments containing various parasiticides are available for disinfestation. They are applied every night for several nights, but overuse should be avoided because of the danger of injury to the tender tissues of the genital and anal region. Some doctors recommend soaking the infested part of the body several times daily in a mild solution of potassium permanganate. Lice on the eyebrows and eyelashes may have to be removed individually with a pair of tweezers. Clothing and other con-taminated materials must be carefully cleaned to prevent reinfestation.

Complications of an infestation of pubic lice include intense itching (known medically as *pruritus*) and secondary infections from scratching. These may require special medical care and administration of antibiotics, corticosteroid creams, or other appropriate remedies.

DISORDERS OF THE URINARY SYSTEM

Both men and women are subject to disorders of the urinary system, but there are a few disorders that affect women chiefly or women only, for reasons related to anatomical structure. See also *Diseases of the Urinogenital System*, p. 1248.

Inflammation of the Bladder

Any inflammation of the bladder is known medically as *cystitis*. Factors such as urinary tract stones, injury, and obstructions to the normal flow of urine can aggravate or cause cystitis in either sex. Cystitis due to infectious organisms, however, is much more common in women than men. This is understandable in view of the relative shortness of the female urethra—the tube through which urine is discharged from the bladder and through which infectious organisms can reach the bladder from the outside. In addition, the anus and the vagina, both of which may frequently be sources of infection, are situated relatively close to the external opening of the female urethra.

In women generally, the symptoms of cystitis may include a burning sensation around the edges of the vulva. There is usually a frequent urge to urinate and difficulty

THE FEMALE URINARY SYSTEM

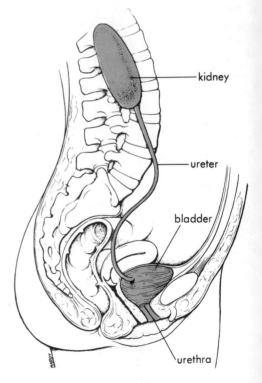

kidney

ureter

bladder

urethra

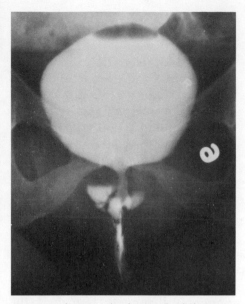

An X-ray photograph of a urethral diverticulum, visible as a spreading light area just below the balloon-shaped bladder.

or pain *(dysuria)* associated with urination. Urinary retention and dehydration, which are generally under the control of the individual, can contribute to the spread of infection once it begins. The lining of the urinary bladder is relatively resistant to infection by most microorganisms as long as the normal flow of liquids through the urinary tract is maintained. In cases that do not yield quickly to copious fluid intake, there are medications that may be prescribed to cure the infection. Where urinary frequency or difficulty is accompanied by the appearance of blood in the urine, a doctor should be consulted immediately.

HONEYMOON CYSTITIS: One type of cystitis tends to occur mostly in young women during the first few weeks of frequent sexual activity, to which it is attributed. This so-called honeymoon cystitis may re-

sult in swelling of the urethra and the neck of the bladder, making urination difficult. The inflammation of these tissues can in turn make them more susceptible to infection. A treatment recommended specifically for honeymoon cystitis is to drink large quantities of water or other fluids and to empty the bladder before and after engaging in sexual intercourse. Adequate lubrication, such as petroleum jelly, is also important. Medical care should be sought if the condition persists.

Urethral Disorders

The urethra is perforce involved in the inflammation of cystitis, since it is the route by which infectious organisms reach the bladder. In addition, there are disorders that are essentially confined to the urethra.

Urethral Caruncle

Urethral caruncle is a rather uncommon urinary-tract disorder that tends to be confined to women after the menopause. A *caruncle* (not to be confused with *carbuncle*) is a small, red, fleshy outgrowth. It may be visible near the opening of the urethra. A caruncle growing from the cells of the urethra may be a sign of a bacterial infection, a tumor, or any of several other possible conditions. Symptoms may include vaginal bleeding, pain, tenderness, painful sexual intercourse (dyspareunia), a whitish, viscid discharge, and difficulty in urinating. A doctor should be consulted when such symptoms are present. A tissue biopsy and Pap smear may be taken to diagnose the condition. Caruncles are easily treated and of no long-term consequence.

Urethral Diverticulum

Another disorder of the urethra is a *urethral diverticulum*, or outpocketing of the urethra. The problem can be due to a developmental malformation, an injury, inflammation, a cyst, a urinary stone, or a venereal disease. Stones are a common cause, and in some patients there may be more than one diverticulum. The symptoms may include discomfort and urinary difficulty as well as dys-pareunia. The disorder can be diagnosed with the help of X-ray photographs of the region of the urethra and bladder after they have been filled with a radiopaque substance that flows into any diverticula that may be present.

Treatment of a urethral diverticulum includes antibiotics to stop infection, medications to relieve pain and discomfort, and douches. In some cases, surgery is needed to eliminate the diverticula.

STRUCTURAL ANOMALIES

Various kinds of injury may be sustained by the female reproductive system and other abdominal organs, chiefly as a result of childbearing. The structural damage can generally be repaired by surgical measures.

Fistula

An abnormal opening between two organs or from an organ to the outside of the body is known as a *fistula.* Fistulas may involve the urinary and reproductive systems of a woman. Damage to the organs during pregnancy or surgery, for example, can result in a fistula between the urethra and the vagina, causing urinary incontinence. A similar kind of fistula can develop between the rectum and the vagina as a result of injury, complications of pregnancy, or surgery. Disorders of this sort must be repaired surgically.

Prolapsed Uterus

The uterus normally rests on the floor of the pelvis, held in position by numerous ligaments. Damage to the ligaments and other supporting tissues permits the uterus to descend, or *prolapse*, into the vagina. There are various degrees of prolapse, ranging from a slight intrusion of the uterus into the vagina to a severe condition in which the cervix of the uterus protrudes out of the vaginal orifice. Prolapse of the uterus resembles a hernia but is not a true hernia because the opening through which the uterus protrudes is a normal one.

Backache and a feeling of heaviness in the pelvic region may accompany the condition. Many women complain of a "dragging" sensation. An assortment of complications may involve neighboring organ systems; bleeding and ulceration of the uterus are not uncommon. Coughing and straining can aggravate the symptoms.

Like the various types of hernia, a prolapsed uterus does not improve without treatment, but tends instead to worsen gradually. The only permanent treatment is surgical repair.

In mild cases, a woman may get relief from symptoms through exercises intended to strengthen the muscles of the pelvic region. Supporting devices, such as an inflatable, doughnut-shaped pessary, are available as temporary methods of correcting a prolapse. Preventive exercises may be recommended for childbearing women who want to avoid weakened muscles and ligaments leading to prolapse.

Tipped Uterus

The uterus may be out of its normal position without being prolapsed. A malpositioned uterus may be "tipped" forward, backward, or otherwise be out of alignment with neighboring organs. A malpositioned uterus may cause no symptoms, or it may be associated with dysmenorrhea or infertility. If a malpositioned uterus causes pain, bleeding, or other problems, the condition can be corrected surgically, or a pessary support may relieve the symptoms. Displacement of the uterus occasionally is the result of a separate pelvic disease that requires treatment.

Hernias of the Vaginal Wall

The wall of the vagina may be ruptured in childbirth, especially in a multiple delivery or birth of a larger-than-average baby. The kind of hernia depends on the exact site of the rupture and what organ happens to lie against the vaginal wall at that point. The condition may be further complicated by a prolapsed uterus. Careful examination of the patient and X-ray pictures may be necessary to determine whether just one or several of the urinary, reproductive, and gastrointestinal organs in the pelvic cavity are involved.

CYSTOCELE: *Cystocele* is a hernia involving the bladder and the vagina. Structurally, part of the bladder protrudes through the wall of the vagina. The symptoms, in addition to a feeling of pressure deep in the vagina, may be urinary difficulties such as incontinence, a frequent urge to urinate, and inability to completely

PROLAPSED UTERUS

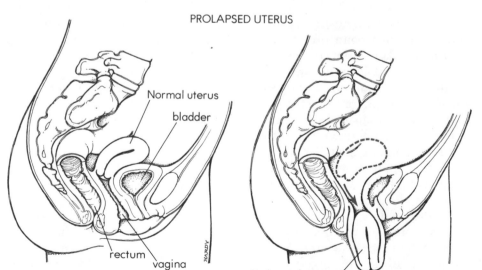

Normal uterus
bladder
rectum
vagina

Prolapsed uterus

HERNIAS OF THE VAGINAL WALL

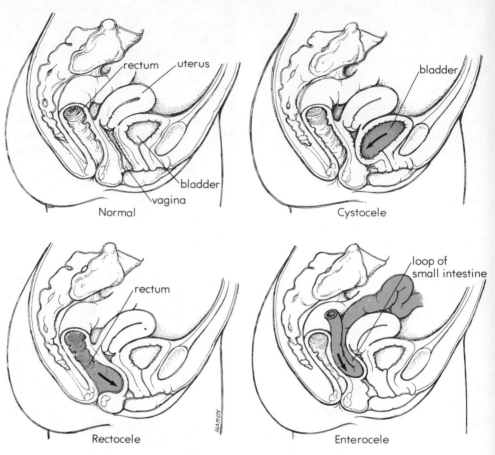

Normal

Cystocele

Rectocele

Enterocele

empty the bladder. Residual urine in the bladder may contribute to infection and inflammation of the bladder. Treatment includes surgery to correct the condition, pessaries if needed to support the structures, and medications to control infection.

RECTOCELE: A hernia involving the tissues separating the vagina and the rectum, behind the vagina, is called a *rectocele*. The symptoms are a feeling of fullness in the vagina and difficulty in defecating. Enemas or laxatives may be needed to relieve constipation because straining, or even coughing, can aggravate the condition. Surgery is the only per-

manently effective treatment. Special diets, laxatives, and rectal suppositories may be prescribed pending surgery.

ENTEROCELE: A herniation of the small intestine into the vagina is called an *enterocele*. Some of the symptoms are similar to those of other hernias involving the vaginal wall, and in addition, a patient with an enterocele may experience abdominal cramps shortly after eating. An enterocele can be dangerous as well as uncomfortable, since a segment of the small bowel can become trapped and obstructed, requiring emergency surgery.

Varicose Veins

Varicose veins of the vulva, vagina, and neighboring areas are another possible effect of pregnancy, although the legs are more often affected. Obesity, reduced physical activity during pregnancy, and circulatory changes associated with pregnancy can contribute to the development of varicose veins. The symptoms generally are limited to discomfort although there can be bleeding, particularly at the time of childbirth. Varicose veins that occur in the vulva and vagina during pregnancy and cause discomfort can be treated surgically during the early months of pregnancy. Some drugs and supportive therapy can be used to help relieve symptoms. But many doctors recommend that surgical stripping of veins be delayed until after the pregnancy has been terminated. A complication of untreated varicose veins can be development of blood clots in the abnormal blood vessels. For a discussion of varicose veins of the legs during pregnancy, see p. 580. See also p. 1124.

BENIGN NEOPLASMS

The word *neoplasm* refers to any abnormal proliferation of tissue that serves no useful function. There are numerous kinds of neoplasms, but just two main groups—cancerous, or *malignant;* or noncancerous, or *benign.* In ordinary speech the word *benign* suggests some positive benefit, but a benign neoplasm, though noncancerous, may in fact be harmful to health or at least worrisome. Benign neoplasms that are of particular concern to women are discussed below.

Cysts

A *cyst* is a sac containing a gaseous, fluid, or semisolid material. (Certain normal anatomical structures, like the urinary bladder, are technically known as cysts—hence the term *cystitis* for inflammation of the bladder.) Abnormal, or neoplastic, cysts can develop at several sites within the urinary and reproductive systems.

Vaginal Cysts

A cyst may develop in a gland at the opening of the vagina as a result of infection with a venereal or other disease. Such a cyst can block the flow of secretions from the gland and produce swelling and pain. Dyspareunia, or painful intercourse, is sometimes a symptom. A vaginal gland cyst usually is treated with antibiotics and hot packs. In some cases, it may be necessary for a doctor to make an incision to drain the cyst.

Ovarian Cysts

Cysts in the ovaries may be caused by a malfunction of physiological process or by a pathological condition. Some pathological cysts are malignant. The cysts in the ovaries generally are filled with fluid that may range in color from pale and clear to reddish brown, depending upon the source of the fluid. Some cysts are too small to be seen with

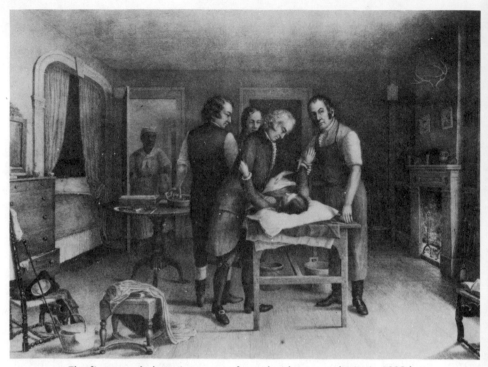

The first recorded ovariotomy, performed without anesthetics in 1809 by the American surgeon Ephraim McDowell. A 20-pound tumor was removed from the patient, who recovered and survived for another 30 years.

the naked eye, whereas others may be four or five inches in diameter when symptoms begin to cause discomfort. There are several different kinds of ovarian cysts.

FOLLICULAR CYST: A *follicular*, or *retention*, cyst, is a physiological cyst and is one of the most common types. It develops in an old follicle in which an ovum for some reason has failed to break out of its capsule during the ovulation process. Ordinarily, the contents of such a follicle are resorbed, but sometimes a cyst develops. It rarely grows larger than about two inches in diameter. It may rupture but usually disappears after a few months. The symptoms may include pain with some uterine bleeding and dyspareunia. Treatment consists of warm douches, analge-

sics, and hormone therapy designed to restore normal ovarian activity. If the symptoms persist or the cyst continues to increase in size, or if serious complications occur, the doctor may recommend exploratory surgery.

Occasionally such cysts, whether or not they rupture, produce symptoms that mimic those of appendicitis, with severe abdominal pain. The abdomen may become so tender that a doctor cannot palpate the organs in order to distinguish between an ovarian cyst and appendicitis, particularly if the right ovary is involved. The symptoms occur at the time that ovulation would be expected. If the doctor cannot be certain that the cause of the abdominal pain is indeed a cyst, for which surgery is not needed, he may recommend surgery anyway—just to be on the safe side.

Multiple follicular cysts, involving the ovaries on both sides (*bilateral polycystic ovaries*) can result in a syndrome (or group of symptoms) that includes infertility, obesity, and abnormal growth of body hair. All of these effects are related to a disruption of normal sex-hormone activity; they generally occur in young women, from teen-agers to those in their 20s. The therapy includes both medical and surgical efforts to restore normal menstrual function, a diet to control obesity, and the use of various depilatory techniques to remove unwanted body hair.

CORPUS LUTEUM CYST:This kind of cyst may develop in the ovary following ovulation or during the early part of a pregnancy. The corpus luteum is a small, temporary gland that forms in the empty follicle after the ovum has been released from the ovary. Its function is to produce the hormone progesterone, which is important in preparing the endometrium, the lining of the uterus, to receive a fertilized ovum. However, the corpus luteum also can be overproductive of a brownish fluid which fills the former follicular space, causing it to swell to a diameter of two or three inches. The cyst causes symptoms of pain and tenderness and may also result in a disruption of normal menstrual cycles in a woman who is not pregnant.

Most corpus luteum cysts gradually decrease in size without special treatment, except to relieve the symptoms. There may, however, be complications such as torsion, or painful twisting of the ovary, or a rupture of the cyst. A ruptured corpus luteum cyst can result in hemorrhage and peritonitis, requiring immediate surgery.

CHOCOLATE CYST: So called because of their brownish-red color, chocolate cysts consist of misplaced endometrial tissue growing on the ovary instead of in its normal position lining the uterus. Chocolate cysts are among the largest of the ovarian cysts, ranging up to five or six inches in diameter. They cause symptoms associated with a variety of disorders of the reproductive system, including infertility, dyspareunia, and dysmenorrhea. Surgery usually is a favored method of therapy, the precise procedure depending upon the amount of ovarian tissue involved. A small chocolate cyst can be cauterized but a large cyst may require removal of a portion of the ovary. See also *Cancer of the Ovary*, p. 1026.

Cysts of the Breast

Cysts may form in the milk glands or the ducts leading from the glands. They are caused by imbalances in ovarian hormones and they tend to develop in mature women approaching the menopause. The cysts tend to fluctuate in size, often enlarging just before or during menstruation, and there may be a discharge from the nipple. Pain and tenderness are usually present, although painless cysts are sometimes discovered only when a woman examines her breasts for possible lumps. Cysts may be almost microscopic in size or as large as an inch or more in diameter. It is not uncommon for more than one cyst to occur at the same time in one breast or both.

A medical examination is recommended when any kind of lump can be felt in the breast tissue. This is particularly important for women who have passed menopause. The doctor frequently can determine whether a lump is a result of a cyst or cancer by the patient's history and by physical examination, especially when repeated at intervals of several weeks. Mammography and biopsy study of a small bit of tissue are used to confirm the diagnosis.

Women who are troubled by breast cysts may be helped by wearing a good brassiere at all times, even during sleep, to protect tender areas. The only medications available are those that relieve pain and discomfort—symptoms that usually subside when the menopause is reached.

OTHER NONCANCEROUS MASSES: A benign lump in the breast can be caused by either a fat deposit or an abscess. A fatty mass frequently forms if an injury to the breast damages adipose tissue. Because of a similarity of the symptoms to those of breast cancer, a biopsy is usually required to distinguish the lesion from a cancer. The involved tissue may in any case be removed surgically.

An abscess of the breast as a result of an infection, although a rare problem, may produce a lump that requires treatment with antibiotic medications or by an incision to drain the pus. Breast infections leading to abscesses are most likely to occur in nursing mothers but can also develop in women who are not lactating. When an infection develops in a breast being used to nurse a baby, nursing has to be discontinued temporarily while the infection is treated. See also *Cancer of the Breast*, p. 1027.

Polyps

A *polyp* is a strange-looking growth, even for an abnormal growth of tissue. It has been described as having the appearance of a tennis racket or a small mushroom. Polyps are found in many parts of the body, from the nose to the rectum. Usually they are harmless. But a polyp can result in discomfort or bleeding and require surgical excision. A polyp on the breast, for example, can become irritated by rubbing against the fabric of a brassiere. Although polyps generally are not cancerous, it is standard procedure to have the polyp tissue, like any excised tissue, tested in the laboratory. If malignant cells accompany a polyp, they are usually found at the base of the growth, which means that some of the tissue around the polyp must be excised along with the growth itself. Once a polyp is removed it does not grow again, although other polyps can occur in the same region.

CERVICAL POLYP: Polyps in the cervix are not uncommon, occurring most frequently in the years between menarche and menopause. A cervical polyp may be associated with vaginal bleeding or leukorrhea; the bleeding may occur after douching or sexual intercourse. In some cases, the bleeding is severe. Cervical polyps can usually be located visually by an examining physician and removed by minor surgery.

ENDOMETRIAL POLYP: Endometrial polyps, which develop in the lining of the uterus, usually occur in women who are over 40, although they can develop at any age after menarche. They are frequently the cause of nonmenstrual bleeding. They tend to be much larger than polyps that grow in other organs of the body: an endometrial polyp may be rooted high in the uterus with a stem reaching all the way to the cervix. Such a polyp is usually located and removed during a D and C procedure. As in the case of a cervical polyp, the growth and a bit of surrounding tissue are studied for traces of cancer cells.

Benign Tumors

Tumors are rather firm growths that may be either benign or malignant. In practice, any tumor is regarded with suspicion unless malignancy is ruled out by actual laboratory tests. Even a benign tumor represents a tissue abnormality, and if untreated can produce symptoms that interfere with normal health and activity.

Fibromas

Among the more common of the benign tumors is the *fibroma,* commonly known as a *fibroid tumor,* composed of fibrous connective tissue. About one of every 20 ovarian tumors is a fibroma, and a similar growth in the uterus is the most common type of tumor found in that organ. Fibromas also occur in the vulva.

OVARIAN FIBROMA: Ovarian fibromas are usually small, but there are instances in which they have grown to weigh as much as five pounds. A large fibroma can be very painful and produce symptoms such as a feeling of heaviness in the pelvic area, nausea, and vomiting. The growth may crowd other organs of the body, causing enlargement of the abdomen and cardiac and respiratory symptoms. The only treatment is surgical removal of the tumor, after which there is usually a quick and full recovery.

UTERINE FIBROMA: Fibroid tumors of the uterus can also grow to a very large size, some weighing many pounds. Like ovarian fibromas, they can press against neighboring organs such as the intestine or the urinary bladder, producing constipation or urinary difficulty. More commonly, there is pain and vaginal bleeding, along with pelvic pressure and enlargement of the abdomen. It is possible in some cases for a fibroid tumor to grow slowly in the uterus for several years without causing serious discomfort to the patient. If the tumor obstructs or distorts the reproductive tract, it may be a cause of infertility.

Treatment of fibroid tumors varies according to their size, the age of the patient and her expectations about having children, and other factors. If the tumor is small and does not appear to be growing at a rapid rate, the doctor may recommend that surgery be postponed as long as the tumor poses no threat to health. For an older woman, or for a woman who does not want to bear children, a hysterectomy may be advised, especially if symptoms are troublesome. If the patient is a young woman who wants to have children, the doctor is likely to advise a *myomectomy,* a surgical excision of the tumor, since a fibroid tumor of the uterus can cause serious complications during pregnancy and labor. It can result in abortion or premature labor, malpresentation of the fetus, difficult labor, and severe loss of blood during childbirth. While fibroid tumors of the uterus are not malignant, special tests are made of the endometrial tissue as part of any myomectomy or hysterectomy to rule out the possibility that cancer cells may be involved in the disorder.

Endometriosis

Endometriosis is the medical term for a condition in which endometrial tissue, the special kind of tissue that lines the uterus, grows in various areas of the pelvic cavity outside the uterus. Endometrial cells may invade such unlikely places as the ovaries (the most common site), the bladder, appendix, Fallopian tubes, intestinal tract, or the supporting structure of the uterus. The external endometrial tissue may appear as small blisters of endometrial cells, as solid nodules, or as cysts, usually of the ovary, which may be four inches or more in diameter, like the chocolate cysts of the ovaries. Such a mass of sometimes tumorlike endometrial cells is called an *endometrioma*.

The misplaced endometrial tissue causes problems because it goes through menstrual cycles just as the endometrium does within the cavity of the uterus. The endometrial tissue proliferates after ovulation and may cause almost constant pain, wherever it is located, for a few days before the start of menstruation. The symptoms subside after the menstrual flow begins. The effects may include dyspareunia, rectal bleeding, backache, and generalized pain in the pelvic region as sensitive tissues throughout the pelvic cavity are irritated by monthly cycles of swelling and bleeding.

Since infertility is associated with endometriosis, which can become progressively worse, young women who want to bear children are sometimes encouraged to begin efforts to become pregnant as early as possible if they show signs or symptoms of the disorder. Treatment includes hormone medication and surgery to remove the lesions of endometriosis or the organ involved. For patients with extensive spread of endometrial tissue outside the uterus, the doctor may recommend removal of one or both ovaries. Destruction of the ovaries surgically or by radiation therapy may be employed to eliminate the menstrual cycle activity that aggravates the symptoms of endometriosis. These procedures cause sterility and premature menopause, but some women prefer this to the discomfort of endometriosis. The hormone therapy inhibits the ovulation phase of the menstrual cycle. Without ovulation, the endometrial tissue does not proliferate. For this reason, pregnancy often eliminates or eases the symptoms of endometriosis during parturition and for a period of time thereafter.

Dyspareunia

Dyspareunia, or painful intercourse, is often associated with endometriosis and is attributed to irritation of nerve fibers in the area of the cervix from the pressure of sexual activity. There are many other possible causes of painful intercourse, some functional and some organic in nature. In addition to endometriosis, the problem may be due to a vaginal contracture, a disorder involving the muscles of the pelvic region, inflammation of the vagina or urethra, prolapsed or malpositioned uterus, *cervicitis* (inflammation of the cervix), or a disorder of the bladder or rectum. A cause of dyspareunia in older women may be a degeneration of the tissues lining the vagina, which become thin and dry. Temporary therapy for dyspareunia may include water-soluble lubricants, anesthetic ointments, steroid hormones, analgesics, and sedatives. In appropriate cases, surgery is effective in correcting an organic cause of painful sexual intercourse. Functional or psychogenic (of psychological origin) causes of dyspareunia usually require psychological counseling for the patient and her sexual partner.

Backache

Still another effect of endometriosis that can mimic symptoms of other disorders is backache. When endometrial tissue invades the pelvic region, there may be a fairly constant pain in the back near the tailbone or the rectum. Usually the backache subsides only after the cause has been eliminated. Temporary measures include those advised for other kinds of backache: sleeping on a firm mattress, preferably reinforced with a sheet of plywood between springs and mattress; application of dry heat or warm baths; sedatives to relieve tension, and analgesics to relieve the pain.

A backache that radiates down the back and into a leg, following the path of a sciatic nerve, can be due to a disorder of the ovaries or uterus. An ovarian cyst or infection of the Fallopian tubes can produce a backache that seems to be centered in the lumbosacral area of the spinal column. Such backaches, sometimes called gynecologic backaches, tend to occur most frequently during a woman's childbearing years and affect women who have had several children more often than women who have not been pregnant. Tumors also can produce backache symptoms. X-ray pictures, myelograms, and laboratory studies may be required in order to rule out the possibilities that the back pain may be caused by a tumor, a herniated or "slipped" disk, or a deformity of the spinal column that might have been aggravated by one or more pregnancies. Most backaches, however, relate to poor posture or muscle tension. Anxiety or other kinds of emotional stress can aggravate the symptoms. See also *Backaches,* p. 835, and *Back Pain and Its Causes,* p. 1068.

CANCERS OF THE REPRODUCTIVE SYSTEM

Cancer of the Cervix

The cervix of the uterus is the second most common site of cancers affecting the reproductive system of women. As compared with all cancers affecting women, it rates third, after breast cancer and colon and rectum cancer. It has been estimated that about 20,000 cases of cervical cancer are found among American women each year, and approximately 7,500 deaths every year are due to this disease.

Though it is not considered a venereal disease, cancer of the cervix seems to be closely related to past sexual activity. Statistically, women who began sexual intercourse at an early age or who have had many

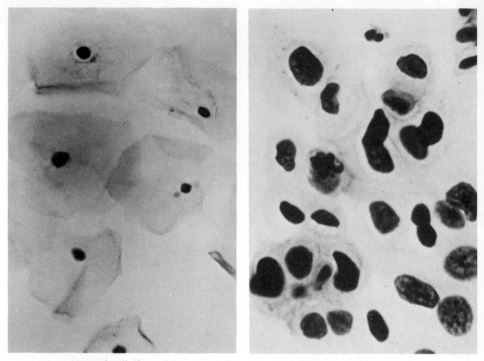

Normal cells from the cervix *(left)* contrasted with cancer cells *(right)*.

partners are much more likely to have cervical cancer than women who have never engaged in sexual activity or who have had one or very few sexual partners. There is also statistical evidence that intercourse with uncircumcised men increases the probability of cervical cancer and that the incidence of cancer of the penis is increased in men whose sexual partners have developed cancer of the cervix, and vice versa. Studies also indicate that cancer of the cervix is less likely to occur when the male partner habitually wears a condom. However interesting these statistical associations may be, the actual causes of cervical cancer are still unknown. Current medical thinking suggests that there is no causal relationship between cervical cancer and the use of oral contraceptives.

PREINVASIVE STAGE: The earliest signs of cervical cancer tend to appear between the ages of 25 and 45. At this early, *preinvasive* stage, the cancer is described as *in situ*—confined to its original site. If the cancer is not treated at this stage, the disease spreads and becomes a typical invasive cancer within five to ten years. Signs of bleeding and ulceration usually do not appear until this has occurred. However, because of the relatively slow growth of cervical cancer in the early stage, the disease usually can be detected by a Pap smear test before it becomes invasive.

Diagnostic Methods

PAP SMEAR TEST: The *Pap smear* test (named for Dr. George Papanicolaou, who developed the technique in 1928) is a quick and simple

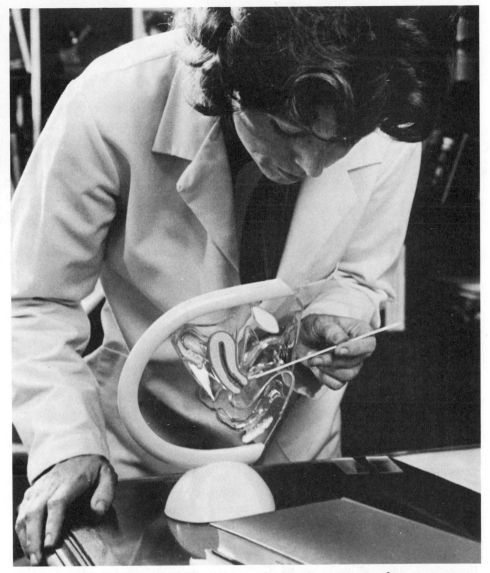

A demonstration of the technique of taking Pap test smears from
the cervix, using a plastic model of the female reproductive system.

method of detecting cancerous cells in secretions and scrapings from mucous membrane. It requires the collection of small samples of cells from the surface of the cervix and from the cervical canal. Such samples are obtained by inserting a plastic spatula or a cut wooden tongue depressor into the vagina, in- to which a speculum has been placed previously. The device is scraped gently over the areas of the cervix in which a cancer is most like-ly to develop, or from any other sur-face of the cervix that appears abnor-mal during visual inspection. The doctor may collect also a sample of vaginal secretions, which may con-

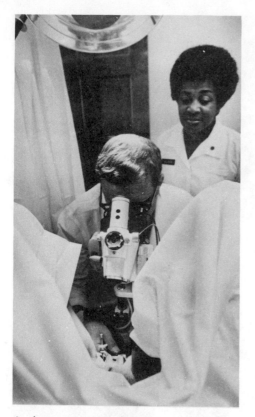

A doctor uses a colposcope, a magnifying instrument, to make a biopsy test for possible cervical cancer. The test is said to be virtually painless and does not require hospitalization.

mal), suspicious, or positive. If the findings are negative, the woman will be advised to return in one year for another Pap smear test. If the findings are suspicious, the woman usually will be asked to return for a second test either immediately or within six months. A report of suspicious findings generally indicates the presence of unusual or abnormal cells, which may be due to an infection or inflammation as well as to a cancerous condition. If a specific disease organism is found in a sample—such as a trichomonas organism, for example—the laboratory report includes that information.

OTHER DIAGNOSTIC TESTS: A positive Pap smear is one containing cells that are probably or definitely cancerous. When a report of positive findings is returned by the laboratory, the doctor immediately arranges for further studies. These involve examination of the cervix visually by a special microscopic technique known as *colposcopy* and the removal of small tissue samples. These studies are usually done in the doctor's office. In some cases a biopsy is necessary. This requires that the woman enter a hospital where she can receive an anesthetic. The biopsy sample is taken when possible from the same location on the cervix as the Pap smear that resulted in positive findings. Other tests, including X-ray films of the chest and bones, can be made during the hospital stay to determine whether the cancer, if verified by biopsy, has extended to nearby areas or spread to other areas of the body by metastasis. Treatment ordinarily is not started until all of the studies have verified that there is cancer in the tissues of the cervix; other disorders such as

tain possibly cancerous cells not only from the cervix but from the ovaries and uterus as well. (This is the only way a Pap smear test can be done if a woman has had a complete hysterectomy and has no cervix.) All cell samples are placed (smeared) on microscope slides and treated with a chemical preservative. The slides are sent to a laboratory for study and a report is made to the examining physician, usually within a few days, on the findings.

The laboratory report may classify the cell samples as negative (nor-

cervicitis, venereal infection, and polyps can mimic symptoms of cervical cancer.

Therapy

The kind of treatment recommended for a case of cervical cancer generally depends upon several factors, such as the stage of cancer development and the age and general health of the patient. For a young woman who wishes to have children despite cancer in situ, which is limited to the cervix, surgeons may excise a portion of the cervix and continue watching for further developments with frequent Pap smears and other tests. The treatment of choice for cervical cancer in the early stage, however, is surgical removal of the body of the uterus as well as the cervix—a procedure called a *total hysterectomy*. This is the usual treatment for women over the age of 40 or for those who do not wish to have children. Sometimes more extensive surgery is necessary.

Radiation treatment may be advised for women who are not considered to be good surgical risks because of other health problems. Radiation may be recommended along with surgery for women with advanced cervical cancer in order to help destroy cancer cells that may have spread by metastasis to other tissues.

The five-year cure rate for cervical cancer is about 99 percent when treatment is started in the early preinvasive stage. The chances of a cure drop sharply in later stages, but the five-year cure rate is still as high as 65 percent if treatment is started when the cancer has just begun to spread to the vagina or other nearby tissues.

Cancer of the Body of the Uterus

Cancer of the body of the uterus, or *endometrial cancer,* is less common than cancer of the cervix. Cervical cancer primarily affects women before middle age; endometrial cancer occurs more frequently among women beyond the menopause, with its highest rate occurring among women between the ages of 60 and 70. A statistical association has been found between the increased use of estrogen hormones and the increasing rate of cancer of the uterus among middle-aged women since the 1960s. It has been suggested that the uterine lining (endometrium) in some women is particularly sensitive to the effects of estrogens.

Diagnostic Methods

Early symptoms usually include bleeding between menstrual periods or after menopause, and occasionally, a watery or blood-stained vaginal discharge. Most patients experience no pain in the early stages although pain is a symptom in advanced uterine cancer or when the disease is complicated by an infection. Unfortunately, there is no simple test, like the Pap smear for cervical cancer, that provides a good diagnostic clue to the presence of endometrial cancer. The Pap smear does occasionally pick up cells sloughed off by the endometrium, and laboratory tests can tell if they might be malignant. But a doctor who is suspicious of symptoms of endometrial cancer must depend upon more direct methods to confirm or rule out the disease. The usual method is a D and C, during which a small sample of uterine lining will

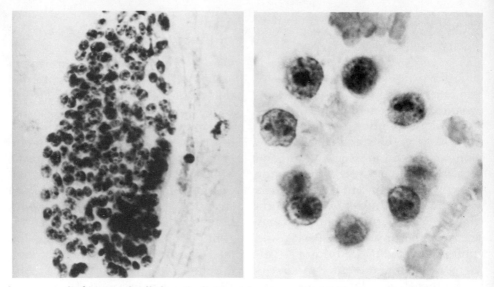

(Left) Normal cells from the lining of the uterus. *(Right)* Uterine cells taken in an aspiration smear, showing a rosettelike pattern indicating cancer.

be removed for biopsy, or a sample may be withdrawn by suction (aspirated) from the uterine cavity. Aspiration can be done in the doctor's office with local anesthesia of the cervix or with no anesthesia. There is little or no discomfort following aspiration.

Therapy

If the diagnostic D and C is done when the abnormal bleeding associated with uterine cancer first begins, the chances of a cure are very good. The first step, if the general health of the patient permits surgery, is complete removal of the uterus, ovaries, and Fallopian tubes—a procedure called a *radical hysterectomy*. Radiation may also be administered to control the spread of cancer cells in the pelvic region.

Since 90 percent of the women affected by endometrial cancer are past childbearing age, removal of the reproductive organs is usually less traumatic for them than it would be if they were young women with hopes of raising families. For premenopausal women, the natural ovarian hormones that are lost with the ovaries may be artificially replaced by prescription in order to ease the sudden transition to a menopausal condition.

A hysterectomy should not affect a woman's normal sexual activity. Sexual relations usually can be resumed about six to eight weeks after the operation, or when the incision has healed. If the incision is made through the pubic region or vagina, there should be little or no visible scar.

A number of possible causes of uterine cancer have been suggested. High blood pressure, diabetes, and obesity are believed to increase the risk of developing endometrial cancer. There is some evidence that the disease tends to occur in families, particularly among women who experience a greater-than-average degree of menstrual difficulty.

Estrogen and Cancer

There is a higher incidence of cancer of the uterus among women who have tumors of the ovary that produce estrogen as well as among women whose menopause begins later than the usual age (and hence who have produced estrogen naturally for a longer-than-usual period). Because of the statistical associations between uterine cancer and estrogen-producing tumors, as well as other factors, the American Cancer Society has cautioned that doctors should exert "close supervision of women on estrogen, with an awareness that sustained use [of estrogens] may stimulate dormant factors in the body and lead to development of endometrial cancer."

Among the conditions for which estrogen has been prescribed for women of middle age and beyond are uncomfortable effects of menopause, such as itching and irritation caused by dryness of the vagina. However, there are available hormone creams that help relieve dryness of the vaginal tissues; the creams may contain estrogen, but not enough to cause concern about their possible carcinogenic properties.

Diethylstilbestrol

An estrogenlike synthetic compound has definitely been implicated in the development of a type of cancer (*adenocarcinoma*) which primarily affects epithelial tissue. The synthetic hormone known chemically as diethylstilbestrol (DES) or stilbestrol was taken for the most part in the late 1940s and through the 1950s by pregnant women, primarily for the treatment of such complications as bleeding and threatened miscar-

riage. Around 1971, doctors became aware that some of the daughters whose mothers had taken DES during their pregnancy had developed an unusual cell formation in vaginal tissue, vaginal and cervical cancers, and some anatomical abnormalities. Cancers have been discovered in daughters as young as seven years of age. An unknown but substantial number of women in the United States alone received DES while pregnant, but only about 200 of their daughters have been found to be afflicted with cervical or vaginal cancers. The National Cancer Institute has urged that all mothers and daughters who may have been exposed to DES during the mother's pregnancy arrange to be examined by a physician for possible effects of the drug.

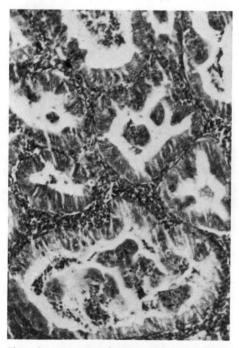

This photomicrograph shows invasive adeno-carcinoma of the endometrium, or lining of the uterus.

The use of DES for pregnant women has been discontinued, although the compound is still available for treating certain cases of breast cancer and menopausal symptoms in nonpregnant women.

Cancer of the Ovary

Cancer of the ovary is not as common as cervical and endometrial cancers, but ovarian cancer does account for nearly one out of every six malignant tumors of the female reproductive system. The disease is responsible for a greater number of deaths because an ovarian cancer can remain symptomless until it has spread. There are several different kinds of malignant tumors of the ovary; some originate in the ovaries and others are caused by cells that have metastasized from a cancer at some other site, such as the uterus.

There are no age limits for cancer of the ovary, although most cases are detected in women between 50 and 70. A physician at a routine pelvic examination may notice a lump or other abnormal growth in the abdominal region. The symptoms reported by patients usually include abdominal discomfort or digestive problems, possibly because ovarian cancers often grow large enough to press on neighboring organs and cause urinary difficulties, constipation, or other digestive disorders. A

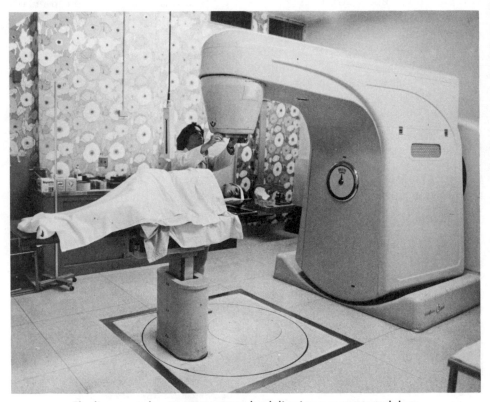

The linear accelerator treats cancer by delivering a concentrated dose of radiation to the tumor, with minimal effect on surrounding tissues.

clue is given in some cases by endometrial bleeding as a result of abnormal hormone production by the affected ovary. However, the more common kinds of ovarian cancers do not produce hormones. Occasionally, cancer cells from an ovarian tumor will be found in a Pap smear sample. But there are no direct, simple tests for cancer of the ovary.

Treatment for ovarian cancer varies with the individual case. As with cancer at other sites, surgery is generally necessary. The extent of the surgery depends upon the type of lesion and other factors. In an advanced case of an older woman, total hysterectomy along with removal of the ovaries and Fallopian tubes would be. the treatment of choice. But if the patient is a young woman and the cancer is not extensive, the surgeon may excise the affected ovary and leave the remainder of the reproductive system intact. Radiation and chemotherapy are commonly applied in addition to surgery. The cure rate for ovarian cancers depends upon the type of tumor and the stage at which treatment started; the five-year survival chances range upward to about 65 percent.

CANCER OF THE BREAST

Cancer of the breast is one of the oldest and best-known types of cancer. It is described in an ancient Egyptian papyrus of 5,000 years ago. The hormonal factors involved in the physiology of breast cancer have been studied by doctors for more than 100 years. But it remains the most common of cancers affecting woman. It kills more women than any other kind of cancer, and more people of both sexes (a minuscule number are men) than only two other cancers—lung cancer and cancer of the colon and rectum. About 90,000 women in the United States develop breast cancer each year, and more than a third die of the disease. Nearly everyone knows a friend or relative who has been stricken by breast cancer. Yet the cause of breast cancer is still unknown.

Breast cancer is less common in the Orient than in America and Western Europe, but Asian women who move to America seem to increase their risk of developing breast cancer—indicating that there may be a dietary factor or some other environmental influence. Women whose female relatives have had breast cancer are more likely to be victims than women from families in which breast cancer is not present. The disease appears to be linked statistically also to women who do not have children before their 30s or who do not have any children; to mothers who do not nurse their babies; to women who reach the menopause later than normal; and to women who began menstruation earlier in life than normal. There is increasing evidence also that ovarian activity may play an important role in the development of breast cancer. Women with ovarian tumors and women who use supplementary estrogen have been shown by some studies to be at increased risk, while the process of having many children and nursing them, which suppresses estrogen hormone activity, is associated with a decreased risk of developing breast cancer.

Cancer of the breast may occur as early as the teens, but this is rare. It is generally not found before the age of 30, and the incidence peaks around the time of menopause. Then there is a second period after the age of about 65 when the incidence of breast cancer rises again.

Breast cancer usually begins in the ducts of the milk glands; the first noticeable sign is a lump in the breast. The lump may appear anywhere in the breast, but the most common site is the upper, outer quadrant. Such lumps are not necessarily or even usually cancerous, but a biopsy (described below) must be performed to check the tissue involved.

In a typical case of breast cancer, a small tumor half an inch in diameter, large enough to be detected during careful self-examination, can grow to a cancer two inches in diameter in six months to a year. The lump generally causes no pain; pain is rarely associated with early breast cancer. If the tumor is allowed to grow unchecked, it may cause pulling of the skin from within. This effect may appear as a flattening of the breast or a dimpling of the skin, or a sinking, tilting, or flattening of the nipple. Less frequently, the tumor begins in a duct near the nipple, causing irritation of the skin of the nipple and a moist discharge. In such cases a scab eventually forms at that site. In time, cancer cells spread to the nearby lymph nodes and the danger becomes very serious of metastasis to any part of the body.

Detection of Breast Cancer

Fortunately, breast cancer can be treated effectively if it is detected early enough. Some 95 percent of breast cancers are discovered by the patient herself when she notices a lump. In all too many cases the discovery is made by chance and the lump may be quite large. The cure rate for breast cancer could be greatly improved if all women made a routine of monthly self-examination and then consulted a physician immediately if they found the least indication of a thickening or lump. Most such lumps are benign, but it is most important that the ones that are malignant be identified without delay.

The American Cancer Society and the National Cancer Institute recommend that every woman follow a prescribed method of self-examination just after the menstrual period, continuing every month after the menopause. The procedure consists of carefully looking at and feeling the breasts, and takes only a few minutes. A detailed description of the proper procedure is available in pamphlet form from the Superintendent of Documents, U.S. Government Printing Office, Washington, D.C. 20402 for 40 cents. Ask for Public Health Service Publication No. 1730. A film entitled "Breast Self-Examination," produced by the American Cancer Society and the National Cancer Institute, is also available.

If a tumor can be detected as even a small lump it must have been developing for some time. There is a truism about breast cancer to the effect that a cancer that is undetectable is curable—leaving unspoken the

SELF-EXAMINATION OF THE BREASTS

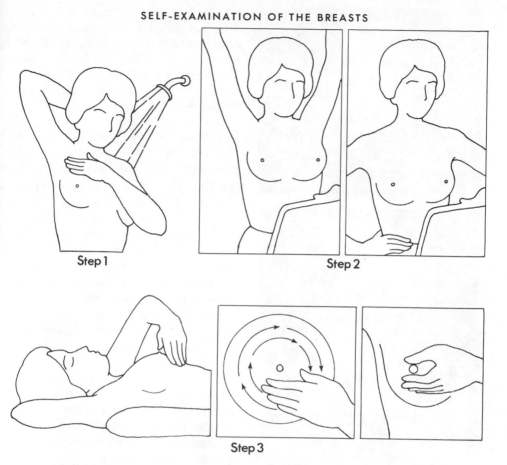

Step 1

Step 2

Step 3

Self-examination of the breasts as recommended by the American Cancer Society. *(Step 1)* Examine breasts during a shower or bath; hands glide easier over wet skin. With fingers flat, move the left hand gently over every part of the right breast, then the right hand over the left breast. Check for any lump, hard knot, or thickening. *(Step 2)* Before a mirror, inspect the breasts with arms at the sides, then with arms raised. Look for any changes in the contour of each breast, a swelling, dimple of skin, or changes in the nipple. Then rest palms on hips and press down firmly to flex the chest muscles. Left and right breasts will not match exactly—few women's breasts do. But regular inspection will show what is normal for you. *(Step 3)* While lying down with a pillow or folded towel under the right shoulder and with the right hand behind the head, examine the right breast with the left hand. With fingers flat, press gently in small circular motions around an imaginary clock face. Begin at 12 o'clock, then move to 1 o'clock, and so on around back to 12. A ridge of firm tissue in the lower curve of each breast is normal. Next, move in an inch toward the nipple and keep circling to examine every part of the breast, including the nipple. This requires at least three more circles. Then repeat the procedure slowly on the left breast with the pillow under the left shoulder and left hand behind the head. Notice how the breast structure feels. Finally, squeeze the nipple of each breast gently between thumb and index finger. Any discharge, clear or bloody, should be reported to a doctor immediately.

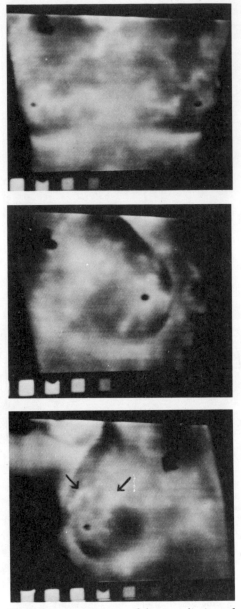

Thermograms, pictures of heat radiation of body tissues, can sometimes reveal the presence of a breast tumor that could not be discovered by touch. The tissue of tumors has a distinctively higher temperature than normal tissue. *(Top)* A typical thermogram, with lightest shades reflecting warmest areas. The other thermograms show an abnormal pattern of temperature elevation in both breasts. Arrows point to a hot quadrant and a dilated vein produced by the lesion.

implication that a cancer that is detectable may not be curable. In recent years, methods of early detection have been refined to the point that tumors once undetectable can now be detected before any lump becomes palpable.

THERMOGRAPHY: One early warning detection technique involves the use of *thermography*, which is based on the fact that tumor cells produce slightly more heat than normal tissue. Hence a device that is sufficiently heat-sensitive can detect and pinpoint the location of an incipient tumor. A harmless tumor, too, would have a higher-than-normal temperature. Further tests would be needed to determine the true cause of the "hot" tissue reading.

MAMMOGRAPHY: *Mammography* is an X-ray technique developed specifically for examination of breast tissue. A tumor shows up on a mammogram as an opaque spot because of mineral concentrations associated with the growth. However, like thermography, mammography cannot determine whether a tumor is benign or malignant or if the opaque spot on the film is due to some other mineral-rich tissue rather than a tumor. The examining physician uses mammography only as one among other diagnostic tools.

Mammography has been widely used by cancer detection centers throughout America in past years. Since 1976, the National Cancer Institute and the American Cancer Society have cautioned doctors and patients about the routine use of mammography, particularly for women under 50 years of age and if older types of X-ray equipment are used. Studies have shown that exposure of the breasts to X rays, especially at

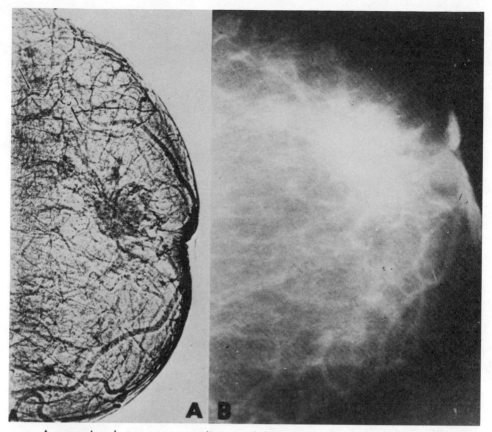

A comparison between a xeroradiogram *(left)* and a mammogram *(right)* of the same breast. The specklike area of cancer shows more clearly in the xeroradiogram.

the dosages produced by the older equipment, and perhaps even by the newer low-intensity equipment, increases the chances of breast cancer by about one percentage point. This means that a woman at low risk who has, say, a six percent chance of developing breast cancer would increase her risk to seven—by a factor of almost 17 percent—by exposure to X-ray mammography. A woman originally at higher risk would suffer a smaller-percentage increment. Hence cancer experts continue to approve the use of X-ray mammography only for high-risk groups—women who have a history of breast cancer or who have had lumps in

their breasts, women above the age of 50, and younger women in the high-risk categories outlined above.

XERORADIOGRAPHY: *Xeroradiography* is a method that, like mammography, uses X rays, but it entails only about half the exposure to radiation. The pictures are developed by xerography, the process made familiar by Xerox copying machines. The picture consists of dots in varying shades of blue. The process produces a sharp picture, making interpretation simpler and more accurate than is possible with X-ray photographs. When performed by experienced medical technicians, xeroradiography can detect from 85 to 95 percent of all breast cancers, including those too small to be located by palpation. The xeroradiography examination and the doctor's examination of the breast usually take only about 20 minutes.

BIOPSY: When a doctor believes there is good evidence of a cancer in a breast as a result of thermography, xeroradiography, mammogra-phy, palpation of lumps, and other factors, the next step is a biopsy study. The suspected lesion is located for the biopsy procedure and the exact position and extent of the planned incision is marked on the skin. The patient is then wheeled into the operating room and the tissue sample is excised while the patient is anesthetized. An entire nodule of

A complete checkup for possible breast cancer involves thermography (recording the heat generated by the breast) and mammography (X rays).

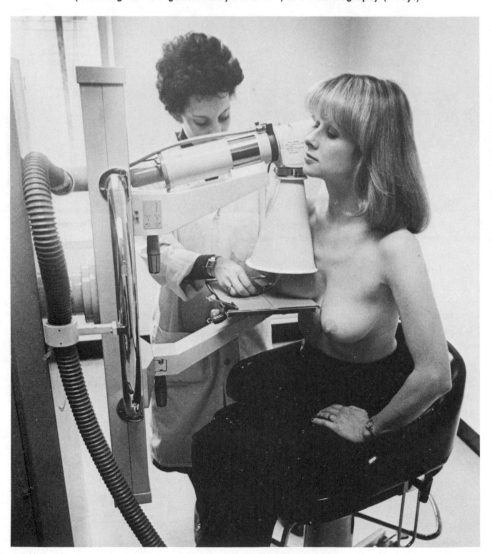

breast tissue is removed for microscopic examination of the tissue cells. It is sent to the pathology department, which usually reports within 90 minutes whether the tissue is noncancerous or malignant. Provisional preparations are made for a mastectomy. If the lesion is not cancerous—and between 60 and 80 percent of biopsies of breast lumps are not—the patient is taken back to the recovery room and reassured that the tumor was benign. The incision made for the biopsy leaves an almost indiscernible scar.

THE TWO-STEP PROCEDURE: Because of the psychological and physical problems associated with breast cancer, approaches to surgery have changed drastically in recent years. The patient today has a choice: if she desires, she can request that the test and operation take place in two separate stages. To make that choice, the woman simply does not sign a form granting permission to perform both the biopsy and the *mastectomy*, or breast removal, on the same day.

In many cases, it may be necessary to perform both operations on the same day. In such cases, experts say, the woman should insist that her surgeon refer her for pre-surgical *staging*.

Staging involves administration of various tests that are carried out before a mastectomy. The tests show whether the cancer has already spread, or metastasized, to other parts of the body outside the breast and local lymph node regions. Staging is widely regarded as a necessary procedure in all cases of breast cancer. A mastectomy has the single purpose of preventing the spread of cancer; the patient has to

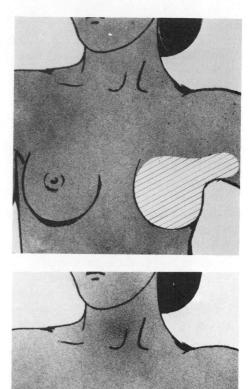

The striped areas show the tissue removed in a radical (above) and a simple (below) mastectomy, including the axillary lymph nodes in the former case.

know, for her own peace of mind, whether it has already spread.

A two-step procedure involves other choices. Where the biopsy is to be carried out separately, the patient may ask to have it done under local anesthesia as an outpatient. That possibility can be explored with the surgeon. If a general anesthetic appears preferable, the patient may have to spend a night in the hospital. But the *diagnostic biopsy*—involving surgical removal of the entire tumor—and mastectomy can still be performed separately. After a biopsy specimen is removed, the specimen may be subjected to an estrogen-receptor assay. The assay tells the surgeon whether or not the cancer depends on the female hormone estrogen for its growth. That information provides a clue to possible future treatment.

Following the biopsy, the patient receives the pathologist's report on whether the finding is positive or negative. If positive, precise information will usually be given on the type of cancer and where it is located in the breast. Then the patient may want to obtain a second opinion on the permanent-section pathology report and slides. The second opinion is also given by a pathologist. It helps materially in making decisions on appropriate surgery.

Mastectomy

If the lesion is malignant, the surgeon proceeds with the mastectomy. Depending on the seriousness of the case and the procedure recommended by the surgeon and pathologist, the operation may be a *simple mastectomy*, a *radical mastectomy*, a *modified radical mastectomy*, or any of a number of other forms of breast operation. In the United States until recently, radical mastectomy was the usual procedure for breast cancer treatment. Today, at least seven different types of mastectomy, some more widely accepted than others, may be performed. All may be recommended in different cases depending on the type of cancer, its invasive potential, or ability to spread, and other factors. The seven:

Engravings from a surgery manual show how primitive breast surgery was in 1750. Few could have undergone or survived such treatment.

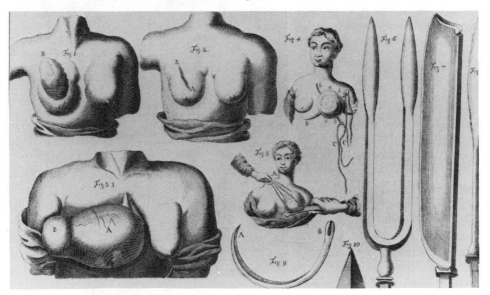

• *Wedge excision, lumpectomy,* or *segmental resection*: the tumor is removed along with some surrounding tissue

• *Simple mastectomy*: the breast alone is removed

• *Simple mastectomy* accompanied by *low axillary dissection*: the breast is removed along with some of the underarm nodes or glands

• *Modified-radical mastectomy* accompanied by *full axillary dissection*: the breast is removed along with all the lymph glands under the arm

• *Halsted-type radical mastectomy*: the breast is removed along with all the underarm lymph glands and the chest muscles

• *Radical mastectomy* with *internal mammary node biopsy*: the same procedure as the Halsted-type radical mastectomy, except that the lymph nodes that lie under the ribs, next to the breastbone, are also sampled for biopsy

• *Super-radical mastectomy*: the same as the above, but all of the internal mammary nodes are removed

Most patients have deep concern about many aspects of breast surgery, including the cosmetic effects. For that reason, it is important to select the appropriate type of surgery. The rates of survival appear to depend as much on timely use of pre- and post-operative radiotherapy and post-operative chemotherapy as on the type of operation. But the kind of operation may determine whether the patient will be able to function normally in a relatively short period of time.

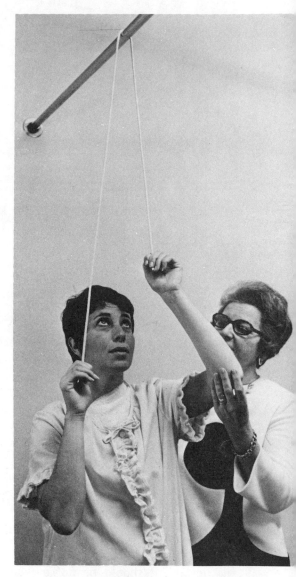

A mastectomy patient doing muscle-strengthening exercises in the American Cancer Society's "Reach to Recovery" program.

Post-Operative Chemotherapy and Immunotherapy

Immunotherapy after breast surgery has also become more common (see "Relief from Allergies: Immunotherapy," p. 871).

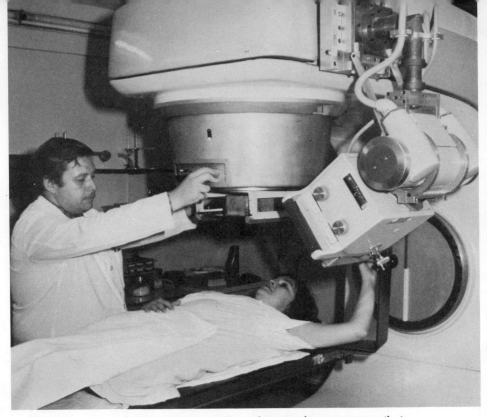

Radiation therapy is frequently used to treat breast cancer patients, sometimes in combination with surgery and other times with drugs.

Immunotherapy, or immunization therapy, seeks to strengthen the patient's own body defenses against cancer. In one form of immunotherapy, a vaccine known as *BCG (bacille Calmette-Guerin)* is administered. The vaccine, ordinarily used to prevent tuberculosis, stimulates the production of antibodies that are believed to destroy cancer cells. Immunotherapy, it should be noted, was still somewhat experimental in the early 1980s.

Other Therapeutic Measures

In some cases of breast cancer, surgeons may recommend excision of the ovaries in addition to removal of breast tissue. Because of the relationships between ovarian function and breast cancer, some doctors believe that elimination of estrogen production by means of surgery or radiation can increase the chances of long-term cure.

Radiation therapy frequently is recommended for cases of breast cancer when the disease is so far advanced that surgery is not feasible, or when the patient's health is too poor to risk surgery. In addition, radiation treatment may be effective in reducing the pain in bones or areas of the central nervous system that may have been invaded by metastasized cancer cells. Radiation also may be used in addition to chemotherapy in certain cases because X rays, or similar radiation, can reach areas where chemical medications cannot penetrate. When administered immediately after surgery, radiation appears to reduce by as much as 50 percent the chances of recurrence of breast cancer.